Phase I Oncology Drug Development

Timothy A. Yap • Jordi Rodon • David S. Hong
Editors

Phase I Oncology Drug Development

Springer

Editors
Timothy A. Yap
University of Texas MD
Anderson Cancer Center
Houston
TX
USA

Jordi Rodon
University of Texas MD
Anderson Cancer Center
Houston
TX
USA

David S. Hong
University of Texas MD
Anderson Cancer Center
Houston
TX
USA

ISBN 978-3-030-47681-6   ISBN 978-3-030-47682-3 (eBook)
https://doi.org/10.1007/978-3-030-47682-3

This Springer imprint is published by the registered company Springer Nature Switzerland AG
The registered company address is: Gewerbestrasse 11, 6330 Cham, Switzerland

Foreword

The Times—They Are A-Changin'
—Bob Dylan
Nobel Laureate for Literature 2016

It is certainly no longer "the bad old days" in the field of oncology phase I clinical trials.

The days of treating patients with advanced refractory cancer when all prior treatments *have failed them* with just the next phase I agent coming off the drug development assembly line are thankfully over. Potential new therapeutic entities are becoming available for phase I clinical trials at a rapid clip. Whether we are referring a patient for a possible phase I trial or consenting a patient for a phase I study, we must make sure we are offering our patients the best possible chance they will actually benefit from that new agent.

In the "bad old days," only about 1 in every 15 or so new agents tried actually had evidence of helping someone in a phase I trial. Today, it is thankfully at least 1 in every 3 new agents (that will provide clinical benefit for a patient). In fact, with better science, better patient selection, etc., if no participant in a phase I trial derives benefit from the new agent, one quickly wonders whether there is any future at all for that drug. Therefore, now, more than ever, it is critical that physicians trying to do their very best for their oncology patient be familiar with the very latest information on strategies for the most efficient ways to develop a new anticancer agent. Presently, it can make a real difference for patients, e.g., they have a greater chance of achieving clinical benefit in the phase I trial. Done properly, a patient's participation in a phase I clinical trial has a much higher likelihood of helping them (30% today versus 3% in the past). Therefore, in this day and age, to do the best for our patients with advanced cancer, our patients should be offered participation in a phase I clinical trial.

In this volume *Phase I Oncology Drug Development*, three of our most outstanding physician investigators (Timothy Yap, David Hong, and Jordi Rodon) have done all of us a service by assembling a most important perspective on what we all should know about present-day phase I clinical trials.

The authors in this volume cover perspectives from multiple distinguished multinational experts. They, first of all, remind us not to forget the basics like good pharmacokinetic/pharmacodynamic principles and how a great biomarker wins the day for giving our patients the best chance for clinical benefit. They also give the best chance for FDA approval.

Other very helpful topics covered in this volume include:

(a) Differences in interactions required with different regulatory agencies (for the USA and for the European Union)
(b) What pharmacokinetic and pharmacodynamic data should look like in various preclinical models before proceeding to a phase I clinical trial
(c) Strategies for the selection of patients most likely to benefit from a phase I agent
(d) Dose–response relationships for new molecularly targeted immuno-oncology agents or epigenetic modifying agents
(e) Tips on how state-of-the-art preclinical studies (e.g., CRISPR/Cas9, organoids) can be used for target discoveries and for the validation of that target as a driver. These techniques can "de-risk" a compound and give our patients the best chance for clinical benefit
(f) How to set up an outstanding phase I unit so patients do not have to travel far away from home
(g) Novel trial designs: for studying dose escalation (including Bayesian optimal interval (BOIN) design) and selecting the proper dose to take forward into expansion cohorts
(h) The critical area of attribution and management of toxicities
(i) Important consideration for situations that might alter pharmacokinetics. This includes designs with consideration for food effects, drug–drug interactions, and organ impairment
(j) Beautifully detailed description of the development of biomarkers, including imaging and regulatory requirements
(k) Discussion of various new endpoints for detecting early signs of efficacy in the phase I trial
(l) Special consideration for the development of novel technologies (e.g., antibody–drug conjugate, novel formulations)
(m) A unique discussion of phase I combinatorial drug development strategies
(n) How molecular profiling of patients in a phase I setting can inform unexpected results of finding an actionable target, which is incredibly helpful for their care, and which may have implications for their relatives (e.g., germline mutations)
(o) Special strategies for phase I trials for immunotherapeutics, including unique patient selection and agent-specific designs (e.g., with STING agonists, Toll-like receptor agonists), as well as combination strategies for such agents
(p) Novel phase I trial designs involving multiple types of radiation
(q) Special consideration for phase I trials for patients with hematologic malignancies

Throughout the volume, there are multiple successful and unsuccessful examples of therapeutic development. These are very helpful examples. There are also some incredibly helpful tables and diagrams to emphasize important points.

In summary, this is a must-read volume for all those who want to provide the very best possibilities for their patients with advanced cancer. The editors and authors have given us their very best. Yes, the times in phase I trials, they are a-changin'.

Daniel Von Hoff
Translational Genomics Research Institute
Phoenix, AZ
USA

Contents

Chapter 1
The Development of a Drug: A Pharmaceutical Drug Development Perspective

Michael Lahn

Abstract Clinical investigation of New Molecular Entities (NME) in oncology is changing. Drivers of this transformation are advances in pharmacological platforms, such as antibody technology, changes in the regulatory framework to accelerate approval of new treatments, and rapid scientific discovery. As a result of this transformation the established drug development process is being modified and continues to adapt. Today significant resources are being moved towards early clinical development and NME have to show early promise of therapeutic activity. The ideal NME targets specific pathways, for which diagnostic tools can be developed to select or enrich patients for the treatment with NME. This chapter reviews the critical steps enabling the early phase clinical development from the perspective of a pharmaceutical drug developer. The required steps include non-clinical pharmacokinetic (PK) studies, pharmacokinetic/pharmacodynamic (PK/PD) models, pharmacology and toxicology studies, and biomarker development plans.

Keywords Drug development · First in human dose studies · Immuno-oncology · Kinase inhibitors · Targeted agents · Regulatory approval · Antibody · Biomarkers

Key Points

1. Drug Development in Oncology is undergoing adaptation in response to new scientific discoveries.
2. Resources are invested earlier in clinical development to reduce attrition for new molecular entities (NME).
3. Success for identifying NME early appears to depend on the selection of specific targets that can be readily assessed in patients
4. Regulatory framework is evolving to respond to the changes in the clinical investigation of NME.
5. Pharmaceutical drug development continues to search for the right model that will allocate the relevant resources in the overall drug development in a timely manner.

M. Lahn (✉)
iOnctura SA, Geneva, Switzerland
e-mail: m.lahn@ionctura.com

T. A. Yap et al. (eds.), *Phase I Oncology Drug Development*,
https://doi.org/10.1007/978-3-030-47682-3_1

1.1 Introduction

Today the drug development process for oncology NME is undergoing a significant change. Drivers for this change include the evolving science, operational complexities for trials and the need to develop NME in a financially sustainable manner. Given the number of NME in clinical development, in particular for immune-oncology NME [1], it is important to share the perspective of the industry with academic partners to successfully manage this change [2]. While the pharmaceutical industry and academic research are struggling to find efficient and sustainable ways to develop NME [3], the development costs of NME are staggering given the low output [4]. In 2003, the cost of launching a NME was estimated to be over 1 billion US dollars with an expected approval rate of about 7% [5]. Researchers look for reasons to explain the low output of this clinical research. For example, the European Science Foundation commissioned a review on drug development during the twentieth century to uncover the drivers of successful drug development, but this review was not able to pinpoint a single factor that predicted successful drug development [6]. Reviews of recently approved NME found that biomarker-driven programs have a higher success rate of about 13% compared to 7% when no biomarkers are included [7]. Other researchers suggested that the organizational structures of today's pharmaceutical companies delay innovation. In fact, small biotech companies developed over 60% of recently approved NME [8–11]. Today pharmaceutical companies have to answer to diverse shareholder interests and are subject to increasing scrutiny from analysts or day traders, some of which have little or no knowledge of the complexity of drug development [12]. By contrast, small biotech companies may collaborate with large pharmaceutical companies at the risk of failing if they do not produce innovation attractive to larger pharmaceutical firms. Academic partners should be prepared for the eventuality that a small pharmaceutical company may be acquired by a larger pharmaceutical firm during the course of a clinical development. Hence, a standardized process in clinical development is needed and should be encouraged to allow the necessary flexibility to transfer data from one sponsor to another without interrupting the clinical trial.

Given this background, the following chapter will focus on the biomedical approaches that have shown useful in reducing attrition in drug development such as (a) leverage pre-existing information including bioinformatics approaches; (b) integrating non-clinical information to predict clinical properties of NME and (c) optimize the operational costs to gain timely information in early trials [13, 14]. This chapter will discuss the critical components leading to the early phase studies of NME and how these should be integrated to justify the early investment in clinical development.

1.2 Non-clinical Pharmacokinetic Studies

The role of non-clinical pharmacokinetic (PK) studies is particularly critical for oral NME, which make up a third of all NME in clinical development. Provided an appropriately selective oral NME has been identified, the next step is to assess its properties of absorption, distribution, metabolism and excretion (ADME). Such ADME studies can be helpful in predicting the behavior of an NME in humans [15, 16]. The PK profile in animals is often first used to optimize subsequent formulation for oral or intravenous NME. Once the desired profile is achieved, the NME is ready to be explored in non-clinical pharmacology and toxicology studies. The extent of early ADME work depends not only on scientific but also on strategic merits. Consequently, the development team needs to weigh early investments for comprehensive ADME work with the possibility that a NME may not progress beyond initial non-clinical toxicology studies. Thus, the costs for an early comprehensive ADME work may be misplaced. Before embarking on costly non-clinical ADME and toxicology studies it is important that the development team determines the general strategy of a NME. For example, early and comprehensive investment may be warranted if the development team is convinced that the NME will have a unique profile differentiating itself from other NME. Notwithstanding these strategic considerations, without the desired PK properties, subsequent research in non-clinical pharmacology and toxicology studies risk repetitive work and delays, both of which can significantly impact the future development of a NME.

1.3 Non-clinical Pharmacology Models

Non-clinical pharmacology models are often desirable to justify the clinical evaluation of a NME. However, standard non-clinical cell line derived xenograft (CDX) models have limited value to predict activity in humans [17]. The use of patient-derived xenografts (PDX) promises to improve the prediction of antitumor activity in humans than CDX, mainly because PDX retain the original histopathological phenotype and consequently reflect the diversity of tumors [18]. Today the use of PDX has become an integral part of functional assessment of NME [19]. If the NME is targeting immune-related targets, then models with immune-competent animals are preferred. Such immune-competent animal models assess not only the involvement of the immune system, but also the complexities of the tumor microenvironment [20]. While these three model systems provide information that the NME targets a physiologically important mechanism, they are not as predictive for future activity in patients as desired by drug developers. One reason why immune-competent rodent models do not predict behavior in humans may be attributed to the differences of the species-specific immune system. For example, mice have different immune systems from humans in both innate and adaptive immunity, such as leukocyte subsets, Toll receptors, NK cells, T and B cells [21, 22]. Therefore, it is important to appropriately interpret results from animal studies and ensure that these models are not used as predictors for antitumor activity in patients. Because of these limitations, there is an increasing interest in human organoids [23]. These in vitro 3D cultures can be grown from embryonic and adult stem cells and display self-organizing capacities, phenocopying essential aspects of the organs they are derived from. Genetic modification of organoids allows disease modeling in a setting that approaches the physiological environment. Organoids

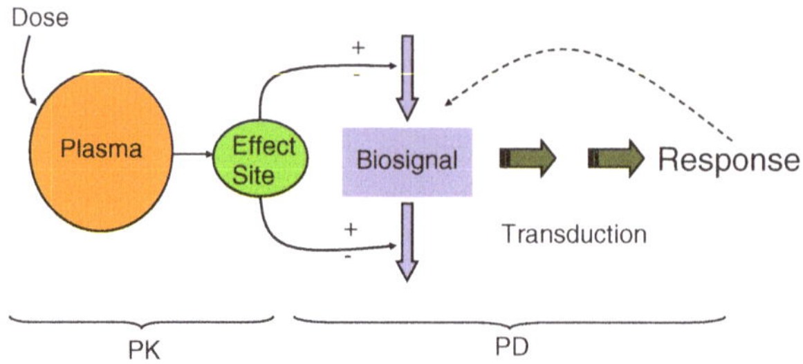

Fig. 1.1 Relating pharmacokinetics (PK) and pharmacodynamics (PD) to establish a PK/PD model for estimating antitumor responses in humans. NME is administered to animals (generally rodent species) to deliver a dose estimated to produce a response (for example antitumor response in a xenograft model). The PK is characterized and related to the effect site. The degree of biosignal at the effect site and its transduction to the expected responses represents the PD effect, which ideally should be measured at multiple time points. The PK/PD model should include a dose range study to understand the degree of response in relationship to drug concentration. (Reference: Derendof H, Meibolm B. Modeling of PK/PD relationships: Concepts and Perspectives. Pharmaceutical Research, Vol 16 (2), 1999)

can also be grown from patient-derived healthy and tumor tissues, potentially enabling patient-specific drug testing and the development of individualized treatment regimens.

For purposes of drug development non-clinical pharmacology models are particularly useful if they are used to estimate drug levels and exposure. Analyzed appropriately, PK studies in animals have shown to be predictive for PK profiles in humans [16]. Non-clinical pharmacology models provide important pharmacodynamic information, which can be correlated with exposure information of a NME (Fig. 1.1) [24]. Such pharmacokinetic/pharmacodynamic (PK/PD) models are helpful to estimate clinical dose and dose schedules in patients [25]. Today, this concept originally developed for chemotherapies is being used for many NME, including monoclonal antibodies [26]. Pharmaceutical companies use information derived from PK/PD models to design: (a) non-clinical toxicology studies in animals, (b) determine of drug requirements for Chemistry, Manufacturing and Controls (CM&C); (c) time points for blood sampling to assess pharmacokinetics and measurements of ADME in humans. In conjunction with animal ADME/toxicology studies, PK/PD models are also helpful to estimate the safe starting dose in an early phase study and thus have become valuable in assessing the benefit/risk for a NME (Fig. 1.2). This is particularly important if the NME is considered to have potentially non-reversible toxicities and thus the drug exposure must be below an anticipated toxicity level. One such example was successfully developed for a small molecule inhibitor targeting the Transforming Growth Factor beta Receptor Type I (TGF-βRI), where the PK/PD model predicted cardiovascular toxicity if an exposure threshold were to be exceeded [27]. Using the PK/PD model a safe therapeutic window was predicted and later confirmed in clinical trials [28, 29].

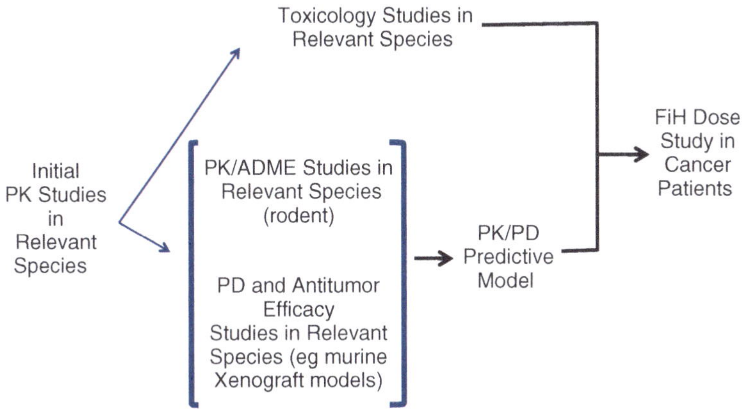

Fig. 1.2 Non-clinical studies to estimate the benefit/risk prior to First-in-human (FiH) dose study. Initial pharmacokinetic (PK) studies are conducted to understand the ADME properties (absorption, distribution, metabolism and excretion, ADME) of a New Molecular Entity (NME) to inform non-clinical toxicology study design, detailed PK/ADME studies, pharmacodynamics (PD) and antitumor efficacy studies, development of a PK/PD predictive model. Using the combined information from non-clinical toxicology studies (risk assessment) and PK/PD model (benefit assessment), a safe starting dose can be determined for the First-in-human (FiH) dose study

1.4 Non-clinical Toxicology Studies

Non-clinical toxicology studies for oncology NMEs are conducted based on the ICH S9 guidance [30]. The most relevant species, generally a rodent and non-rodent species, are selected to estimate the potential risk of a NME and to determine the no-observed adverse effect level (NOAEL). The debate continues in finding alternatives to current animal-based toxicology studies, but to date even "big data" approaches have not been able to supplant the standard animal toxicology studies [31]. In reviewing data from various therapeutic areas and the subsequently observed adverse events in patients, the concordance between animal and human toxicity was examined [32]. Data from 12 pharmaceutical companies and 150 compounds were reviewed and the true positive concordance rate was 71% when a NME was assessed in both rodent and non-rodent species. This observation was confirmed in a recent study, in particular the prediction of cardiovascular arrhythmia and risk of QTc prolongation [33].

1.5 Therapeutic Vaccines

The clinical development of therapeutic vaccines and NME targeting immune cells, such as oncolytic virus, requires a different approach of drug development [34, 35]. The vaccine development assumes that the host will mount an immune responses and thus will not have an immediate antitumor effect. Consequently, vaccine drug development requires the participation of patients that are able to undergo long treatment times to assess the anticipated antitumor effect. Because of this mechanism of action, there has been an ongoing debate which type of patients should be selected for a First-in-human (FiH) dose study. Patients with a high tumor burden and refractory to prior treatments are likely to be immune suppressed. Such patients are generally considered for FiH dose studies, because their benefit/risk assessment is favorable for such a FiH dose study, but they are less likely to respond to vaccines. On the other hand, patients with low tumor and antigen burden are considered to be more likely to respond to vaccines, but they are at a higher potential risk to develop an autoimmune response if the vaccine is potent. This last group has also a different benefit/risk profile and the risks must be carefully weighed. Furthermore, the classical dose-response paradigm generally observed with small molecules or antibodies cannot be expected with vaccines. Monitoring immune responses is therefore not only a measure of efficacy, but also an assessment of safety. Currently, there is no agreement on the extent and type of immune monitoring needed in such a FiH dose study [36]. The recommendation ranges from measuring lymphocytes subsets, measurements of functional responses of the immune cells (such as function of humoral and cellular immunity) as well as degree of antigen processing, presentation and responses.

1.6 Translational Research Plan: The Importance of Patient Selection

Previous successful developments of NME imply that patient selection is a key component in reducing attrition in oncology drug development [7]. With the development of the non-clinical pharmacology models, it is useful to start incorporating pharmacodynamics measures that can be serially examined in patients. A recent example is related to inhibitors of the Fibroblast Growth Factor Receptor (FGFR) pathway [37]. Hyperphosphatemia and increase of Fibroblast Growth Factor 23 (FGF23) levels are PD markers after administration of FGF receptor (FGFR) inhibitors. Both markers are associated with activity in non-clinical models and are used in the clinic for safety monitoring and response measurements [38]. Another example is the use of Epidermal Growth Factor Receptor (EGFR) inhibitors in targeting EGFR mutations in NSCLC [39]. As with the FGFR inhibitors, targeting specific driver mutations of the EGFR pathway are associated with clinical activity and durable responses. The EGFR inhibitor osimertinib was specifically developed to target the mutation T790M in NSCLC. During the FiH dose study, patients were asked to submit to biopsy in order to provide tumor tissue to measure the T790M mutation [40]. Using this approach and observing durable responses surpassing 9 months, especially in patients with T790M mutation, osimertinib was approved in about 4 years from the start of the FiH dose study. These two examples show how patient selection can reduce attrition in clinical development. Admittedly, biomarker-based patient selection will not be possible for many NME and such biomarkers will have to be developed during the clinical development. In such situations drug developers may benefit from interrogating large tumor banks or cell lines [41].

1.7 Planning for the First-in-Human (FiH) Dose Study

As exemplified by the drug development of osimertinib, FiH dose studies are no longer just safety and PK studies, but include design elements which may accelerate the drug development [40]. This is especially true if the drug target is clearly defined and the NME proves to predictably engage the target throughout all stages of non-clinical and clinical development. Thus, the FiH dose study should be designed with sufficient decision points, each of them associated with investment triggers so that clinical development of NME can either be accelerated or expand the clinical investigation with increased translational research. Also, clinical developers must define stopping rules (for example if the PK profile is unpredictable and associated toxicity profile cannot be monitored and/or is not reversible). A project may also be stopped if the NME shows insufficient innovation along with unpredictable PK profiles as demonstrated by a multi-kinase inhibitor program [42]. For pharmaceutical companies this "early kill" allows them to focus on the most promising drugs in their pipeline.

Today most companies wish to stage the clinical development in such a way that if data in the early phase program are encouraging, the NME can be moved quickly towards registration. However, this general concept comes at an investment cost that often is difficult to justify. A company may decide to invest early in the development of an NME if the company is convinced the NME holds a high treatment potential.

In addition to making such early strategic decisions, companies need to select the appropriate centers to conduct clinical trials. Based on a research conducted by Batelle Technology Partnership Practice in 2015, oncology trials are the costliest trials among all therapeutic areas at US$60,000 per patient [43]. The reasons for this high cost are complexity of oncology trials (including the cost for recruiting patients), administrative staff costs for managing the trial and case report forms, complex medical procedures (e.g., biopsies and imaging), and site monitoring costs [44]. Once opened, nearly half of the selected centers either do not enroll patients or enroll less than the projected number. It is therefore understandable that drug developers are careful not only in their design but also in the operational aspects of an early phase trial.

Reducing attrition requires the following prerequisites: (a) anticipated biologically efficacious dose and dose schedule based on PK/PD models; (b) safe starting dose based on non-clinical toxicology studies; (c) biomarker plan to identify or enrich for patients to respond; (d) reduce operational uncertainties by selecting and collaborating with trial centers; (e) well trained staff across all parts of the study. Assuming these prerequisites are met, FiH dose studies consist of two parts: the first part employs a standard dose escalation design and the second part comprises of expansion cohorts (Fig. 1.3). In the first part, the main objective is to confirm the predicted toxicity, PK and, ideally, the PD profile of the NME. Provided a moderate or low variability of the PK profile the first 3–6 patients may confirm the prediction of the biological active dose. If the biological active dose is identified subsequent steps may be triggered, including allowing CM&C to start additional drug campaigns to support future expansion cohorts or Phase 2/3 studies (Fig. 1.4). If antitumor activity is observed during the dose escalation and the antitumor activity is associated with durable responses, the developer of the NME will seek accelerated approval, as exemplified by the development of osimertinib: dose extension and expansion cohorts were started to gain deeper knowledge of the benefit/risk profile and help with the initial development of a companion diagnostic for the EGFR mutation T790M [40]. Based on these cohorts and the initiation of additional studies, approval and marketing authorization was sought. The timeline from FiH dose study was under 4 years compared to the typical development of approximately 7 years. Also the PD1 inhibitor pembrolizumab used a complex FiH dose study (Keynote 001), where receptor occupancy on circulating T cells and functional assays for T cell activation were used to define the biological effective dose (BED) [45]. It is noteworthy, that Keynote

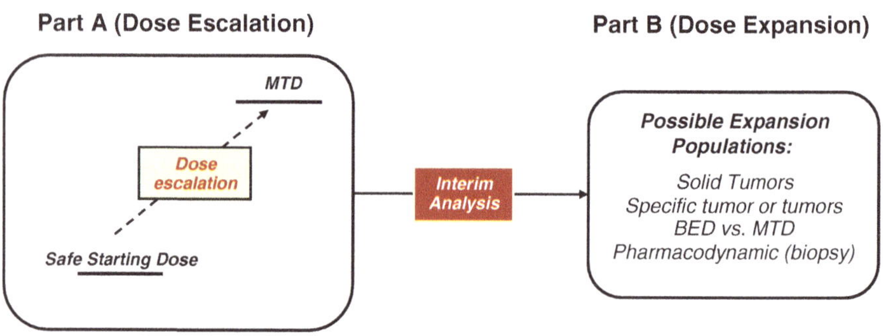

Fig. 1.3 Example of First-in-human (FiH) dose study consisting of a Part A (dose escalation) and a Part B (dose expansion). The safe starting dose is generally based on the non-clinical toxicology studies (often referred to as GLP toxicology studies), but more recently may also include a pharmacokinetic/pharmacodynamic (PK/PD) model. The dose escalation should establish the biologically effective dose (BED) and explore the full dose range of the drug up to the maximum tolerated dose (MTD). The Part B (dose expansion) is generally specific solid tumor types to gain signals of antitumor activity at either the BED (the preferable concept) or the MTD (the traditional concept for chemotherapies). In this part, a particular emphasis on pharmacodyanmic readouts is placed if this has not been integrated in the dose escalation

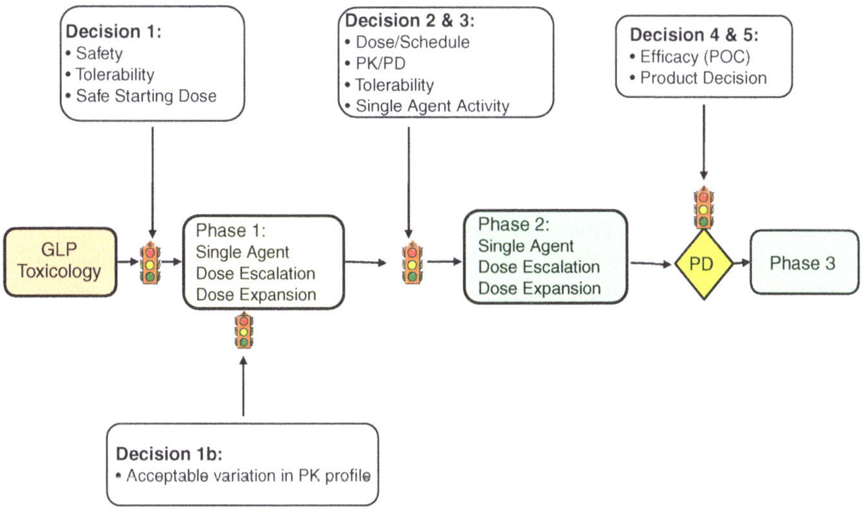

Fig. 1.4 Simplified development path with corresponding standard go/no-go decisions. After determining the benefit/risk using non-clinical GLP toxicology studies and pharmacokinetic/pharmacodynamic (PK/PD) modeling (Decision 1), the Phase 1 study (or First-in-human dose study) is initiated. During the dose escalation in the Phase 1 study the drug must show acceptable variation in PK profile (Decision 1b). Once the drug has shown an acceptable safety profile, acceptable dose schedule at the biologically active dose, confirmed the PK/PD relationship and shown signals of single agent activity (Decisions 2 and 3), the agent may proceed to Phase 2 or 3, where proof-of-concept (POC) or even significant antitumor activity must be demonstrated (Decisions 4 and 5). This is the basis for the initiation of the last milestone with significant investment for a global launch strategy (Product Decision, PD)

001 used an adaptive design and thus facilitated an accelerated approval, including the development of a companion diagnostic for PDL1 expression in tumor tissue [46]. When the expansion cohorts of Keynote 001 were initiated, pembrolizumab was evaluated in a wide range of tumors from patients who had at least 1% of PDL1 expression according to histological analysis of tumor biopsies [47]. This Phase 1b study (Keynote 028) laid the foundation for subsequent Phase 2/3 studies. These examples of osimertinib and pembrolizumab illustrate how a flexible design of early phase studies can accelerate the approval of NME in a cost efficient manner.

Lastly, many studies will combine the NME with another drug to determine whether the combination is superior to historic antitumor responses observed with the combination partner. The risk of moving NME quickly to combination studies is the lack of comparison and thus responses may be over-interpreted. A renewed debate on the value of randomized Phase 2 or Phase 1b studies is needed given the increase in single-arm combination studies in expansion cohorts of FiH dose studies [48].

1.8 Additional Clinical Studies to Facilitate Accelerate Approval

Approval of an NME requires additional supportive studies, which are often not widely published or rarely acknowledged by the wider academic community. These studies are often part of discussions between the drug developer and regulatory agencies. For example, stability studies are critical and without which an approval can be delayed. Because of the time requirements for such stability studies, it is important to initiate stability studies as early as possible. Hence, stability studies are often initiated before the FiH dose study, which in turn requires a strategic decision by the pharmaceutical developer.

In addition to the CM&C-based studies for stability, there is generally a need to conduct clinical pharmacology studies. These additional studies can either be incorporated in ongoing studies or require stand-alone studies in either patients or healthy volunteers. For example, drug-drug-interaction (DDI), food studies, electrophysiological studies (QTc), renal or hepatic insufficiency studies are often needed. Electrophysiological studies in patients (in order to measure QTc prolongation) are often conducted to assess the risk in the intended indication. In such studies or cohort of patients EKGs should be conducted along with PK sampling in approximation to the E14 guidance [29, 49]. In such PK-matched EKG studies it is possible to associate the QTc prolongation with exposure, which in turn helps to differentiate the QTc risk of the NME from co-medication generally known to cause QTc changes (such as antibiotics). In order to isolate a possible QTc prolongation risk, the drug developer may need to also conduct a special QTc study in healthy volunteers. Furthermore, if there is a change in formulation the earlier formulation should be compared to the latest in a bio-equivalence or relative bioavailability study, especially if the most recent formulation is intended for final use in patients. Such studies can also be conducted in particular cohorts with cancer patients [50]. Most of these clinical pharmacology studies are started when the final or pre-final formulation is developed. Otherwise the clinical drug developer risks to repeat such pharmacology studies because they are meant to support the final drug product. Finally, pediatric indication studies should be started as early as possible. Ideally these studies can be started when the recommended Phase 2 dose is established at the time of or immediately after the FiH dose study in adults. In summary, it is important to prepare all the pharmacology or special indication studies as soon as possible in the development cycle of an NME.

1.9 Regulatory Implications

In the past years drug developers have attempted to optimize drug development and to reduce attrition in oncology. Biomarker-driven clinical development have shortened time to registration and in some instances also reduced the need for large numbers of patients within trials [51, 52]. If this approach of biomarker-based drug development is broadened, the medical and pharmaceutical community will need to intensify research on pharmacodynamics markers that are combined with NME. Recent advances in measuring circulating tumor DNA (ctDNA) and re-evaluating standard laboratory tests may facilitate the development of such pharmacodynamic markers.

While medical science progresses, the regulatory framework between European Medicines Agency (EMA) and United States (US) Food Drug Administration (FDA) remains different despite strives to standardize the regulations (Table 1.1). Approval processes for diseases with unmet medical seem to become similar between the two health regulatory organizations [53]. For example, the European Union (EU) recently introduced the "Prime" designation, which provides a more

Table 1.1 Important interactions with health authorities of the European Union (EU), the European Medicines Agency (EMA) and the United States of America (USA) Food and Drug Administration (FDA) and differences in approval

	EMA	FDA
Important interactions with health authorities		
Pre-investigational new drug	No	Yes
Scientific advice	Yes	No
Clinical Trial Application (CTA)	Yes	No
End-of Phase-1 (EOP1) and End-of-Phase 2 (EOP2) meeting	No	Yes
Scientific advice	Yes	No
Need of companion diagnostic	No	Yes
Special Protocol Assessment (SPA)	No	Yes
Scientific Advisory Group (SGA)	Yes	No
Advisory Committee	Yes	Yes
New Drug Application (NDA) or Biological License Agreement (BLA)	No	Yes
Marketing Authorization (MAA)	Yes	No
Type of approvals		
Standard approval	Yes	Yes
Orphan drug designation and approval	Yes	Yes
Expedited approval programs	Yes	Yes
Priority review	No	Yes
Accelerated Assessment	Yes	No
Accelerated approval (need to demonstrate evidence of clinical benefit and in need to be converted to standard approval with appropriate Phase 3 trials)	No	Yes
Conditional approval (need to demonstrate evidence of clinical benefit and requires renewal until full approval)	Yes	No
Prime designation	Yes	No
Breakthrough (BT) designation	No	Yes
Fast track (FT) designation	No	Yes
Rollover new drug application	No	Yes
Exceptional circumstances	Yes	No
Companion diagnostic (requirement of prior in vitro diagnostics approval for NDA)	No	Yes

rapid approval in the EU and is perhaps similar to the "accelerated approval" regulated by the US FDA [54]. In a recent review by the EMA, the Prime designation has been requested and granted mainly for oncology and hematology NME [54]. Another area of recent convergence is the use of patient-reported outcomes in clinical trials, which was historically important to many EU member states and where FDA has recently shown an increased interest. Independent of these approval processes, the EU and US allow approvals for NME targeting rare diseases under the orphan drug designation. One area where EU and US differ is related to the biomarker-based development, which may have an impact on the timely approval of a NME. The US FDA regulation requires a companion diagnostic if treatment decisions are based on the results of a diagnostic test. The EU has focused more on ensuring that the diagnostic test is reliable and thus can be used in the general laboratory setting. One example for this different approach is the use of the PDL1 immunohistochemistry assay to detect PDL1 in tumor tissue: companion diagnostics were developed for each PD1/PDL1 inhibitor to measure the expression of the same target (that is PDL1) without determining whether the tests could be interchanged. Only subsequent comparative studies were able to clarify this uncertainty [55]. The EU has been concerned with strengthen the comparability of the testing across its member states and regions. Hence, the EU has streamlined the use for companion diagnostic to support such comparability of tests in the general diagnostic setting [56].

Key Expert Opinion Points

1. Leveraging non-clinical information as early as possible will allow for the selection of better NME. One such example is the use of pharmacokinetic/pharmacodynamics modeling.
2. Ability to select patients for the right NME appears to reduce attrition and accelerate the approval of NME.
3. The focus on identifying the Biologically Effective Dose/Dose range in early clinical trials will likely accelerate the approval of a NME. It likely will lead to hybrid protocols, where two phases of classical drug development are merged into one (for example, a Phase I study may merge into an accelerated registration study without a Phase II).
4. Standardization of the clinical development process must include close collaboration between regulatory, commercial and academic contributors.

References

1. Tang J, Shalabi A, Hubbard-Lucey VM. Comprehensive analysis of the clinical immuno-oncology landscape. Ann Oncol. 2018;29(1):84–91.
2. Petrova E. Chapter 2: Innovation in the pharmaceutical industry: the process of drug discovery and development. In: Ding M, editor. Innovation and marketing in the pharmaceutical industry international series in quantitative marketing, vol. 20. New York: Springer Science+Business Media; 2014.

3. Dollery CT. Clinical pharmacology – the first 75 years and a view of the future. Br J Clin Pharmacol. 2006;61(6):650–65.
4. Booth B, Glassman R, Ma P. Oncology's trials. Nat Rev Drug Discov. 2003;2(8):609–10.
5. DiMasi JA, Hansen RW, Grabowski HG. The price of innovation: new estimates of drug development costs. J Health Econ. 2003;22(2):151–85.
6. Bonah C. Harmonizing drugs: standards in 20th century pharmaceutical history. Paris: Editions Glyphe; 2009.
7. Wong CH, Siah KW, Lo AW. Estimation of clinical trial success rates and related parameters. Biostatistics. 2018.
8. Munos B. A forensic analysis of drug targets from 2000 through 2012. Clin Pharmacol Ther. 2013;94(3):407–11.
9. Munos BH, Orloff JJ. Disruptive innovation and transformation of the drug discovery and development enterprise. NAM Perspectives Discussion Paper. Washington, DC: National Academy of Medicine; 2016.
10. Partners H. Trends in US new drug approvals: 2017 FDA new drug approvals (and multi-year trends). News Res. 2018.
11. Paul SM, Mytelka DS, Dunwiddie CT, Persinger CC, Munos BH, Lindborg SR, et al. How to improve R&D productivity: the pharmaceutical industry's grand challenge. Nat Rev Drug Discov. 2010;9:203.
12. Cuatrecasas P. Drug discovery in jeopardy. J Clin Invest. 2006;116(11):2837–42.
13. Burgess M, de Alwis DP. The true face of the revolution in oncology drug development: a personal reflection. Curr Clin Pharmacol. 2007;2(1):31–5.
14. Hughes JP, Rees S, Kalindjian SB, Philpott KL. Principles of early drug discovery. Br J Pharmacol. 2011;162(6):1239–49.
15. Jones HM, Mayawala K, Poulin PJTAJ. Dose selection based on physiologically based pharmacokinetic (PBPK) approaches. 2013;15(2):377–87.
16. Van den Bergh A, Sinha V, Gilissen R, Straetemans R, Wuyts K, Morrison D, et al. Prediction of human oral plasma concentration-time profiles using preclinical data. 2011;50(8):505–17.
17. Johnson JI, Decker S, Zaharevitz D, Rubinstein LV, Venditti JM, Schepartz S, et al. Relationships between drug activity in NCI preclinical in vitro and in vivo models and early clinical trials. Br J Cancer. 2001;84(10):1424–31.
18. Fiebig HH, editor. Comparison of tumor response in nude mice and in patients. Berlin: Springer; 1988.
19. Perez M, Navas L. Carnero A. Patient-derived xenografts as models for personalized medicine research in cancer. 2016;2(6):197–202.
20. Day C-P, Merlino G, Van Dyke T. Preclinical mouse cancer models: a maze of opportunities and challenges. Cell. 2015;163(1):39–53.
21. Haley PJ. Species differences in the structure and function of the immune system. Toxicology. 2003;188(1):49–71.
22. Mestas J, Hughes CC. Of mice and not men: differences between mouse and human immunology. J Immunol. 2004;172(5):2731–8.
23. Drost J, Clevers H. Organoids in cancer research. Nat Rev Cancer. 2018;18(7):407–18.
24. Derendorf H, Meibohm B. Modeling of pharmacokinetic/pharmacodynamic (PK/PD) relationships: concepts and perspectives. Pharm Res. 1999;16(2):176–85.
25. Simeoni M, De Nicolao G, Magni P, Rocchetti M, Poggesi I. Modeling of human tumor xenografts and dose rationale in oncology. Drug Discov Today Technol. 2013;10(3):e365–e72.
26. Schroeder P. Pharmacokinetic/pharmacodynamic modeling in drug discovery: a translational tool to optimize discovery compounds toward the ideal target-specific profile. Predictive ADMET2014.
27. Bueno L, de Alwis DP, Pitou C, Yingling J, Lahn M, Glatt S, et al. Semi-mechanistic modelling of the tumour growth inhibitory effects of LY2157299, a new type I receptor TGF-beta kinase antagonist, in mice. Eur J Cancer. 2008;44(1):142–50.

28. Gueorguieva I, Cleverly AL, Stauber A, Sada Pillay N, Rodon JA, Miles CP, et al. Defining a therapeutic window for the novel TGF-beta inhibitor LY2157299 monohydrate based on a pharmacokinetic/pharmacodynamic model. Br J Clin Pharmacol. 2014;77(5):796–807.
29. Rodon J, Carducci MA, Sepulveda-Sanchez JM, Azaro A, Calvo E, Seoane J, et al. First-in-human dose study of the novel transforming growth factor-beta receptor I kinase inhibitor LY2157299 monohydrate in patients with advanced cancer and glioma. Clin Cancer Res. 2015;21(3):553–60.
30. ICH harmonised tripartite guideline: nonclinical evaluation for anticancer pharmaceuticals S9 – current step 4 version. 2009.
31. Burden N, Chapman K, Sewell F, Robinson V. Pioneering better science through the 3Rs: an introduction to the national centre for the replacement, refinement, and reduction of animals in research (NC3Rs). J Am Assoc Lab Anim Sci. 2015;54(2):198–208.
32. Olson H, Betton G, Robinson D, Thomas K, Monro A, Kolaja G, et al. Concordance of the toxicity of pharmaceuticals in humans and in animals. Regul Toxicol Pharmacol. 2000;32(1):56–67.
33. Clark M, Steger-Hartmann T. A big data approach to the concordance of the toxicity of pharmaceuticals in animals and humans. Regul Toxicol Pharmacol. 2018;96:94–105.
34. Finn OJ, Khleif SN, Herberman RB. The FDA guidance on therapeutic cancer vaccines: the need for revision to include preventive cancer vaccines or for a new guidance dedicated to them. Cancer Prev Res (Phila). 2015;8(11):1011–6.
35. Guidance for industry – clinical considerations for therapeutic cancer vaccines. 2011.
36. Rahma OE, Gammoh E, Simon RM, Khleif SN. Is the "3+3" dose-escalation phase I clinical trial design suitable for therapeutic cancer vaccine development? A recommendation for alternative design. Clin Cancer Res. 2014;20(18):4758–67.
37. Porta R, Borea R, Coelho A, Khan S, Araújo A, Reclusa P, et al. FGFR a promising druggable target in cancer: molecular biology and new drugs. Crit Rev Oncol Hematol. 2017;113:256–67.
38. Chae YK, Ranganath K, Hammerman PS, Vaklavas C, Mohindra N, Kalyan A, et al. Inhibition of the fibroblast growth factor receptor (FGFR) pathway: the current landscape and barriers to clinical application. Oncotarget. 2016;8(9):16052–74.
39. Hirsh V. Turning EGFR mutation-positive non-small-cell lung cancer into a chronic disease: optimal sequential therapy with EGFR tyrosine kinase inhibitors. Ther Adv Med Oncol. 2018;10:1758834017753338.
40. Jänne PA, Yang JC-H, Kim D-W, Planchard D, Ohe Y, Ramalingam SS, et al. AZD9291 in EGFR inhibitor–resistant non–small-cell lung cancer. N Engl J Med. 2015;372(18):1689–99.
41. Zehir A, Benayed R, Shah RH, Syed A, Middha S, Kim HR, et al. Mutational landscape of metastatic cancer revealed from prospective clinical sequencing of 10,000 patients. Nat Med. 2017;23(6):703–13.
42. Wacheck V, Lahn M, Dickinson G, Füreder W, Meyer R, Herndlhofer S, et al. Dose study of the multikinase inhibitor, LY2457546, in patients with relapsed acute myeloid leukemia to assess safety, pharmacokinetics, and pharmacodynamics. Cancer Manag Res. 2011;3:157–75.
43. Practice BTP. Biopharmaceutical industry-sponsored clinical trials: impact on state economies. 2015.
44. Sertkaya A, Wong H-H, Jessup A, Beleche T. Key cost drivers of pharmaceutical clinical trials in the United States. Clin Trials. 2016;13(2):117–26.
45. Patnaik A, Kang SP, Rasco D, Papadopoulos KP, Elassaiss-Schaap J, Beeram M, et al. Phase I study of pembrolizumab (MK-3475; anti-PD-1 monoclonal antibody) in patients with advanced solid tumors. Clin Cancer Res. 2015;21(19):4286–93.
46. Kang SP, Gergich K, Lubiniecki GM, de Alwis DP, Chen C, Tice MAB, et al. Pembrolizumab KEYNOTE-001: an adaptive study leading to accelerated approval for two indications and a companion diagnostic. Ann Oncol. 2017;28(6):1388–98.
47. Merck. Phase IB study of pembrolizumab (MK-3475) in subjects with select advanced solid tumors (MK-3475-028/KEYNOTE-28). 2014.

48. Tang H, Foster NR, Grothey A, Ansell SM, Goldberg RM, Sargent DJ. Comparison of error rates in single-arm versus randomized phase II cancer clinical trials. J Clin Oncol. 2010;28(11):1936–41.
49. ICH harmonised tripartite guideline – the clinical evaluation of QT/QTC interval prolongation and proarrhythmic potential for non-antiarrhythmic drugs – current step 4 version E14. 2005.
50. Gueorguieva I, Cleverly A, Desaiah D, Azaro A, Seoane J, Braña I, et al. Relative bioavailability of three formulations of galunisertib administered as monotherapy in patients with advanced or metastatic cancer. Drugs Context. 2016;5:1–8.
51. Blumenthal GM, Kluetz PG, Schneider J, Goldberg KB, McKee AE, Pazdur R. Oncology drug approvals: evaluating endpoints and evidence in an era of breakthrough therapies. Oncologist. 2017;22(7):762–7.
52. Postel-Vinay S, Soria J-C. Phase I trials in oncology: a new era has started. Ann Oncol. 2015;26(1):7–9.
53. Senderowicz AM, Pfaff O. Similarities and differences in the oncology drug approval process between FDA and European Union with emphasis on in vitro companion diagnostics. Clin Cancer Res. 2014;20(6):1445–52.
54. Agency EM. PRIME: priority medicines European Medicines Agency. 2018. https://www.ema.europa.eu/human-regulatory/research-development/prime-priority-medicines.
55. Rimm DL, Han G, Taube JM, Yi ES, Bridge JA, Flieder DB, et al. A prospective, multi-institutional, pathologist-based assessment of 4 immunohistochemistry assays for pd-l1 expression in non–small cell lung cancer. JAMA Oncol. 2017;3(8):1051–8.
56. Union E. The new regulations on medical devices. 2017. https://ec.europa.eu/growth/sectors/medical-devices/regulatory-framework_en.

Chapter 2
Paradigms in Cancer Drug Development: A Universe with Many Galaxies

Cinta Hierro and Jordi Rodon

Abstract Cytotoxic chemotherapeutics (CHTs) have been the backbone cancer therapy for many years. Recently, a rapidly growing body of evidence has demonstrated the interdependence of cancer genetics, epigenetics, and immunology, giving rise to the generation of new promising compounds. The development of new molecularly targeted agents (MTAs), immune checkpoint-targeted monoclonal antibodies (ICT mAbs), and epigenetic drugs (EPDs) has increased the ready-to-use arsenal for patients with different cancers, but at the same time, has resulted in many substantial changes in clinical trial design, altering the early drug development (EDD) landscape. Despite sharing common developmental principles, the significant differences in their mechanisms of action (MoAs) have led researchers to reconsider previous assumptions regarding the design and execution of Phase I clinical trials (Ph1), leading to the recognition of four established paradigms in oncology. In this chapter, we review drug development evolution with a broad view of the major differences in EDD between these four paradigms, namely CHTs, MTAs, ICT mAbs, and EPDs, addressing many of the controversial issues and challenges that helped shape them. Only a comprehensive view of their main characteristics will enable successful design of future therapeutic options.

Keywords Cytotoxic chemotherapeutics (CHTs) · Molecularly targeted agents (MTAs) · Immune checkpoint-targeted monoclonal antibodies (ICT mAbs) Epigenetic drugs (EPDs) · Novel mechanisms of action (MoAs) · Early drug development (EDD) · Phase I clinical trials (Ph1) · Oncology paradigms

C. Hierro
Medical Oncology Department, Catalan Institute of Oncology (ICO)-Badalona; Badalona-Applied Research Group in Oncology (B-ARGO), Badalona, Barcelona, Spain

Molecular Therapeutics Research Unit, Vall d'Hebron Institute of Oncology (VHIO), Universitat Autònoma de Barcelona (UAB), Barcelona, Spain
e-mail: chierro@iconcologia.net

J. Rodon (✉)
Division of Cancer Medicine, Institute for Personalized Cancer Therapy, The University of Texas MD Anderson Cancer Center, Houston, TX, USA
e-mail: JRodon@mdanderson.org

T. A. Yap et al. (eds.), *Phase I Oncology Drug Development*,
https://doi.org/10.1007/978-3-030-47682-3_2

Key Points

1. Molecularly targeted agents (MTAs), immune checkpoint-targeted monoclonal antibodies (ICT mAbs) and epigenetic drugs (EPDs) represent the new paradigms in cancer therapy after traditional cytotoxic chemotherapeutics (CHTs).
2. The novel mechanisms of action that characterize these MTAs, ICT mAbs and EPDs entail new dose-response relationships. Integration of pharmacokinetics (PK), pharmacodynamics (PD), and other markers of effect, has proven to be crucial to define the optimal efficacious dose of these drugs.
3. Preclinical models have limitations to predict toxicities in humans. Novel toxicity profiles have been described during the development of new anticancer agents, thus early recognition measures and management guidelines have been implemented to adequately treat emerging adverse events.
4. Distinct reliable endpoints must be carefully defined in clinical trials, according to the type of drug developed, since suboptimal designs can mislead the development of new anticancer agents.
5. The success of new drugs in oncology relies on our capacity of better selecting those patients more likely to respond. Finding validated predictive biomarkers is a priority that should be adequately addressed.

2.1 Introduction

Over the last few decades, cytotoxic chemotherapeutics (CHTs) have been the backbone systemic therapy for treating cancer, relying on its innate ability to kill rapidly-dividing cancer cells. Based on these underlying principles, traditional Phase I clinical trials (Ph1) involving the assessment of CHTs focused primarily on safety objectives, and served to establish the principles of early drug development (EDD). These initial Ph1 were designed using a 3+3 dose escalation methodology, strictly ruled by the emergence of observed acute toxicities. Assuming a direct single dose-response relationship, with limited efficacy at lower doses and increased secondary effects at higher doses, only refractory heavily pre-treated patients with limited or no antitumor therapeutic options were recruited. The concomitant optimization of supportive medications (e.g., anti-nausea drugs, granulocyte-colony stimulating factors (G-CSFs), recombinant human erythropoietin) paralleled the development of CHTs, improving their safety profile and drastically contributing to the widespread use of cytotoxic drugs for a variety of cancers. However, in the early 1990s, the imperative need to reduce systemic toxicities related to CHTs, parallel to the discovery of the hallmarks of cancer [1, 2], contributed to the incorporation of a new class of drugs into the therapeutic arsenal for oncology patients, leading to a shift from this first paradigm of CHTs towards the molecularly targeted agents (MTAs) era [3].

Promising early and prolonged responses were observed among patients with advanced cancers treated with MTAs, although this was soon tempered by a series of challenges. The specific mechanism of action (MoA) and toxicity profile of these

MTAs, the selectively targeting some of the signaling pathways involved in human carcinogenesis, mandated a rethink of some of the EDD assumptions dominated by previous experiences with CHTs. As the classic dose-response-toxicity model was not applicable, oncology Ph1 had to evolve accordingly. Additional information became necessary to further delineate the biological MoAs of these agents, carefully integrating pharmacokinetic (PK) and pharmacodynamic (PD) data, and also incorporating long-term toxicities to fine-tune the final recommended dose for a specific MTA. Novel dose-escalation schemes and innovative statistical methodologies that had started with CHTs became widely used in MTA development. Together with revisited response evaluation criteria, unprecedented modifications were implemented to circumvent the limitations of previous Ph1 designs, leading to a marked change in the populations eligible to participate in early clinical trials [4].

But if MTAs represent a revolutionary new chapter in the history of the EDD, immunotherapy (IT) has gained its own title as the third paradigm following CHTs and MTAs. Understanding of antitumor immune responses has vastly improved during the last decade, to the point that IT was considered the scientific breakthrough of the year in 2013. Since then, a large and heterogeneous family of IT strategies has emerged, amongst which immune checkpoint-targeted monoclonal antibodies (ICT mAbs) have been the most frequently approved therapies so far. Obvious major differences observed between CHTs or MTAs and ICT mAbs have led to profound changes in most EDD areas, but especially in clinical trial design [5]. The uncertainty of novel immune regulation mechanisms, the lack of accurate preclinical models that could predict unexpected immune-related adverse events (irAEs), the difficulty in finding robust immune-predictive biomarkers, or the need to redefine trial designs, are some of the controversial points of this third paradigm in oncology [6].

Epigenetic modulation is another promising area of cancer drug development. Despite almost every cell in our body sharing the same DNA sequence, humans have evolved as complex organisms composed of specialized tissues hierarchically organized in different organs. Just like an orchestra can play the same piece of music in many different ways, cells use their DNA code differently by modulating gene expression depending on their needs. In this context, epigenetic drugs (EPDs) have emerged as an interesting option, aiming to regulate the changes in DNA expression that occur in cancerous cells [7]. Of note, the epigenetic targets may have different expression patterns and roles throughout the body, and this ubiquitous pattern might make it difficult to effectively deliver EPDs to their targeted cells, avoiding undesired damage in normal cells. Whilst the "first generation" of EPDs have shown limited efficacy as monotherapies in solid tumors, promising results have recently suggested roles as sensitizers to other anticancer agents [8]. Epigenetics can be considered the fourth paradigm in EDD after CHTs, MTAs and ICTs, and future well-designed clinical trials should pursue an improvement in the selectivity of these compounds, whilst identifying molecular determinants of response and elucidating the benefits of combined strategies.

In this chapter, we will review drug development evolution with a broad view of the major differences across these four paradigms, positioning some of the

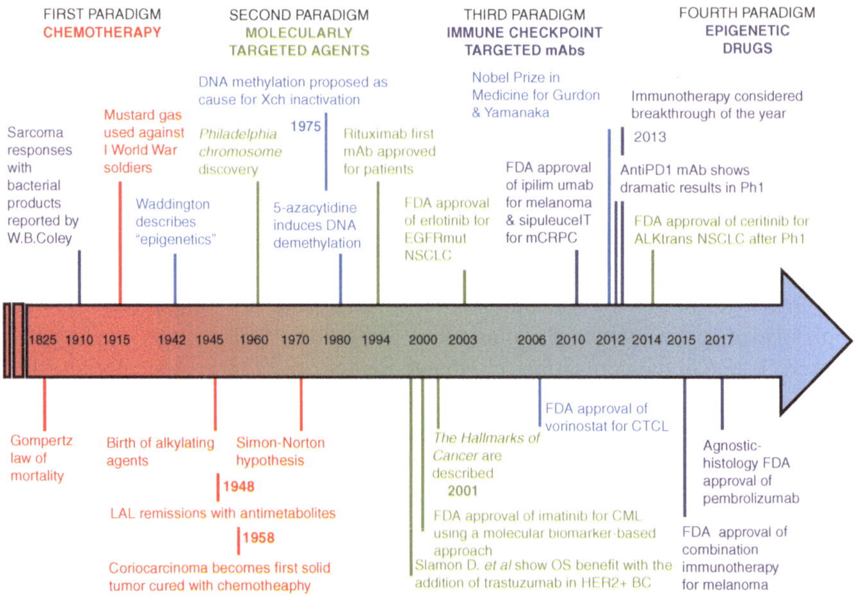

Abbreviations: LAL (Lymphoblastic Acute Leukemia); CML (Chronic Myeloid Leukemia); OS (Overall Survival); HER2+ (Human Epidermal growth factor Receptor 2 positive); BC (Breast Cancer); Xch (X chromosome); EGFR (Epidermal Growth Factor Receptor-mutant); NSCLC (Non-Small Cell Lung Cancer); CTCL (Cutaneous T Cell Lymphoma); mCRPR (metastic Castration Resistant Prostate Cancer); ALKtrans (ALK-translocated)

Fig. 2.1 Milestones of the different paradigm shifts in the timeline of oncology EDD

milestones that contributed to define them in the timeline of oncology EDD history (Fig. 2.1) and addressing many of the controversial issues that helped shape them. In the universe of EDD, one size does not fit all. These four paradigms represent generalities based on their underlying mechanisms of action, which mainly serve as a reference, for understanding the differences and hurdles that are faced when developing any new drug, rather than representing a rigid classification. Since the EDD arena is becoming increasingly complex, the type of drug will have to be carefully considered when designing a Ph1, to accelerate approval and ensure that we continue to do more good than harm to patients. Table 2.1 summarizes the main characteristics that have shaped these four paradigms in oncology EDD [6, 9, 10].

2.2 Cytotoxic Chemotherapeutics (CHTs): The Traditional First Paradigm in Oncology EDD

During World War II, observations of low blood cell counts in soldiers exposed to sulfur mustard (mustard gas) led to the birth of cytotoxic drugs. Sulfur was replaced by nitrogen to give nitrogen mustard, a predecessor of the alkylating agents. Following this, many more drugs that blocked cell replication were discovered: antimetabolites, antitumor antibiotics, adrenal steroids, tubulin-binders, and topoisomerase inhibitors.

Table 2.1 Main differences between the four established paradigms in oncology EDD

Key differences	First paradigm	Second paradigm	Third paradigm	Fourth paradigm
Type of drug	Cytotoxic chemotherapies (CHT) 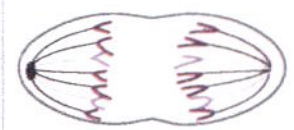	Molecularly-targeted agents (MTA) 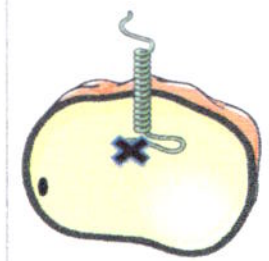	Immune-checkpoint targeted monoclonal antibodies (ICT mAbs) 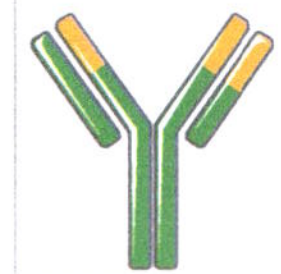	Epigenetic drugs (EPD) 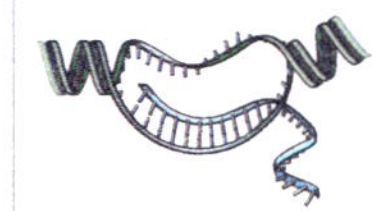
Example	Cisplatin	Erlotinib	Pembrolizumab	Vorinostat
Mechanism of action	Non-selective anti-proliferative	Modulation of a signaling pathway selective target	Agonist or antagonist of immune-induced checkpoints	Inhibition of chromatin modifiers
Patient populations in Ph1	Heavily pretreated refractory patients	– Advanced cancers with/without other treatment options – Healthy volunteer studies – Window-of-opportunity studies – Phase 0 studies – Molecularly-selected populations	Immune-enriched populations defined with a reliable predictive biomarker (e.g., MSI-H/dMMR or CPS PD-L1 positive)	– Slow growing tumors – Small populations based on an oncogene-addicted model (e.g., NUT midline carcinomas) – Need for an epigenetic-enriched enrollment strategy (e.g., DNAmet)
Number of patients in typical Ph1	30–50 unselected patients	30–200 patients	100–10,000 patients	50–100 patients
Formulation	Intravenous > Oral	Oral > Intravenous	– Intravenous – Possibility of new routes (intra-tumoral injection)	Oral

(continued)

Table 2.1 (continued)

Key differences	First paradigm	Second paradigm	Third paradigm	Fourth paradigm
Schedule	Often intermittent	Usually continuous	Intermittent	Intermittent and continuous
Toxicity profile	Usually affecting tissues with high turnover (e.g., bone marrow, hair, gastrointestinal epithelium)	Both on-target and off-target toxicities	Immune-mediated toxicities focused on skin, gastrointestinal, endocrine and liver systems	Myelosuppression, gastrointestinal toxicity
Toxicity assessment	– Linear dose-toxicity relationship – Predictable AEs – CTCAE v.4.03 assessment	– Modified dose-toxicity curves – Relative safer drugs – Need for a revisited CTCAE version in light of new toxicities	– No clear dose-toxicity relationship – Unpredictability of acute and chronic irAEs – Consider delayed toxicities – Need for an immune-CTCAE grading system	– Linear dose-toxicity relationships – Ubiquitous distribution of the target may cause damage in all normal tissues – CTCAE v.4.03 may apply – Possibility of delayed toxicities – Slow recovery from toxicities, once the epigenetic profile is reprogrammed
Toxicity management	– Dose reductions and delays – Supportive medication (e.g., GCSF, antiemetics)	– On-target effects: address directly (e.g., antihypertensive for anti-VEGFR MTA) – Off-target effects: dose reduction (e.g., chronic fatigue)	Role for immunosuppressants, to attenuate the triggered immune system	To be defined, but until then, wait and support
Ph1 design	Traditional 3+3 escalation design	– 3+3 escalation design with large expansion cohorts in molecularly-selected populations – Basket and umbrella trials in small and difficult-to-find molecularly-defined populations	– New escalation designs to capture the effect of late-onset toxicities: accelerated titration with Bayesian designs – Need for adapted endpoints (irOS, irPFS, composite ORR/DoR)	Traditional 3+3 escalation design followed by expansion cohorts in epigenetic-selected populations

Ph2 dose recommendation	– Linear dose-response relationship – Fine-tuning dosage based on acute toxicities during DLT period – MTD definition based on dose-response observations – MTD almost-systematically reached	– No clear dose-response relationship – Optimal BED mandatory – Incorporation of chronic toxicities – MTD inconstantly reached	– Less clear dose-response relationship – Need for an imBED – DLT periods extended – Toxicities beyond DLT period should be incorporated – MTD rarely reached	– Difficult-to-define dose-response relationship – Different RP2D may be considered for monotherapy versus combination purposes – MTD usually reached
PK/PD data	– Exploratory biomarkers – Additional information for defining schedule and RP2D	– Research of PD biomarkers of for BED correlation – PD-driven studies for biomarker assay validation and subsequent molecular enrichment	– Need for integrating validated measures of immune-modulation (immune-biomarkers) – PK/PD modeling for recommendation of final RP2D	– Research of differential epigenetic PD biomarkers in cancerous cells versus normal cells – Need for repeated clinical validation of potential biomarkers
Antitumor activity	Tumor shrinkage	Incorporation of tumor stabilizations and changes in density or metabolism	Patterns of pseudo-progressions, delayed and dissociate responses	Tumor shrinkage
Response evaluation	– WHO evaluation – RECIST v.1.1.	– mRECIST criteria – Choi criteria	– irRC criteria (1D) – irRECIST criteria (2D)	– RECIST v.1.1. in monotherapy – Adapted criteria according to each partner in combinations: mRECIST/Choi in EPD+MTA irRC/irRECIST in EPD+ICTmAbs

Abbreviations: *MSI-H* microsatellite instability-high, *dMMR* mismatch repair deficient, *CPS* PD-L1 combined positive score programmed death-ligand 1, *CTCAE* common terminology criteria for adverse events, *irAEs* immune-related adverse events, *irOS* immune-related overall survival, *irPFS* immune-related progression-free-survival, *composite ORR/DoR* composite overall response rate/duration of response, *DLT* dose-limiting toxicities, *MTD* maximum-tolerated dose, *RP2D* recommended phase 2 dose, *BED* biologically effective dose, *imBED* immune-biologically effective dose, *PK/PD* pharmacokinetics/pharmacodynamics, *WHO* World Health Organization, *RECIST* response evaluation criteria in solid tumors, *mRECIST* modified response evaluation criteria in solid tumors, *irRC* immune-related response criteria, *irRECIST* immune-related response evaluation criteria in solid tumors, *Ph3* phase III clinical trials, *Ph2* phase II clinical trials, *Ph1* phase I clinical trials

The objective of CHTs is to eradicate tumor cells, characterized by their limitless replicative potential. The therapeutic effect with CHTs is achieved by actively killing rapidly-growing cells, interfering with the most vulnerable points of the cell cycle, such as DNA synthesis or mitosis.

Modern understanding of malignant growth originated in the nineteenth century, when the mathematician Benjamin Gompertz postulated that biological growth rates of populations are not constant. According to Gompertzian kinetics, a growth curve in a semi-logarithmic plot would have a sigmoid shape tumor, meaning that smaller tumors grow faster: at first, cells number increases slowly because of the small number of cells, then-rapidly, and then slow again due to anoxia and a significant fraction of cells entering in G0 [11].

The efficacy seen with traditional CHTs follows also a sigmoid dose-response relationship, meaning that the higher the dose administered, the greater the benefit expected (except at very low and very high doses) [12]. However, this relationship also translates to a sigmoidal dose-toxicity effect, i.e., greater toxicities with increasing doses, especially among tissues with a continuously dividing population of cells (e.g., bone marrow or gastrointestinal epithelium) [13]. Therefore, the definition of an optimal safe dose was deemed the key point to be addressed by the EDD of CHTs. In 1970, Norton and Simon established a fundamental principle for developing CHTs, using a mathematical approach for integrating the information of in vitro biological growth into the definition of treatment scheduling: as tumors follow Gompertzian functions, lesions given less time for regrowth between treatments are more likely to be destroyed [14]. This hypothesis is considered one of the greatest advances in the EDD, because it highlighted that dose, timing, duration, and scheduling of a certain compound are meaningful variables to consider in clinical trial design.

In this context, Ph1 emerged as the necessary arena for finding the therapeutic window of a certain CHT, the range between a toxic and a therapeutic dose. Aiming to define the maximum tolerated dose (MTD) that would subsequently be used in a Phase II trial (recommended Phase II dose, RP2D), clinical researchers implemented escalation strategies in Ph1 using the observed toxicity to guide fine-tuning dosage. Conventionally, a safe starting dose derived from one tenth of the lethal dose in 10% of mice (LD10) or from one-sixth of the highest non-severely toxic dose (No observed adverse effect level or NOAEL) in non-rodent species is used [15]. Assuming that dose-limiting toxicity (DLT) is the unacceptable toxicity towards normal cells, an average probability of DLT of 20–33% has been considered acceptable within a trial. In 1989, Storer described the conservative 3+3 escalation method, where three-patient cohorts are enrolled per level, expanding them to a total of six if one of these three patients presents a DLT [16]. Although the 3+3 scheme continues to dominate the Ph1 practice, new escalation designs have lately emerged. Accelerated titration designs advocate for single-patient cohorts at early dose levels, in an attempt to reduce the number of patients treated at infra-therapeutic levels [17], and the continual re-assessment method proposes a pre-specified dose-toxicity curve which is continuously re-shaped as patient toxicity data becomes available [18].

The development of CHT combinations has represented a major challenge in the EDD of this first paradigm. Combinatorial drug regimens significantly increase the chance of remission, taking advantage of the synergistic effects of different MoAs.

Usually, agents that differ in their toxicity profile have been tested either in sequential or additive schemes, using cyclic regimens that allow appropriate intervals for the regeneration of critical healthy tissues (e.g., bone marrow). The parallel development of many chemoprotectors (e.g., folinic acid for methotrexate) and supportive medications (e.g., anti-nausea drugs such as 5-HT3 or neurokinin 1 antagonists), has been crucial for the successful progress of CHTs [19]. The Intergroup 0148/CALGB 9344 adjuvant trial in breast cancer illustrates the layers of complexity that must be considered when integrating different CHTs into a single study: the rational use of different MoAs to increase efficacy and overcome resistances (doxorubicin (A), cyclophosphamide (C), and paclitaxel (P)), the dose adjustment (three different doses of A tested), the feasibility of sequentiality (P following CA), the optimization of timing and duration schedule (four CA cycles followed by four cycles of P), and the determination of required supportive medications (concomitant G-CSFs and ciprofloxacin given routinely at higher A doses) [20]. Despite the advances in this field, new schemes of CHTs and innovative delivery strategies are currently under development, in an effort to design novel approaches that ensure a desired rate of tumor killing without unacceptable toxicity.

Nearly 70 years after the initial development of chemotherapeutics, we are witnessing a re-interpretation of the potential uses of cytotoxic drugs, thanks to antibody-drug conjugate (ADC) technology. ADCs are complex immunoconjugates, designed to selectively deliver toxic molecules that have been conjugated to a mAb via a stable chemical linker. ADCs have repurposed mAbs into very efficient delivery vehicles for many potent cytotoxic drugs, widening the therapeutic window of some molecules previously considered too toxic to be administered systemically [21]. Figure 2.2 depicts the dose-response and dose-toxicity curves that have traditionally limited the therapeutic window of CHTs. However, despite successful approved examples, such as trastuzumab emtansine for breast cancer [22] or brentuximab vedotin for Hodgkin's lymphoma [23], there are still many considerations that will need to be addressed to ensure the implementation of ADCs: (1) the rational selection of target antigens, expressed in normal cells at very low levels (e.g., carcinoembryonic antigen); (2) the careful modification of the mAb (e.g., selective mutations to improve linker and payload distribution); (3) the improvement in antibody-engineered delivery systems (e.g., immunoliposomes); (4) the consideration of different payloads according to each tumoral context (e.g., tubulin polymerization inhibitors for breast cancer); or (5) the definition of its optimal stoichiometry (e.g., ratio of CHT molecules per antibody), among others [24].

2.3 Molecularly Targeted Agents (MTAs): The (R)evolution of a Second Paradigm of Precision Medicine

In the 2000s, Hannahan and Weinberg published two thorough reviews summarizing our current understanding of tumorigenesis and its core traits. They attempted to describe *"the hallmarks"* of cancer: insensitivity to anti-growth signals, self-sufficiency in growth signals, limitless replicative potential, apoptosis evasion,

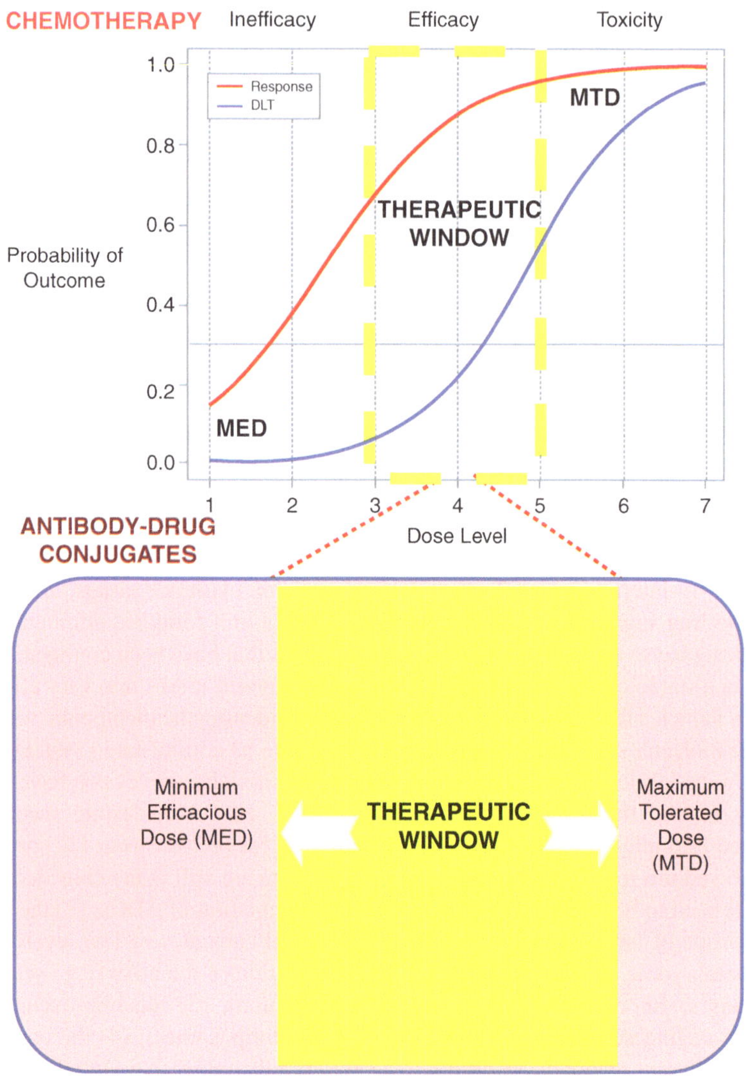

Fig. 2.2 Dose-response-toxicity relationship curves and therapeutic window for CHTs. The dose-response curve for traditional CHTs follows a sigmoidal shape, slowly rising until a minimum efficacy threshold is met (minimum efficacious dose, MED), followed by a linear phase that then reaches a plateau. The antitumor activity occurs in the linear phase, although extreme doses of CHT do not translate into higher activity rates once the plateau phase is reached; on the contrary, they might correlate with toxicity towards normal tissues (maximum tolerated dose, MTD). The therapeutic window is the range of doses comprised in the area where the curves separate, and comprises those doses that achieve the greatest therapeutic benefit without resulting in unacceptable side effects. ADC technology offers the possibility of widening this therapeutic window and efficaciously targeting selected antigen-expressing cancer cells

sustained angiogenesis, tissue invasion and metastasis, instability and mutation, immune response evasion, reprogramming of energy metabolism, and tumor-promoting inflammation [1, 2]. The understanding of the cancer biology illuminated our knowledge of the behavior of malignant cells, and led to the development of a whole new set of anticancer agents, the MTAs. This class of agents emerged as highly-specific compounds rationally designed to modulate different altered cellular components linked to the development of cancer.

These MTAs significantly altered the landscape of EDD, forcing researchers to reconsider some of the entrenched CHTs principles, especially regarding the dose-response-toxicity relationships. Given the mechanism of action of MTAs, traditional Ph1 designs based on toxicity-dosing seemed invalid, as MTAs challenge the underlying assumption that the mechanism resulting in toxicity is similar to the mechanism leading to efficacy. The basis for a certain MTA is the modulation of a cellular target that could translate into anti-tumoral activity, while at higher doses, efficacy may not increase and selectivity may even be lost, with off-target toxicities becoming evident. Finding the MTD was not always considered the only goal of this second paradigm, and these observations brought into the equation the need to define a biologically effective dose (BED) by evaluating markers of drug effect [10]. Figure 2.3 shows the changes in dose-response-toxicity curves associated with MTAs, and encompasses the different levels of drug effect biomarkers that should be integrated into the design of these MTA Ph1.

In this context, MTA Ph1 progressively focused on demonstrating the modulation of the putative target in tissues of interest, by identifying pharmacodynamic biomarkers, as a readout that indicates the effect that a certain MTA has in the body ("a proof-of-mechanism") [25]. U S Food and Drug Administration (FDA) approval of vismodegib in 2012, the first marketed sonic hedgehog inhibitor for the treatment of basal cell carcinoma, exemplifies this strategy. In a Ph1, vismodegib was tested at different doses without establishing an MTD. Detailed evaluation in non-malignant skin biopsies demonstrated evidence of GLI1 down-modulation as a PD marker that confirmed that the drug was suppressing the pathway even at the lower level. Hence, the RP2D was established at 150 mg daily based on the tumor responses seen at this dose, the fact that similar PK exposure was observed over 150–540 mg/day, and the evidence of pathway suppression PD data [26]. Using these integrative strategies, well-defined lower doses of MTAs might be efficacious enough when accurately hitting the target, facilitating the adherence of patients to chronic therapy and diminishing the number of dropouts due to long-term toxicities [27].

However, although a PD readout is necessary, it might not be sufficient, as the presence of PD modulation might not fully demonstrate that the MTA is acting via the intended target. The need for an a priori understanding of the biology behind each target and the feasibility of obtaining tissue biopsies may limit the implementation of PD studies, and other measurements of effect markers have been suggested [28]. On top of PD markers, additional effect markers have been increasingly used as a complementary strategy for delineating the BED of MTAs, such as markers of

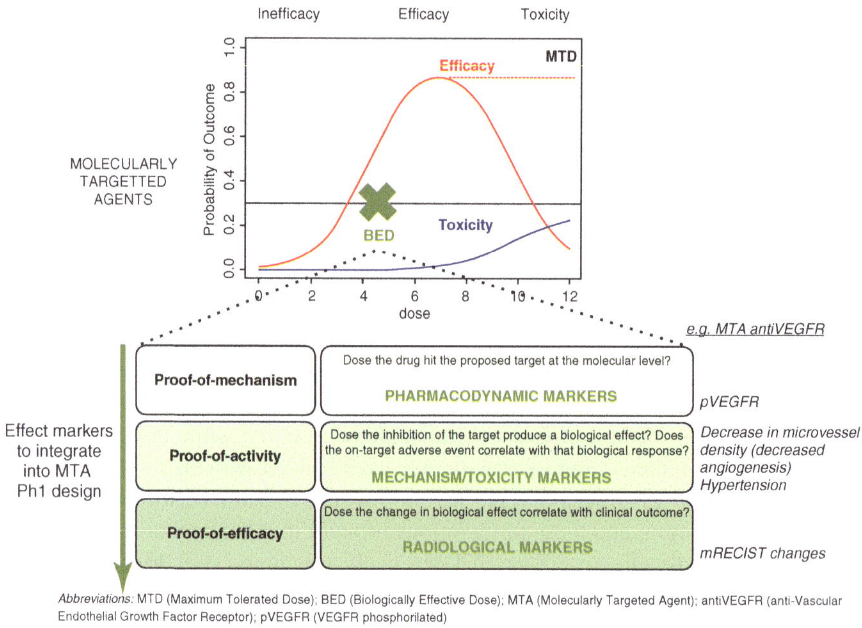

Fig. 2.3 Dose-response-toxicity relationship curves and integration of effect markers for defining the biologically effective dose (BED) of a certain MTA. The traditional CHT dose-response-toxicity sigmoidal curves have been reshaped with this second paradigm in EDD: very low doses of a MTA might be sufficient for hitting the desired target. Two scenarios can occur at higher doses: either sustained efficacy once the target modulation has reached a plateau (dotted red line), or a progressive decrease in clinical benefit due to loss of selectivity (straight red line). Toxicity might occur at very high doses or might never occur, and in certain occasions, the MTD may not be reached with traditional toxicity-guiding escalation designs (blue curve). Hence, to define an optimal BED, many markers of effect, pharmacodynamics, toxicity or radiological markers should be integrated into novel Ph1 designs developing MTAs

target engagement (e.g., toxicity derived from blocking a specific tyrosine kinase receptor) or disease progression markers (e.g., changes in tumor size). Mechanism-based adverse events, such as skin rash with epidermal growth factor receptor inhibitors, can be used as proof-of-activity markers for some MTAs. For others, tumor size, metabolic or radiomic changes (such as changes in density) may also represent an important effect marker for guiding decisions in EDD [28]. In fact, the unique mechanisms of these MTAs made it necessary to revisit some of the traditional response evaluation criteria used with CHTs, resulting in the modified Response Evaluation Criteria in Solid Tumors (mRECIST) [29] and the Choi criteria [30]. For the first time, metabolic changes assessed by positron emission tomography proved to be closely related to clinical benefit of an MTA, and in the case of gastrointestinal stromal tumor patients, even preceded the changes in size seen by simple computed tomography scans by months [31].

The particular toxicity profile of these MTAs changed the participation criteria for early trials, favoring the conduct of studies previously deemed unfeasible in the era of CHTs. Based on their relatively broad safety profile, some MTAs were implemented in healthy volunteer studies, aiming to collect robust PK/PD data from a certain drug in unbiased patient populations. Also, to confirm the hypothetical target modulation of a specific MTA, neo-adjuvant window-of-opportunity studies and Phase 0 studies emerged as an ideal scenario for obtaining tumor biopsies from treated subjects. Finally, the advent of new high-throughput technologies has started revealing specific mutational landscapes of patients, offering a valuable opportunity for guiding personalized strategies in molecularly-selected patient populations, the so-called "Precision Medicine" approach applied to EDD [4]. The FDA approval of imatinib mesylate, a BCR-ABL tyrosine kinase inhibitor for treating patients with chronic myeloid leukemia (CML) in 2001, demonstrated the potential of this model for the development of new anticancer drugs in small patient populations. The BCR-ABL rearrangement—the *Philadelphia chromosome*—was known to be the key clonal hematopoietic stem-cell event that initiates CML, and imatinib exhibited impressive benefits when selectively developed for treating this disease [32].

Some of the MTAs are currently developed in parallel with companion diagnostics that enable identification of patient populations that are most likely to respond favorably. Despite the myriad of molecular discoveries, the validation of predictive biomarkers remains a highly complex area of research, where many challenges may limit the success of certain MTAs [33]. First, it is important to acquire a comprehensive understanding of the tumor biology behind each particular case, assuming the intrinsic existence of both spatial and temporal intra/inter-tumoral heterogeneity. Secondly, the multiple pre-analytical procedures might interfere in the interpretation of the results for validating a specific biomarker (e.g., paraffin versus frozen samples), therefore it is critical to determine the best standard operating procedures for collecting and processing these biological specimens (e.g., selection of primary tumor versus metastatic lesion sample). And lastly, given that rare molecularly-selected populations may be difficult to recruit, we need to evaluate the feasibility of implementing complex screening logistics among several centers for fostering the enrollment into experimental studies. The fast approval of ceritinib for patients with non-small cell lung cancer harboring an ALK rearrangement, solely based on the results of the Ph1, represented a milestone in the history of EDD, and confirmed that well-conducted Ph1 can accelerate the approval of new drugs, especially when they potentially fill a void for poor prognosis cancers [34].

The development of next-generation sequencing tools enabled genomic characterization of solid tumors, promoting the recognition of tumors as genetic diseases, and facilitating the path from the discovery of new biomarkers towards the development and approval of a new family of MTAs [35]. The development of tropomyosin receptor kinase (TRK) inhibitors perfectly illustrates how the advent of biomarker-driven trials transformed oncology EDD. The "seamless" approach where Ph1 investigated dose and activity of TRK inhibitors in a variety of cancers sharing a difficult-to-find molecular aberration ("basket" trial design), became the basis for the development of entrectinib and larotrectinib among NTRK fusion-positive solid tumors [36, 37]. Furthermore, recent well-designed Ph1 have demonstrated that the early implementation of translational studies may also lead to the successful discovery of resistance mechanisms during early trials, guiding the subsequent development of second-generation MTAs that could even be validated in the same cohort of discovery patients [38].

2.4 Immune Checkpoint-Targeted Monoclonal Antibodies (ICT mAbs): A Challenging Third Paradigm of Uncertainties

The treatment of cancer by harnessing immune responses goes back as far as the late nineteenth century, when efforts to use the immune system against sarcomas were made by injecting bacterial products, with anecdotal successful results [39]. Since then, more in-depth knowledge of the biological components involved in orchestrating the immune response has fostered the development of cancer IT. Most of the initial insights into specific antitumor immune responses were obtained in melanomas, when high doses of interleukin 2 (IL-2), a T cell growth factor, showed 16% response rates among studies conducted in metastatic patients, with impressive durable efficacy among those who achieved complete responses [40]. Despite the life-threatening risks associated with this strategy, IL-2 became FDA approved in 1998. However, the immune system has a complex network of escape mechanisms to avoid excessive immune activation, and this hampered the development of further IT strategies. Nonetheless, the unique MoA of a novel class of ICT mAbs designed to selectively block the immune-induced checkpoint surface proteins, namely the cytotoxic T-lymphocyte associated antigen 4 (CTLA-4) [41] and the programmed death 1 (PD-1) receptor and its ligand (PD-L1) [42], provided the impetus for a third paradigm in oncology EDD.

These successes underscored the importance of decoding the basic concepts of tumor immunology. To delineate the underlying basis for cancer immune evasion and design more effective drugs, it was essential to consider some crucial premises in immune-oncology research: a) the capacity of immune adaptability and memory that could produce long-term antitumor effects and increase the response rate, breaking the ceiling of the traditional 16% response rates observed in initial trials (e.g., overall response rate of 57.6% with ipilimumab/nivolumab in melanoma patients [43]); b) unique MoAs expanded the opportunities for testing new combination strategies that may increase antitumor activity (e.g., pembrolizumab plus pemetrexed and platinum salts for non-small cell lung cancer [44]); c) targeting the immune system instead of transformed malignant cells offered the potential to effectively treat multiple tumor types (e.g., avelumab in Merkel cell carcinoma [45]).

Over the last few years, different ICT mAbs, mainly anti-CTLA-4 and anti-PD-1/L1, have been approved for an unprecedented number of indications. But the development of checkpoint inhibitors beyond PD-1/PD-L1 and CTLA4 has not met the high expectations generated, and some of them have already been discontinued due to their lack of efficacy or intolerable adverse events. This advocates for smarter clinical trial design in the early phases of development, carefully reviewing the lessons learned from the initial Ph1 that helped define this third paradigm shift in oncology [6]. One of the major limitations faced by EDD of ICT mAbs is the lack of preclinical studies that represent the human disease. Different in silico and in vitro methods are used for predicting the biological activity and toxicity of a certain new drug; however, immunotoxicology and immunopharmacology assays have not yet been fully optimized for ICT mAbs [46]. In addition, current preclinical animal models are not able to faithfully recapitulate the characteristics of the human immune system, since mice lack some of the human targets, which can in turn translate into an underestimation of serious toxicities and inaccurate safe starting doses [5]. A notable example was the acute development of a life-threatening cytokine release syndrome after a single dose of a CD28 agonist in six healthy volunteers participating in the first-in-human trial of TGN141 in 2006 [47]. This episode, known as the "TeGenero incident", warned the EDD community about the challenges of dealing with the innate unpredictability of immune-modulation and the limitations of animal models due to the particularities of the immune system of each species.

Most of the Ph1 for ICT mAbs have implemented a traditional 3+3 escalation method, although no clear consensus regarding the most suitable escalation design has been reached. Since the dose-efficacy and dose-toxicity curves are less defined for these antibodies, the standard strategy for defining an optimal RP2D does not apply. Low doses of ICT mAbs are equally effective as higher doses, challenging the MTD and RP2D establishment [9]. Of note, none of the six Ph1 that led to FDA approval of ICT mAbs (ipilimumab, nivolumab, pembrolizumab, atezolizumab, avelumab, and durvalumab) declared an MTD, and complementary PK/PD and safety markers were used for fine-tuning their RP2D [5]. In the case of pembrolizumab, the RP2D was selected using an integrative approach that correlated PK/PD relationships with tumor size markers, following a smart Ph1 dosing strategy driven by the understanding of the immuno-biologically effective dose (imBED). First, the imBED was estimated to be 2 mg/kg because IL-2 responses approached saturation levels at exposures consistent with this dose, and posterior clinical studies using this dose demonstrated early clinical responses measured by changes in tumor size [48]. Later exposure-response analysis showed similar antitumor response over doses ranging from 2 to 10 mg/kg, leading to the approval of a RP2D of 2 mg/kg [49]. Final population PK modeling assessed that a weight-based dosing of pembrolizumab had no advantages, leading to the final establishment of a 200 mg flat dose [50].

Treatment with ICT mAbs can last for a long time, therefore Ph1 designs should consider the unpredictability of irAEs, which can occur outside a traditional DLT-evaluation period, usually restricted to one treatment cycle. As ICT mAb-related irAEs can appear at any time during their administration, those lower adverse events lasting throughout multiple cycles, or isolated harmful grade 3/4 events that occur beyond the DLT-evaluation period, should be integrated into the final RP2D definition. Figure 2.4 illustrates the typical Kaplan Meier curve for overall survival (OS) observed among trials testing ICT mAbs, positioning the probability of appearance of some of the commonest G3-5 irAEs.

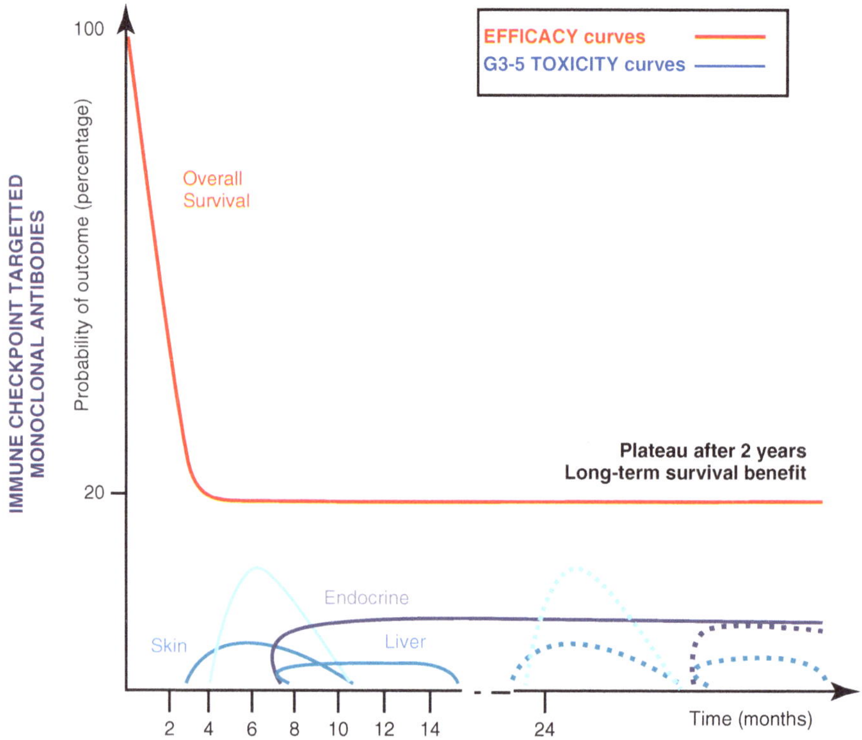

Fig. 2.4 Overall survival (OS) curve and probability of severe G3-5 immune-related adverse events (irAEs) with ICT mAbs. In the case of rapidly progressing malignancies with high tumor growth rates, Kaplan Meier curves for OS with ICT mAbs typically show a rapid decrease during the first months of therapy, then enter a slowly descending curve (red line). Those patients who benefit from the ICT mAb and survive beyond 24 months tend to reach a plateau and may represent a tail of long-term survivors [51]. Most of the G3-5 irAEs described with ICT mAbs appear within the first 3–6 months of the start of therapy, with no clear linear dose-dependent relationship. ICT mAbs are generally safe, although gastrointestinal colitis or diarrhea (light blue line), endocrine toxicity (lilac line), skin-rash or pruritus (dark blue line), and liver toxicity (turquoise line) are among the most common irAEs, with maximum reported rates for all tumor types in the main clinical trials for anti-CTLA-4, anti-PD-1, and anti-PD-L1 ICT mAbs of around 12%, 4%, 2%, and 1%, respectively. Although irAEs are unpredictable and can occur at any time during the administration of these drugs, a peculiar pattern has been observed, as illustrated in this figure. Although most of these severe irAEs can be solved completely with early detection and adequate medication, a delayed response to the ICT mAb cannot be excluded even 1 year after starting administration, and oncologists must keep such responses in mind during the follow-up of exposed patients (dotted lines). Immune-related endocrine disorders (hypothyroidism, hypophysitis, adrenal insufficiency) tend to occur later during the treatment, but in most of cases, patients will require permanent hormone replacement [52–54]

One of the most challenging differences that ICT mAbs brought to the EDD field was a new toxicity profile [55]. Second-generation ICT mAbs developed beyond the initial inhibitory molecules, such as novel co-stimulatory antibodies targeting CD40, OX40, inducible co-stimulator of T-cells (ICOS), or glucocorticoid-induced tumor necrosis factor receptor (GITR), made it necessary to revisit the way in which Ph1 were conducted, as there were concerns regarding the possibility of triggering a life-threatening cytokine release syndrome, hyper-immune stimulation, or uncontrolled autoimmune reactions [56]. These new types of side effects moved investigators to reconsider study designs, leading to the implementation of measures for minimizing risks. These include staggering the inclusion of patients among the first cycles or hospitalizing patients during the first 24 h after administration. In fact, first-in-human Ph1 testing ICT mAb agonists require a new skill set for recognizing and managing these toxicities, so they should be run in EDD units with experience of managing irAEs and close access to intensive care units. As early recognition and initiation of treatment for these irAEs are crucial for reducing potential sequelae, great efforts have been undertaken to characterize the most frequent ICT mAb-related irAEs and to develop management guidelines [52, 53].

Corticosteroids and immunosuppressants have been routinely used for managing irAEs, although it is unclear whether these drugs should be avoided in patients treated with ICT mAbs, based on the hypothesis that steroids and immune-modulators could antagonize the desired effect of experimental immunotherapies [57]. This particular toxicity profile has made it necessary to revisit some of the Ph1 patient eligibility criteria, to avoid enrolling unfit candidates or those harboring pre-existing conditions that indicate a degree of immune activation, such as gastro-intestinal autoimmune diseases (e.g., Crohn's disease). However, employing such strict criteria may bias the results obtained with the initial studies testing ICT mAbs, as they do not truly reflect the real-world patient population [58]. Many advocate for a redefinition of the exclusion criteria based on a stronger biological rationale, which we will certainly gather as we progressively gain more experience from large cohorts of ICT mAb-treated patients [59].

In addition to the safety considerations, the development of ICT mAbs has opened an intense debate regarding the suitability of the RECIST criteria v.1.1. for evaluating the efficacy of these antibodies. Unusual and unexpected response patterns have been reported with ICT mAbs, ranging from pseudo-progressions, delayed or even dissociated responses. Wolchok et al. summarized these response patterns into the immune-related response criteria (irRC) in an attempt to reflect the complexity of the biological processes involved between tumor cells and the immune system of the host. The aim was to help recognize patients who may benefit from an ICT mAb and who should not be prematurely shifted to another drug despite not presenting clear radiological evidence of efficacy [60]. However, these irRC were developed in parallel with anti-CTLA-4 antibodies in melanoma, and their extrapolation to other ICT mAbs and in other histologies should be approached with caution. Also, it is worth noting that these criteria can be considered much more subjective than the traditional RECIST criteria, therefore the investigator's own assessment might bias the progression free survival (PFS) evaluation.

Alternative strategies, such as the immune-related RECIST (irRECIST) [61] criteria have also been proposed. Whichever the criteria used, it seems crucial that they should be a reliable tool for capturing the dynamic changes of the immune response, as delayed efficacy could in part explain the discrepancies seen between OS and PFS rates among ICT mAb-treated patients.

The novel pattern of responses seen with ICT mAbs revolutionized several Ph1 statistical concepts for the assessment of efficacy. The infrequent although possible phenomenon of pseudo-progression might impact the PFS assessment, which had been considered a reliable surrogate endpoint for OS with CHTs and MTAs. Attention has focused on the non-responder subgroups, as pseudo-progressions wrongly labeled as true progressions could lead to patient withdrawal from the study, negatively impacting the PFS evaluation and not reflecting the true benefit of a certain ICT mAb [62]. As an example, the randomized Phase III study in renal carcinoma comparing nivolumab with everolimus demonstrated a benefit in OS favoring the IT arm, but not in PFS [63]. On the other hand, continuing treatment in true progressors (which, in melanoma, for example, account for 90% of cases of increased targeted lesions) could hamper future treatment options of these patients. Also, these antibodies re-shaped the traditional Kaplan-Meier curves. Since ICT mAb responses can be delayed for several months, the early comparison between survival curves might underestimate differences in long-term efficacy [51]. All these observations have led researchers to consider the need for new statistical models to provide reliable outcome measures, taking into consideration that hazard ratios between curves are not constant over time [64]. In view of these limitations, we must eagerly await the future development and prospective validation of specific endpoints for ICT mAb trials, such as new immune-related OS (irOS) or PFS (irPFS) endpoints, or composite endpoints of overall response rate and duration of response, that could better predict the effect of IT on long-term survival [65].

Finally, early development of IT has revealed the importance of finding appropriate predictive immune-biomarkers to define those patients whose cancers are likely to respond. Several potential biomarkers are under investigation, although the strongest evidence relies on the expression of PD-L1 [66], the presence of tumor-infiltrating lymphocytes (TILs) at the invasive tumor margin [67], the existence of a high tumor mutation burden (TMB) with a specific neo-antigen signature [68, 69], or the detection of microsatellite instability-high (MSI-H)/mismatch-repair-deficient (dMMR) tumors [70]. The lack of standardized methods for defining the presence of these immune-biomarkers has long resulted in inconsistencies in the selection of ideal candidates.

In the case of PD-L1 expression, the variety of immunohistochemistry (IHC) assays and PD-L1-positive thresholds developed [71] highlights the heterogeneity used for the approval of ICT mAbs in different histological settings, although several efforts have been made for validating novel PD-L1 scoring methods [72]. As an example, the PD-L1 combined positive score (CPS), defined a reproducible IHC scoring algorithm that supported the accelerated approval of pembrolizumab in third line PD-L1 CPS $\geq$ 1 metastatic gastric cancer patients and facilitated the investigation in other indications [73]. In the case of MSI-H tumors, they share common predictive features of immunotherapy response, such as PD-L1 expression, high TMB, and TILs [74]. Fortunately, when the ICT mAb development focused on this population, IHC testing or PCR-based assays were already validated for detecting MSI patients in clinics [75]. On May 23, 2017, the FDA approved pembrolizumab for the treatment of adult and pediatric patients with MSI-H or dMMR solid tumors, irrespective of their origin [76]. This indication has represented a milestone in the development of ICT mAbs, linking personalized medicine based on cancer genomics with immunotherapy, and the first indication of a drug for the treatment of patients regardless of tumor type.

2.5 Epigenetic Drugs (EPDs): The Fourth Paradigm Has Arrived

In 1942, Conrad Waddington defined the term epigenetics as "the branch of biology which studies the causal interactions between genes and their products, which bring the phenotype into being" [77]. Initial epigenetics focused on the study of heritable changes in gene functions, describing the dynamic interactions between the genome and the cellular environment that lead to a final phenotype. However, these early principles were anchored in evolutionary theory. Increased understanding of the underlying biochemical mechanisms that tightly control our hierarchically organized human genome led to the development of molecular epigenetics [78]. Since then, many scientific discoveries contributed to describe the main set of actors that play a crucial role in epigenetics, namely DNA, RNA, and their intimately associated proteins [79]. In 2012, the Nobel Prize in Medicine was awarded to JB. Gurdon and S. Yamanaka for their discovery that mature somatic human cells can be successfully reprogrammed into pluripotent cells [80].

It was realized that countless examples of alterations in epigenetic patterns may be behind the development of many human diseases [81]. Histone modification by different enzymes—histone acetyltransferases (HATs) and deacetylases (HDACs), histone methyltransferases (HMTs) and demethylases (HDMs)—has been recognized as a fundamental epigenetic mechanism, as has the methylation of CpG islands. CpG islands are regions with a high frequency of CpG dinucleotides that tend to overlap with gene promoters. The methylation of cytosines in CpGs, which is performed by several DNA methyltransferases (DNMTs), results in a condensed state of chromatin, inactive for transcriptional purposes. In addition to these two major epigenetic modifiers, ATP-dependent complexes involved in chromatin remodeling, such as the switch/sucrose non fermentable (SWI/SNF) complex, have recently highlighted the relevant role of this multi-subunit in the positioning of nucleosomes, thereby regulating transcription [82]. Finally, recent work has shown the involvement of non-coding RNA interference transcripts (miRNAs) in post-transcriptional RNA silencing mechanisms [83].

In the last decade, different epigenetic changes have been studied in detail, thanks to several high-throughput sequencing and array technologies, such as whole-genome bisulfite sequencing. This work has contributed to the elucidation of the clinical implications of the epigenetic network in a wide range of human tumors [84]. Now, in the wake of cancer-applied 'omics', the mapping of human genome-wide epigenetics has emerged as a new research field, so-called epigenomics [85]. Genomic aberrations in histone variants, promoter hypomethylation patterns, abnormal expression of chromatin-remodeling proteins, or altered microRNA-processing machinery enzymes, account for the epigenetic traits globally displayed by cancers [86]. Envisaging the possibility of modulating the epigenetic regulation, a new class of drugs has been developed, termed epigenetic drugs (EPDs), leading towards a fourth paradigm shift in oncology drug development.

5-Azacytidine, the agent that improved the prognosis of myelodysplastic syndromes, was initially synthetized as a cytotoxic drug, but was readily repurposed at lower doses as one of the first EPDs in light of the discovery that it induces DNA demethylation [87]. In fact, these observations highlighted one of the main controversies under discussion, whether EPDs should be considered part of the CHT family or whether they deserve recognition as a separate entity based on their particular DNA expression modulation-based MoAs. In the past few years, we have witnessed the emergence of several investigational small molecules specifically targeting epigenetic writers, readers, erasers, and chromatin remodelers—inhibitors for HATs/HDACs/HMTs (e.g., enhancer of zeste homolog 2, EZH2, or protein arginine N-methyltransferase 1, PRMT1)/HDMs (e.g., lysine-specific HDM 1, LSD1), DNMT inhibitors, bromodomain extra-terminal (BETinh) and IDH1-2 inhibitors, blockers of transcription factors, or drugs that target miRNAs, among others—[88], culminating in the first FDA approval of the HDAC inhibitor (HDACinh) vorinostat for cutaneous T cell lymphoma in 2006 [89]. Several ideas on the trial design and dosing and schedules have begun to emerge from the initial Ph1 testing EPDs.

One of the major critical points about the use of EPDs in patients is how we can ensure a certain degree of specificity for the target. Most of the epigenetic targets are essential proteins ubiquitously expressed throughout the body. The therapeutic window for EPDs has been empirically defined based on the premise that cancer cells might rely more than normal cells on the epigenetic regulator, to sustain a malignant transcriptional program. However, the fact that many silenced genes might be unintentionally activated by EPDs and cause deleterious effects in normal cells, is a sufficient valid concern that warrants further consideration in designing future Ph1 [82]. Despite these initial concerns, early data suggests that EPDs are relatively well-tolerated drugs, although some of them are particularly myelosuppressant, especially when used at higher doses, as is often the case in Ph1 searching for an MTD. EPDs may take time to efficiently modulate the epigenome and reprogram the targeted cancer cells, therefore patients might need to stay on trial for longer periods of time before any benefit is seen, and in some cases, only stabilization of the tumor growth rate is seen [90]. Longer periods of treatment are accompanied by a greater risk of developing chronic toxicity, although it is worth keeping in mind that the epigenetic modifications are usually reversible. In light of these particularities, DLT definition and efficacy assessment are two major challenges to deal with in the early phases of EPDs clinical development.

Much still needs to be done in selecting the optimal drug dosing and schedule, for example, we will need to obtain a better understanding of where an EPD is engaging its target at the chromatin level in each specific cellular setting, as this will allow for a more appropriate definition of respective PD biomarkers. The use of techniques that profile epigenetic modifications across the genome in early clinical trials will be essential [91]. Interestingly, the use of these PD markers may help in refining the definition of a low-versus-high doses of EPD, giving us a more detailed profile of the broad spectrum of effects that different doses of a certain drug can exert in a cell. A plethora of new next-generation sequencing-based technologies applied to DNA methylation profiling are currently investigating the changes in the epigenetic landscape, such as whole-genome bisulfite sequencing, methylation capture sequencing, or methyl-CpG binding domain sequencing, among others [92]. These massively-parallel methods represent useful tools for decoding the patterns of DNA modifications following epigenetic therapy, offering a great opportunity for unraveling the distinct changes associated with a range of doses.

In the face of modest activity as single agents, a combinatorial regimen with other anticancer agents represents a promising strategy for synergistically exploiting the potential of EPDs [93]. For example, there is increasing evidence that HDACinh can effectively increase antitumor immunity, either by directly upregulating the expression of major histocompatibility complex class I/II proteins and adhesion/co-stimulatory molecules, or by altering cytokine production, supporting their combination with ICT mAbs. Also, as they can lower the apoptotic threshold within a tumor cell, HDACinh have emerged as an ideal partner for CHTs or MTAs, taking advantage of the possibility that EPDs can contribute in reversing epigenetic-modulated mechanisms of resistance to these cancer drugs. Finally, EPDs enhance the tumor-killing effects of radiotherapy. Importantly, empirical combinations of different therapies should be considered with caution, especially when mixing two drugs that can substantially alter the epigenome, because normal and malignant epigenetic regulation is context-cell specific, and they may potentially be detrimental (e.g., combinations of DNMTs and HDACinh) [94]. A greater understanding of the precise MoAs and differential characteristics that define the different members of the EPD family will provide a more robust molecular rationale for further guiding the development of Ph1 with synergistic combinations.

Undoubtedly, gaining more insights into the molecular determinants of resistance to EPDs may provide the basis for optimizing therapeutic combinations to circumvent these resistance mechanisms. Tumor-specific factors, both at the level of malignant cells or tumor microenvironment, or systemic factors like PK, have been linked to failure of treatment with HDAC inhibitors, for example [95]. To date, most of the resistance hypotheses have been drawn from preclinical studies. Hence, the real characterization of these intrinsic resistance mechanisms in a real-world clinical setting will be crucial for identifying patients most likely to respond. So far, most of the EPDs have shown limited success in epithelial solid tumors, revealing the need to improve the selection of sensitive patients for these drugs.

Based on increasing evidence regarding recurrent mutations in chromatin modifiers among different cancer types, one could consider pursuing the development of new compounds in epigenetic-selected populations, following an oncogene-addicted model. In addition, the epigenetic approach has emerged as an interesting option for exploiting the synthetic lethality relationships of certain loss-of-function-mutant tumors [90]. In this direction, some of the newest epigenetic agents are moving into the Ph1 stage enrolling genetically-defined patient populations in order to foster their path from the laboratory to the clinical setting: for example, BETinh and HDACinh focused on rare chemo-resistant NUT midline carcinomas, where the pathognomonic molecular aberration involves a BRD3/4-NUT fusion protein, and EZH2 HMT inhibitors focused on INI1 loss solid tumors with loss of SWI/SNF subunits [82]. A second strategy for an enrichment-based development of EPDs could be the identification of specific patterns of epigenetic modulation in cancers, such as DNA methylation (DNAme) profiles, histone methylation or acetylation markers, or specific miRNA signatures. However, the feasibility of this approach relies on the capacity to standardize adequate companion diagnostics for routine use in clinics, which has proven challenging. As an example, a variety of DNAme assays have been tested, but with clear technical limitations that might have resulted in non-comparable results across different studies [96]. To date, many promising epigenetic candidate markers have been identified, but unfortunately, few of them have found a meaningful application. This inadequate clinical validation urgently needs to be addressed.

2.6 Conclusions

It has almost been a century since CHTs were initially tested, and the insights gained since then into human carcinogenesis have led to the development of a range of new promising drugs. A second, third, and even fourth paradigm in the EDD field can now be recognized, based on the new MoAs that defined the advent of MTAs, ICT mAbs, and EPDs.

The development process of these four paradigms has unveiled the universal fact that the efficient use of any new anticancer drug is best supported by appropriate markers of drug effect. Validation assays that correlate clinical responses with drug-induced efficacy have provided strong support from a mechanistic point of view, and only the ability to measure the expected target engagement of a given drug has successfully facilitated its development. Early in the discovery of any new anticancer agent, researchers should refer to the pharmacological audit trail framework, which comprises a set of critical biomarker-driven questions that support evidence-based decision-making in drug development [97]. Ph1 studies are progressively occupying a more central role in the development plan of new agents, aiming to enrich the participant population according to pre-specified exploratory biomarkers to identify trends and signals that can define responding populations early on. Also, resistance mechanisms to these novel therapies are being described early on as a result of thoughtful translational research performed in parallel to Ph1. We are, therefore, witnessing how clinical, pharmacological, molecular, and translational research have been brought closer together in EDD programs. Certainly, the final success of any strategy will be determined by our ability to overcome many of the obstacles outlined in each of these four paradigms.

Drug classes other than mAbs and small molecules are in the pipeline, which may drastically change the basis of EDD concepts in the coming years. Most of these emergent therapies are based on immune strategies aiming to expand the role of IT for treating cancer: different options of adoptive cellular therapy (TILs, chimeric antigen receptor T cell therapies, dendritic cells), sophisticated cytokine cocktails, viral vaccines (modified proteins from oncolytic viruses), and/or bacteria-engineered therapies (ADC with payloads of bacterial products). In addition, *"pseudo-targeted"* agents are emerging, such as enzyme modulators (e.g., IDO inhibitors), inhibitors of cell cycle-regulating kinases (e.g., aurora kinase inhibitors), or inhibitors of homeostatic pathways (e.g., WNT/β-catenin inhibitors), which all fall into a separate miscellaneous category [98]. Perhaps, if we move forward and succeed with the development of one of these novel modalities of cancer therapy, we shall witness the establishment of another paradigm shift in oncology.

Unfortunately, it is unlikely that any of the drugs discussed here and developed under any of these four paradigms will provide a cure for any solid aggressive cancer as a single agent, and therefore the future seems to drive the field towards strategies involving rational patient selection and thoughtful combination strategies [99]. We are cautiously optimistic that we will witness the establishment of another paradigm for developing combinations among the different classes of agents described here in the near future. Understanding the differences between these agents will be crucial for the future successful design of Ph1 developing new anticancer strategies.

Key Expert Opinion Points

1. Despite the incorporation of several innovative drugs into the therapeutic arsenal for treating cancer, cytotoxic chemotherapeutics (CHTs) remain the mainstay treatment option for oncology patients. Personalized CHT dosing strategies, novel combinatorial drug regimens, optimization of supportive medications and new delivery systems, aim to widen the potential uses of CHTs in forthcoming years.
2. Our understanding of the specific oncogenic drivers on which tumors depend is only beginning to emerge. The critical issue in the development of new molecularly targeted agents (MTAs) relies on clarifying the biology behind the molecular targets of these drugs, to further characterize the on- and off-target effects for understanding their resulting activity and toxicity. Efforts in identifying and selecting a genetically better defined subset of candidate patients will be crucial to run thoughtful biomarker-driven clinical trials and successfully guide the development of new MTAs.
3. Immune checkpoint-targeted monoclonal antibodies (ICT mAbs) have succeeded in triggering the immune system of cancer patients, an approach that has had impressive results in different tumor types. However, the future goal should focus on achieving durable responses with minimal toxicity in a broader population of patients. Optimizing the efficacy of ICT mAbs will probably need targeting multiple levels of the immune system, and this will certainly require a

rational design of synergistic combinations. New selection criteria based on biological premises and reliable immune-biomarkers, but also reflecting the real-world population, seem mandatory to ensure the future success of new ICT mAbs.

4. Early successes in treating hematologic malignancies and discoveries of epigenetic regulators in a wide array of cancers have fostered the development of epigenetic drugs (EPDs). However, understanding how cancer cells exploit epigenetic mechanisms to induce survival, and modulate drug resistance or immune surveillance, will be the key point to exploit the therapeutic potential of EPDs, probably best combined with CHTs, MTAs or ICT mAbs. How genetic alterations in oncogenes or tumor suppressor genes, as well as epigenetic changes, can be used as predictive biomarkers to EPDs, are some of the challenges that should be adequately addressed.
5. While expectations are rising with these four paradigms, a new miscellaneous category of drugs is emerging, comprising alternative immunotherapy strategies or "*pseudo-targeted*" drugs, among others. For researchers to be ready for this new era, it will be crucial to integrate the knowledge in molecular biology and cancer-applied omics into innovative clinical trial designs, since early phases of the development of these novel anticancer drugs.

References

1. Hanahan D, Weinberg RA. The hallmarks of cancer. Cell. 2000;100:57–70.
2. Hanahan D, Weinberg RA. Hallmarks of cancer: the next generation. Cell. 2011;144:646–74.
3. Rodon J. An (only) partially established paradigm of drug development of targeted therapies. Eur J Cancer. 2014;50:2037–9.
4. Hierro C, Azaro A, Argiles G, et al. Unveiling changes in the landscape of patient populations in cancer early drug development. Oncotarget. 2017;8:14158–72.
5. Ochoa de Olza M, Oliva M, Hierro C, et al. Early-drug development in the era of immuno-oncology: are we ready to face the challenges? Ann Oncol. 2018;29:1727–40.
6. Martin-Liberal J, Hierro C, Ochoa de Olza M, Rodon J. Immuno-oncology: the third paradigm in early drug development. Target Oncol. 2017;12:125–38.
7. Cramer SA, Adjei IM, Labhasetwar V. Advancements in the delivery of epigenetic drugs. Expert Opin Drug Deliv. 2015;12:1501–12.
8. Suraweera A, O'Byrne KJ, Richard DJ. Combination therapy with histone deacetylase inhibitors (HDACi) for the treatment of cancer: achieving the full therapeutic potential of HDACi. Front Oncol. 2018;8:92.
9. Postel-Vinay S, Aspeslagh S, Lanoy E, et al. Challenges of phase 1 clinical trials evaluating immune checkpoint-targeted antibodies. Ann Oncol. 2016;27:214–24.
10. Le Tourneau C, Dieras V, Tresca P, et al. Current challenges for the early clinical development of anticancer drugs in the era of molecularly targeted agents. Target Oncol. 2010;5:65–72.
11. Lloyd HH. Estimation of tumor cell kill from Gompertz growth curves. Cancer Chemother Rep. 1975;59:267–77.
12. Heller JR. Cancer chemotherapy, history and present status. Bull N Y Acad Med. 1962;38:348–63.
13. Fernando J, Jones R. The principles of cancer treatment by chemotherapy. Surgery (Oxford). 2015;33(3):131–5.

14. Schmidt C. The Gompertzian view: Norton honored for role in establishing cancer treatment approach. J Natl Cancer Inst. 2004;96(20):1492–3.
15. Hansen AR, Cook N, Ricci MS, et al. Choice of starting dose for biopharmaceuticals in first-in-human phase I cancer clinical trials. Oncologist. 2015;20:653–9.
16. Storer BE. Design and analysis of phase I clinical trials. Biometrics. 1989;45:925–37.
17. Simon R, Freidlin B, Rubinstein L, et al. Accelerated titration designs for phase I clinical trials in oncology. J Natl Cancer Inst. 1997;89:1138–47.
18. O'Quigley J, Pepe M, Fisher L. Continual reassessment method: a practical design for phase 1 clinical trials in cancer. Biometrics. 1990;46:33–48.
19. Lundqvist EÅ, Fujiwara K, Seoud M. Principles of chemotherapy. Int J Gynecol Obstet. 2015;131:S146–9.
20. Henderson IC, Berry DA, Demetri GD, et al. Improved outcomes from adding sequential Paclitaxel but not from escalating Doxorubicin dose in an adjuvant chemotherapy regimen for patients with node-positive primary breast cancer. J Clin Oncol. 2003;21:976–83.
21. Smaglo BG, Aldeghaither D, Weiner LM. The development of immunoconjugates for targeted cancer therapy. Nat Rev Clin Oncol. 2014;11:637–48.
22. Verma S, Miles D, Gianni L, et al. Trastuzumab emtansine for HER2-positive advanced breast cancer. N Engl J Med. 2012;367:1783–91.
23. Younes A, Gopal AK, Smith SE, et al. Results of a pivotal phase II study of brentuximab vedotin for patients with relapsed or refractory Hodgkin's lymphoma. J Clin Oncol. 2012;30:2183–9.
24. Teicher BA, Chari RV. Antibody conjugate therapeutics: challenges and potential. Clin Cancer Res. 2011;17:6389–97.
25. Garralda E, Dienstmann R, Tabernero J. Pharmacokinetic/pharmacodynamic modeling for drug development in oncology. Am Soc Clin Oncol Educ Book. 2017;37:210–5.
26. LoRusso PM, Rudin CM, Reddy JC, et al. Phase I trial of hedgehog pathway inhibitor vismodegib (GDC-0449) in patients with refractory, locally advanced or metastatic solid tumors. Clin Cancer Res. 2011;17:2502–11.
27. Jain RK, Lee JJ, Hong D, et al. Phase I oncology studies: evidence that in the era of targeted therapies patients on lower doses do not fare worse. Clin Cancer Res. 2010;16:1289–97.
28. Sachs JR, Mayawala K, Gadamsetty S, et al. Optimal dosing for targeted therapies in oncology: drug development cases leading by example. Clin Cancer Res. 2016;22:1318–24.
29. Lencioni R, Llovet JM. Modified RECIST (mRECIST) assessment for hepatocellular carcinoma. Semin Liver Dis. 2010;30:52–60.
30. Choi H, Charnsangavej C, Faria SC, et al. Correlation of computed tomography and positron emission tomography in patients with metastatic gastrointestinal stromal tumor treated at a single institution with imatinib mesylate: proposal of new computed tomography response criteria. J Clin Oncol. 2007;25:1753–9.
31. Van den Abbeele AD. The lessons of GIST–PET and PET/CT: a new paradigm for imaging. Oncologist. 2008;13(Suppl 2):8–13.
32. Druker BJ, Talpaz M, Resta DJ, et al. Efficacy and safety of a specific inhibitor of the BCR-ABL tyrosine kinase in chronic myeloid leukemia. N Engl J Med. 2001;344:1031–7.
33. Ileana Dumbrava E, Meric-Bernstam F, Yap TA. Challenges with biomarkers in cancer drug discovery and development. Expert Opin Drug Discov. 2018;13:685–90.
34. Shaw AT, Kim DW, Mehra R, et al. Ceritinib in ALK-rearranged non-small-cell lung cancer. N Engl J Med. 2014;370:1189–97.
35. Chin L, Gray JW. Translating insights from the cancer genome into clinical practice. Nature. 2008;452:553–63.
36. Drilon A, Siena S, Ou SI, et al. Safety and antitumor activity of the multitargeted Pan-TRK, ROS1, and ALK inhibitor entrectinib: combined results from two phase I trials (ALKA-372-001 and STARTRK-1). Cancer Discov. 2017;7:400–9.
37. Drilon A, Laetsch TW, Kummar S, et al. Efficacy of larotrectinib in TRK fusion-positive cancers in adults and children. N Engl J Med. 2018;378:731–9.
38. Drilon A, Nagasubramanian R, Blake JF, et al. A next-generation TRK kinase inhibitor overcomes acquired resistance to prior TRK kinase inhibition in patients with TRK fusion-positive solid tumors. Cancer Discov. 2017;7:963–72.

39. Coley WB. The treatment of inoperable sarcoma by bacterial toxins (the mixed toxins of the Streptococcus erysipelas and the Bacillus prodigiosus). Proc R Soc Med. 1910;3:1–48.
40. Atkins MB, Lotze MT, Dutcher JP, et al. High-dose recombinant interleukin 2 therapy for patients with metastatic melanoma: analysis of 270 patients treated between 1985 and 1993. J Clin Oncol. 1999;17:2105–16.
41. Hodi FS, O'Day SJ, McDermott DF, et al. Improved survival with ipilimumab in patients with metastatic melanoma. N Engl J Med. 2010;363:711–23.
42. Topalian SL, Hodi FS, Brahmer JR, et al. Safety, activity, and immune correlates of anti-PD-1 antibody in cancer. N Engl J Med. 2012;366:2443–54.
43. Larkin J, Chiarion-Sileni V, Gonzalez R, et al. Combined nivolumab and ipilimumab or monotherapy in untreated melanoma. N Engl J Med. 2015;373(1):23–34.
44. Gandhi L, Rodriguez-Abreu D, Gadgeel S, et al. Pembrolizumab plus chemotherapy in metastatic non-small-cell lung cancer. N Engl J Med. 2018;378:2078–92.
45. Kaufman HL, Russell J, Hamid O, et al. Avelumab in patients with chemotherapy-refractory metastatic Merkel cell carcinoma: a multicentre, single-group, open-label, phase 2 trial. Lancet Oncol. 2016;17:1374–85.
46. Kizhedath A, Wilkinson S, Glassey J. Applicability of predictive toxicology methods for monoclonal antibody therapeutics: status Quo and scope. Arch Toxicol. 2017;91:1595–612.
47. Suntharalingam G, Perry MR, Ward S, et al. Cytokine storm in a phase 1 trial of the anti-CD28 monoclonal antibody TGN1412. N Engl J Med. 2006;355:1018–28.
48. Patnaik A, Kang SP, Rasco D, et al. Phase I study of pembrolizumab (MK-3475; anti-PD-1 monoclonal antibody) in patients with advanced solid tumors. Clin Cancer Res. 2015;21:4286–93.
49. Ahamadi M, Freshwater T, Prohn M, et al. Model-based characterization of the pharmacokinetics of pembrolizumab: a humanized anti-PD-1 monoclonal antibody in advanced solid tumors. CPT Pharmacometrics Syst Pharmacol. 2017;6:49–57.
50. Freshwater T, Kondic A, Ahamadi M, et al. Evaluation of dosing strategy for pembrolizumab for oncology indications. J Immunother Cancer. 2017;5:43.
51. McDermott D, Lebbe C, Hodi FS, et al. Durable benefit and the potential for long-term survival with immunotherapy in advanced melanoma. Cancer Treat Rev. 2014;40:1056–64.
52. Michot JM, Bigenwald C, Champiat S, et al. Immune-related adverse events with immune checkpoint blockade: a comprehensive review. Eur J Cancer. 2016;54:139–48.
53. Weber JS, Kahler KC, Hauschild A. Management of immune-related adverse events and kinetics of response with ipilimumab. J Clin Oncol. 2012;30:2691–7.
54. Puzanov I, Diab A, Abdallah K, et al. Managing toxicities associated with immune checkpoint inhibitors: consensus recommendations from the Society for Immunotherapy of Cancer (SITC) Toxicity Management Working Group. J Immunother Cancer. 2017;5:95.
55. Melero I, Hervas-Stubbs S, Glennie M, et al. Immunostimulatory monoclonal antibodies for cancer therapy. Nat Rev Cancer. 2007;7:95–106.
56. Dempke WCM, Fenchel K, Uciechowski P, Dale SP. Second- and third-generation drugs for immuno-oncology treatment-The more the better? Eur J Cancer. 2017;74:55–72.
57. Garant A, Guilbault C, Ekmekjian T, et al. Concomitant use of corticosteroids and immune checkpoint inhibitors in patients with hematologic or solid neoplasms: a systematic review. Crit Rev Oncol Hematol. 2017;120:86–92.
58. Donia M, Kimper-Karl ML, Hoyer KL, et al. The majority of patients with metastatic melanoma are not represented in pivotal phase III immunotherapy trials. Eur J Cancer. 2017;74:89–95.
59. Sun R, Champiat S, Dercle L, et al. Baseline lymphopenia should not be used as exclusion criteria in early clinical trials investigating immune checkpoint blockers (PD-1/PD-L1 inhibitors). Eur J Cancer. 2017;84:202–11.
60. Wolchok JD, Hoos A, O'Day S, et al. Guidelines for the evaluation of immune therapy activity in solid tumors: immune-related response criteria. Clin Cancer Res. 2009;15:7412–20.
61. Bohnsack OHA, Ludajic K. Adaptation of the immune-related response criteria: irRECIST. Ann Oncol. 2014;25(Suppl 4):iv361–72.

62. Flaherty KT, Hennig M, Lee SJ, et al. Surrogate endpoints for overall survival in metastatic melanoma: a meta-analysis of randomised controlled trials. Lancet Oncol. 2014;15:297–304.
63. Motzer RJ, Escudier B, McDermott DF, et al. Nivolumab versus everolimus in advanced renal-cell carcinoma. N Engl J Med. 2015;373:1803–13.
64. Hoos A, Eggermont AM, Janetzki S, et al. Improved endpoints for cancer immunotherapy trials. J Natl Cancer Inst. 2010;102:1388–97.
65. Emens LA, Ascierto PA, Darcy PK, et al. Cancer immunotherapy: opportunities and challenges in the rapidly evolving clinical landscape. Eur J Cancer. 2017;81:116–29.
66. Reck M, Rodriguez-Abreu D, Robinson AG, et al. Pembrolizumab versus chemotherapy for PD-L1-positive non-small-cell lung cancer. N Engl J Med. 2016;375:1823–33.
67. Tumeh PC, Harview CL, Yearley JH, et al. PD-1 blockade induces responses by inhibiting adaptive immune resistance. Nature. 2014;515:568–71.
68. Snyder A, Makarov V, Merghoub T, et al. Genetic basis for clinical response to CTLA-4 blockade in melanoma. N Engl J Med. 2014;371:2189–99.
69. Rizvi NA, Hellmann MD, Snyder A, et al. Cancer immunology. Mutational landscape determines sensitivity to PD-1 blockade in non-small cell lung cancer. Science. 2015;348:124–8.
70. Dudley JC, Lin MT, Le DT, Eshleman JR. Microsatellite instability as a biomarker for PD-1 blockade. Clin Cancer Res. 2016;22:813–20.
71. Udall M, Rizzo M, Kenny J, et al. PD-L1 diagnostic tests: a systematic literature review of scoring algorithms and test-validation metrics. Diagn Pathol. 2018;13:12.
72. Kulangara K, Zhang N, Corigliano E, et al. Clinical utility of the combined positive score for programmed death ligand-1 expression and the approval of pembrolizumab for treatment of gastric cancer. Arch Pathol Lab Med. 2018.
73. Fashoyin-Aje L, Donoghue M, Chen H, et al. FDA approval summary: pembrolizumab for recurrent locally advanced or metastatic gastric or gastroesophageal junction adenocarcinoma expressing PD-L1. Oncologist. 2018.
74. Howitt BE, Shukla SA, Sholl LM, et al. Association of polymerase e-mutated and microsatellite-instable endometrial cancers with neoantigen load, number of tumor-infiltrating lymphocytes, and expression of PD-1 and PD-L1. JAMA Oncol. 2015;1:1319–23.
75. Kawakami H, Zaanan A, Sinicrope FA. Microsatellite instability testing and its role in the management of colorectal cancer. Curr Treat Options Oncol. 2015;16:30.
76. Lemery S, Keegan P, Pazdur R. First FDA approval agnostic of cancer site – when a biomarker defines the indication. N Engl J Med. 2017;377:1409–12.
77. Goldberg AD, Allis CD, Bernstein E. Epigenetics: a landscape takes shape. Cell. 2007;128:635–8.
78. Tronick E, Hunter RG. Waddington, dynamic systems, and epigenetics. Front Behav Neurosci. 2016;10:107.
79. Felsenfeld G. A brief history of epigenetics. Cold Spring Harb Perspect Biol. 2014;6.
80. Takahashi K, Tanabe K, Ohnuki M, et al. Induction of pluripotent stem cells from adult human fibroblasts by defined factors. Cell. 2007;131:861–72.
81. Gibbons RJ, Higgs DR. Molecular-clinical spectrum of the ATR-X syndrome. Am J Med Genet. 2000;97:204–12.
82. Egger G, Liang G, Aparicio A, Jones PA. Epigenetics in human disease and prospects for epigenetic therapy. Nature. 2004;429:457–63.
83. Choudhuri S. From Waddington's epigenetic landscape to small noncoding RNA: some important milestones in the history of epigenetics research. Toxicol Mech Methods. 2011;21:252–74.
84. Heyn H, Esteller M. DNA methylation profiling in the clinic: applications and challenges. Nat Rev Genet. 2012;13:679–92.
85. Jones PA, Baylin SB. The fundamental role of epigenetic events in cancer. Nat Rev Genet. 2002;3:415–28.
86. Esteller M. Cancer, epigenetics and the Nobel Prizes. Mol Oncol. 2012;6:565–6.
87. Jones PA, Taylor SM. Cellular differentiation, cytidine analogs and DNA methylation. Cell. 1980;20:85–93.

88. Mair B, Kubicek S, Nijman SM. Exploiting epigenetic vulnerabilities for cancer therapeutics. Trends Pharmacol Sci. 2014;35:136–45.
89. Mann BS, Johnson JR, Cohen MH, et al. FDA approval summary: vorinostat for treatment of advanced primary cutaneous T-cell lymphoma. Oncologist. 2007;12:1247–52.
90. Morel D, Almouzni G, Soria JC, Postel-Vinay S. Targeting chromatin defects in selected solid tumors based on oncogene addiction, synthetic lethality and epigenetic antagonism. Ann Oncol. 2017;28:254–69.
91. Bolden JE, Peart MJ, Johnstone RW. Anticancer activities of histone deacetylase inhibitors. Nat Rev Drug Discov. 2006;5:769–84.
92. Barros-Silva D, Marques CJ, Henrique R, Jeronimo C. Profiling DNA methylation based on next-generation sequencing approaches: new insights and clinical applications. Genes (Basel) 2018;9.
93. Nolan L, Johnson PW, Ganesan A, et al. Will histone deacetylase inhibitors require combination with other agents to fulfil their therapeutic potential? Br J Cancer. 2008;99:689–94.
94. Thurn KT, Thomas S, Moore A, Munster PN. Rational therapeutic combinations with histone deacetylase inhibitors for the treatment of cancer. Future Oncol. 2011;7:263–83.
95. Fantin VR, Richon VM. Mechanisms of resistance to histone deacetylase inhibitors and their therapeutic implications. Clin Cancer Res. 2007;13:7237–42.
96. Lorincz AT. The promise and the problems of epigenetics biomarkers in cancer. Expert Opin Med Diagn. 2011;5:375–9.
97. Banerji U, Workman P. Critical parameters in targeted drug development: the pharmacological audit trail. Semin Oncol. 2016;43:436–45.
98. Martin-Liberal J, Ochoa de Olza M, Hierro C, et al. The expanding role of immunotherapy. Cancer Treat Rev. 2017;54:74–86.
99. Day D, Siu LL. Approaches to modernize the combination drug development paradigm. Genome Med. 2016;8:115.

Chapter 3
Preclinical Studies to Enable First in Human Clinical Trials

Rajesh Chopra and Florence I. Raynaud

Abstract Drug discovery is a multidisciplinary process which requires a coordinated effort to deliver a drug candidate with appropriate pharmaceutical properties and a clear therapeutic paradigm. Identifying a suitable target for therapeutic intervention requires careful biological and technical assessments to ensure its validity and druggability. Optimal screening strategies must be established to identify tractable hit matter. A robust test cascade enables triage and optimisation of compounds for further evaluation in models of increasing complexity. The ability to relate target engagement and phenotypic effect provides proof of concept in early studies. Investigation of the pharmacokinetic and pharmacodynamic properties in preclinical models facilitates prediction of suitable exposure in patients with an appropriate formulation and scheduling. Toxicology studies establish an acceptable safety margin for the product. Understanding of the clinical context in which to best use the development compound i.e. patient populations, resistance mechanism and combination strategies pave the way for a successful clinical development.

Keywords Target validation · Screening cascade · Pharmacokinetics-pharmacodynamics · Efficacy · Toxicology · Candidate selection · Target product profile

Key Points

- Target selection and validation based on:
  - Biological assessment
  - Technical assessment
- Strategy for obtaining hit matter including the establishment of a screening cascade
- Defining appropriate pharmaceutical properties
  - Drug candidate selection

R. Chopra (✉) · F. I. Raynaud
CRUK Cancer Therapeutics Unit & Division of Cancer Therapeutics, Institute of Cancer Research, London, UK
e-mail: Raj.Chopra@icr.ac.uk; Florence.Raynaud@icr.ac.uk

T. A. Yap et al. (eds.), *Phase I Oncology Drug Development*,
https://doi.org/10.1007/978-3-030-47682-3_3

  - Establishing a Target Product Profile including definition of which disease, which patient populations, dose and schedule, combination strategies, pathways associated with resistance and a differentiated therapeutic impact.
- Clear definition of safety considerations
- Preclinical data to support a First in Human/Patient study

3.1 Introduction

The discovery of new anticancer agents has revolutionised therapy for a broad range of tumors. In 2018 for example, 25% of all new drugs approved by the FDA were anticancer agents (https://www.fda.gov/drugs). Cytotoxic agents were first discovered and clinically used in the 1940s, and in the subsequent 50 years these drugs have been the mainstay of anticancer therapy. Since the late 1990s, with the initial success of Gleevec in targeting the BCR-ABL kinase in chronic myeloid leukaemia (CML) [1], there has been an increasing trend in approval of targeted agents for cancer therapy. Whilst cytotoxic agents continue to play an important role, targeted agents, based on our understanding of the molecular pathology of cancer, are increasingly incorporated into treatment protocols [2]. Currently, tyrosine or serine/threonine kinases, together with transmembrane receptors, ligand-dependent nuclear receptors and G-coupled receptors, constitute the majority of targeted agents. As we move forward in cancer drug discovery there are a number of challenges facing the field, not least that despite major advances in our understanding of the underlying molecular mechanisms associated with the pathogenesis of cancer and billions of dollars invested in technologies, such as high throughput chemistry, structural biology, DNA sequencing and computational biology, attrition rates in the drug discovery process are unacceptably high [3]. Furthermore, there is a large amount of preclinical genomic data, derived through large scale CRISPR/cas 9 or RNA knockdown screens, available on-line (https://depmap.org/portal/, https://www.sanger.ac.uk/, https://cansarblack.icr.ac.uk/; [4]); these data define cancer vulnerabilities and thereby identify potential cancer therapeutic targets. However, validating and prioritising these potential targets for cancer drug discoveries remains a challenge. Determining which networks, pathways or molecules are true drivers of a cancer can be difficult, particularly, if there are limited published data available. Where known drivers have been defined, e.g., c-MYC overexpression, p53 loss, Ras mutations or Wnt pathway dysregulation, these have proven 'difficult to drug' using conventional approaches. This is, in part, due to these targets containing 'shallow pockets', in which inhibitors cannot bind selectively and potently, or protein-protein and protein-DNA/RNA interactions. In addition, with targets that are not kinases, e.g., helicases or ATPases, there is little precedence for drug targeting and these targets therefore present novel challenges.

Table 3.1 Key steps in pre-clinical drug discovery to enable a successful phase 1 outcome

- Target selection
- Target validation based on:
  - Biological assessment
  - Technical assessment
- Strategy for obtaining hit matter
- Establishment of a screening cascade
- Defining appropriate pharmaceutical properties
  - Drug candidate selection
- Establishing a Target Product Profile

The aim of this chapter will be to highlight the state-of-the-art preclinical studies necessary to define the key steps for eventual therapeutic success in the clinic, with a focus on small molecule anticancer discovery. The key steps necessary for successful preclinical drug discovery are summarised in Table 3.1.

3.2 Target Selection and Validation

Target selection in cancer drug discovery and its subsequent validation before entry into a drug discovery project, which may entail a 5- to 10-year programme of work at a considerable human and financial cost, requires a thorough evaluation process. Potential drug targets will often be derived from published data that implicate a particular mutation, RNA species or protein as a driver of cancer. At other times, the target will be derived from high throughput functional genome screens using either Si/ShRNA or CRISPR/cas 9 screens to define targets whose loss of function causes cell death in a broad range of cancers. Targets are often derived from clinical observations in patients. This 'bedside to bench' approach (or reverse translation) requires the study of the molecular pathology of patients that have exceptional responses, or intrinsic/acquired resistance. Each one of these groups of patients are likely to define new therapeutic approaches, including drug targets. Irrespective of where the target has been identified, most drug discovery teams will undertake a full biological and technical assessment of which target should be selected and a thorough evaluation process.

3.2.1 Target Validation

Biological assessment Reproducibility represents a major problem for drug discovery, with experimental data in up to 50–80% publications (many in highly cited journals) failing replication attempts in another laboratory [5]. One reason for this poor reproducibility is the lack of robustness in experimental design, i.e., the inability to reproduce data using orthogonal experimental technology [6].

Another pitfall in target identification is the use of clinical data based on univariate statistical analysis to justify target selection, comparing outcome in patients with low and high target expression. A Kaplan-Meier plot may clearly show a difference in survival between patients with different protein expression levels, but it does not establish causality; this approach is, however, often used to justify the selection of a target. If clinical studies are to be used to define the effect of a particular gene/protein on cancer outcome, and therefore a potential target for drug discovery, prospective studies should be utilised. In addition, the choice of a target for drug discovery does not necessarily have to be linked with a poor outcome. For example, the estrogen receptor (ER), when overexpressed in breast tissue, is linked to good prognosis in breast cancer [7], and targeting ER with receptor antagonists has been a major success [8]. Furthermore, during studies undertaking whole genome/exome sequencing in large numbers of patients, many genetic mutations are now being identified, but often it is unclear whether they represent a gain or loss of function. Therefore, further functional experiments will be important before strategies for inhibiting or enhancing enzymatic function are considered.

In addition to available physiological role of the target and the link of pathway and network information to a specific cancer, target validation for a specific protein will often be undertaken by overexpression studies or knockdown of the target by Si/ShRNA or CRISPR/Cas 9 technologies. It is useful in this context to understand the limitations associated with these approaches. Over expression studies are often confounded by the supraphysiological levels of gene expression from an exogenous viral promoter; these overexpression studies require careful titration of an inducible system, so that the target expression approaches that observed in the cancer of interest. For knockdown studies, off-target effects and inability to detect acute consequence of target knockdown are often observed. Mitigation strategies that take account of these limitations are necessary to increase the robustness of these approaches. It is customary to use at least three siRNA or guide RNA sequences at low nM concentrations, in order to make sure off-target effects are controlled for. The goal of most knockdown experiments is to achieve a knockdown of 80%, although if phenotypic changes are seen in a broad range of cell lines at less than 80% the data can be accepted. The use of a broad range of cell lines to show penetrance or cell context-dependent knockdown of a particular gene is essential. Finally, it is important to rescue any phenotype with SiRNA/gDNA resistant mutants. Another limitation of the use of genomic approaches for target validation is the use of antibiotic selection processes to select for cell clones where the target has been knocked out. This process can take up to 2 weeks, meaning that acute consequences of target knockout cannot be studied. The cells selected will often display functional features of cells adapted to the target knockout, rather than acute perturbations. A number of protein degradation-based technologies, such as the dTAG system, allow the evaluation of the acute loss of selected proteins to be undertaken [9]. This approach will become increasingly common.

Chemical probes, where available, may be a useful tool for target validation. These small molecule modulators of target function should ideally be potent and selective for a protein target, without necessarily having the pharmaceutical properties required for a drug treatment [10–12]. The appropriate use of chemical probes can help to associate the particular target and its biological consequence in both cancer and normal tissues. Furthermore, the use of chemical probes in different cell contexts can reveal new biology. A number of resources, such as the Chemical Probes Portal and Probe Miner (https://www.chemicalprobes.org/, https://probeminer.icr.ac.uk/) should be used to select the appropriate chemical compound [13].

In the context of target validation, it is also important to understand the target distribution in normal tissue, as well as its homology to other proteins; this will enable an understanding of the potential therapeutic window. The availability of a knockout mouse, or ideally a conditional knockout mouse, for the target in tissue of interest may give insights into potential side effects, but it should be noted that the phenotype associated with complete knockout may not mirror chemical modulation of an enzymatic domain.

Technical assessment It is important to establish the ability to drug a specific target protein, either directly via its active catalytic site or at a druggable cavity at a more distant site, including enzymatic function via an indirect allosteric effect, before embarking on a drug discovery campaign. Druggability is the presence of protein structures within a target that enable interaction with chemical compounds [14]. The type of target selected will also define the likelihood of obtaining appropriate pharmaceutical drug-like properties, A generally held dogma is that to be orally bioavailable, small molecules should follow the so-called Lipinski's Rule of 5 [15]: a molecular weight of $\leq$500 Da; Log P (a measure of the compound's hydrophobicity) $\leq$5; H-bond acceptors $\leq$10; and H donors $\leq$5. The 'Rule of 5' is derived from the fact that the parameters derived are multiples of 5. Whilst these rules have been based on historically druggable targets, such as kinases, hormone receptors and ion channels, it is unclear whether these rules will be relevant for new emerging targets that are often in large protein complexes. For this reason, a number of additional approaches to predict ligandability need to be undertaken. These include: precedence-based assessment; knowledge of endogenous ligands for the target; algorithms that predict druggable pockets based on structures found in the protein databases [16], or druggability based on machine learning approaches [4]. The availability of known structures not only enables druggability assessment, but may also enable fragment-based drug design strategies [17].

3.3 Establishing a Screening Cascade

Hit generation strategy It is necessary to be able to define what strategies will be deployed for generating lead compounds for drug discovery. Historically, phenotypic screens, which focus on disease models and biological readouts to define chemical matter, have been used [18]. This approach does not require knowledge of the target or pathways and is usually dependent on a predefined biological (in cell models) or physiological (in in vivo models) response. The target is then deconvoluted using chemical cross-linking approaches or proteomic approaches. In the last few decades, large chemical libraries based on combinatorial approaches, together with high throughput target based screening, have become the mainstay of cancer drug discovery. However, phenotypic screens are making a comeback, particularly in the context of the discovery of drugs that degrade target proteins rather than modulating their function [19]. High throughput target-based screens require assays that exploit the biochemistry of the purified protein complexes or cell-based screens for identifying chemical 'hits'. For kinases and receptors, biochemical approaches have been used, whilst for nuclear receptors, ion channels and membrane transcription factor cell-based assays are preferable.

Screening methodologies and assays for the cascade The identification and optimisation of a selective therapy is dependent on the establishment of a robust test cascade, designed to select for the most promising compounds and remove those with highly unfavourable characteristics early on. Each assay within the cascade helps to build a picture of the overall properties of both individual compounds and compound series, with assays often increasing in complexity and specificity as the cascade progresses. Various screening platforms can be implemented for biochemical or cellular assays, with a focus on cost and resource reduction, for example the miniaturisation of reactions through the use of ultra-high density (384-well and even 1536-well) plates. These homogenous biochemical assays have been used for the development of multiple inhibitors, including inhibitors of kinases, such as the B-Raf inhibitor, sorafenib [20], the lymphocyte selective protein kinase inhibitor, dasatinib [21] and protein kinase B (PKB) inhibitors [22], inhibitors of DNA repair enzymes, such as the PARP inhibitor, olaparib [23] and inhibitors of metabolic enzymes, such as the IDH2 inhibitor enasidenib [24]. More recently, it has become possible to perform high throughput screening reactions in sessile 2D droplet microarrays on planar surfaces. These droplets contain volumes of 0.1–10 nL and can potentially increase the throughput to 6144 reactions per plate [25]. There are currently no registered drugs that have been developed using this technology.

In some instances it is not possible to have the active target in a suitable conformation for a biochemical assay and, instead, cell-based screens have to be developed. An example of this is when the activity of the target relies upon a multiprotein complex that cannot be easily recreated artificially, or when the activated target results from protein fusion e.g. ALK and ceretinib [26].

Cell-based assays can also be used as phenotypic screens whereby effective molecules are identified on the basis of functionality as opposed to direct target engagement (discussed above). The significant deconvolution is required to identify the primary target, which can be a lengthy and risky process, but with potential for novel discovery. For example, phenotypic screens have been fruitful in targeting the Hedghog, WNT and HSF1 networks [27–29]. However, there are several additional parameters which need to be evaluated before a cellular screen is undertaken, including the impact of expressing reporters or overexpressing proteins on cell metabolism, growth kinetics and gene expression at different cell passage numbers. Furthermore, it is essential to counter screen with non-target containing cells, to obtain more selective hit matter. The use of isogenic cell line pairs is useful in this context.

Multiple attempts to generate models that recapitulate human cancer have shown that cells grown in 3D respond differently to treatment compared with cells in 2D cultures [30–33]. It has also been shown that the addition of macrophages or endothelial cells to spheroids generates models that are more representative of tumor biology than single cell models [32]. This has prompted the community to screen libraries of compounds using 3D cell culture [34] or co-culture [35, 36]. Recently, nanotechnologies have allowed cellular assays to be carried out either encapsulating cells in microdroplets or generating microfluidics platforms [37, 38].

A number of complex technologies which may be employed to derive a suitable endpoint and there are various assay endpoints in biochemical and cellular assays, including: fluorescence (fluorescence intensity, polarization, Förster resonance energy transfer [FRET], and time-resolved fluorescence energy transfer [TR-FRET]); absorbance, luminescence, bioluminescence resonance energy transfer (BRET), Alphascreen technology and label-free assay systems. In addition, detection techniques such as mass spectrometry and nuclear magnetic resonance (NMR) can be used, although their throughput is lower than that of the other detection methods [39, 40].

Choice of chemistry approach The target will influence the choice of screening library. For example, antibodies are not usually suitable for intracellular targets where small molecules are more appropriate. The constitution of a library is pivotal and for small molecule libraries, the inclusion of the maximal chemical diversity will increase the chance of finding hit matter. Throughout the program and across all assays, it is essential to have positive controls including endogenous ligands, existing compounds, biologically active natural products or control peptides.

In pilot screens for small molecule drug discovery, compound selection will often be enriched with chemicals already known to interfere with similar targets (i.e. kinase inhibitors). The number of compounds screened may be dictated by the hit rate and the ability to identify tractable chemical matter [41–44]. For instance, difficult targets with low druggability scores may benefit from additional screening platforms to increase the discovery of validated hits. This can include fragment-based approaches combined with crystallography, NMR assays and electron microscopy, all of which can guide the structure-based design [17]. In-silico screens can support the establishment of a pharmacophore to computationally screen libraries of commercially available compounds. The iteration of this approach can help refine the pharmacophore design, which is especially useful in the absence of suitable laboratory technology driving the structure-based design [45].

For cellular assays, it is paramount to focus on compounds with good cellular permeability. Often this can be well predicted based on the physicochemical properties of a compound, and therefore virtual in-silico screens can be implemented, saving both time and resource [46, 47].

Combinatorial libraries of fully human monoclonal antibodies derived from phage display have been utilised in target-based and phenotypic screens [48]. For example, target-agnostic selection strategies for isolating anticancer antibodies paved the way for the identification of the ICAM antibody [49].

Generation of Lead compounds Once hits have been identified, they need to be reconfirmed and an IC50 or GI50 must be established. Additional orthogonal screens confirm activity on the target or discard potential interference with the primary screening assay. For example, a cellular assay or biophysical assay, such as a thermal shift assay, could complement an initial biochemical assay [40]. Correlation between the two types of assay increases confidence, both in the assays and the chemical matter tested [50].

Understanding the relationship between compound potency, target engagement, measured target modulation and the resulting phenotypic effect, is crucial to a successful program. With novel targets, identification of a tool compound that is potent enough to modulate the biomarker and result in antiproliferative effects constitutes an additional validation of the target [10, 51, 52]. Theoretically, the cell line utilised should be driven by target activation (if the target is inhibited). Additional demonstration that the inhibitor has less effect in the context of limited target activation is desirable as it is suggestive of a therapeutic index in normal cells [53].

Finding the target engagement-biomarker-the earlier the better The ability to demonstrate target engagement in order to fulfil a biological function is essential for the development of targeted agents. For well characterised targets, e.g., enzymes with a known endogenous substrate, evaluation of target modulation is relatively easy. For example, protein phosphorylation (AKT for PI3K) for kinases or autophosphorylation (AKT) are well validated proximal biomarkers [51, 54–57]. Downstream effectors, such as ERK phosphorylation for MEK inhibitors or P-PRAS 40 for AKT, are also useful markers to measure on-target activity. It is preferable to have at least one proximal target engagement biomarker, but this is not always achievable [57–62].

Mitotic targets are especially challenging for the identification of target engagement biomarkers, as only a low percentage of non-synchronised cells are in mitosis at any given time and the progression through this cell cycle phase is fairly rapid. For this reason, many programs in this area utilise a proliferation biomarker (P-HH3) [63, 64] and engineered cell lines with reporter assays can be derived to measure target modulation [63]. The potential advantage that these recombinant cell lines confer is that they can be used for in vivo testing, but the target of interest is often massively overexpressed and the model becomes significantly different to the endogenous disease.

When the biology is novel, the biomarker of target engagement may not be identified. Tool compounds may have to be used together with SiRNA or CRISPR technology to discover novel robust biomarkers. These can be obtained from gene expression profiling, proteomics, protein arrays, or metabolomics or a combination of these methods [65–67]. The development of novel robust assays may necessitate production of novel antibodies for ELISA or immunoassays. As a discovery programs matures into late lead optimisation, it is important to generate a quantitative biomarker which allows modelling of PKPD in patients in a robust and reproducible manner. This will be detailed later.

Secondary pharmacology profiling The investigation of specific interactions of a drug at molecular targets distinct from the intended therapeutic molecular target of compound leads must be performed to ensure safety, as many known targets are associated with toxicity [68, 69]. Testing various candidates can potentially guide the selection of the clinical development compound or invoke further testing and evaluations ahead of formal toxicology studies. The International Conference on Harmonization (ICH) S7A recommends a number of targets that can be assessed in vitro [70]. For example, the human ether-a-go-go related gene (hERG) channel is recommended in the ICH S7B [71], but there is no consensus as to when these tests should be performed. A CEREP screen is frequently carried out to unravel additional pharmacology ahead of toxicology studies in vivo (www.cerep.fr). This can highlight potential off-target effects that can be evaluated further in additional in vitro models.

Further in vitro testing—deployment of appropriate efficacy models for patient selection In addition to selected testing to confirm the therapeutic strategy, additional patient populations can be sought by testing large cell panels that are well characterised. For instance, the NCI, Sanger Centre and Broad Institute cell line panels [65, 72–75] can provide sensitivity links to genetics, transcriptomics, proteomics or metabolomics, which can generate novel hypothesis for patient selection. This is required when the original therapeutic hypothesis fails validation in preclinical models, or when additional sensitive patient population are sought ahead of clinical studies. Furthermore, in addition to markers of intrinsic resistance, constant exposure to drugs, or mutagenesis studies, can provide information on potential mechanism of resistance or inform potential drug combinations [64, 76, 77].

Earlier in the chapter, we mentioned the fact that cells grown as spheroids can be used for screening purposes, but they can also be used for compound testing [78]. Organoids derived from patient material are a more complex system, which is even more representative of patient tumors than spheroids [79–81]. For instance, gastrointestinal organoids derived from patients contain many differential features of human intestinal tumors and can mimic the response to current therapy and predict responses [82]. A human intestine model can also be created on a chip, which can be used to study tissues derived from cancer stem cells [83]. Mini-tumor and organ systems can be generated on chips and connected by microfluidics to create a model system of the human body to test drug efficacy [84] and effect on metastatic disease [85, 86], as well as toxicity to normal tissues [87–89] and pharmacokinetics [90]. These systems enable evaluation of cancer and immune cells interactions [91]. Many of these microfluidic devices are in development and validation, but they will undoubtedly become more mainstream in the future. In addition, they can potentially allow evaluation of metabolites as normal liver can be incorporated on the chip [92].

Optimising the PK and predicting the active dose in man The primary aim of pharmacokinetic optimisation is to identify a tool compound or antibody to test in vivo in preclinical models to gain confidence in rationale. Understanding the target requirement from in vitro tests (Fig. 3.1a) is a guide to optimising PK to demonstrate target engagement and efficacy. Once proof of concept is achieved in a PKPD and efficacy experiment (Fig. 3.1b), the search for the clinical development compound consists of balancing and optimising potency on target, selectivity and pharmacokinetic properties. Measurement of target engagement/modulation in vitro and in vivo can inform PKPD modelling, optimise scheduling in preclinical studies and help predict optimal dose and scheduling in man (Fig. 3.1b, c). Two decades ago, 40% of failure in early clinical development of small molecules could be attributed to suboptimal pharmacokinetics [93]. Now understanding of the major

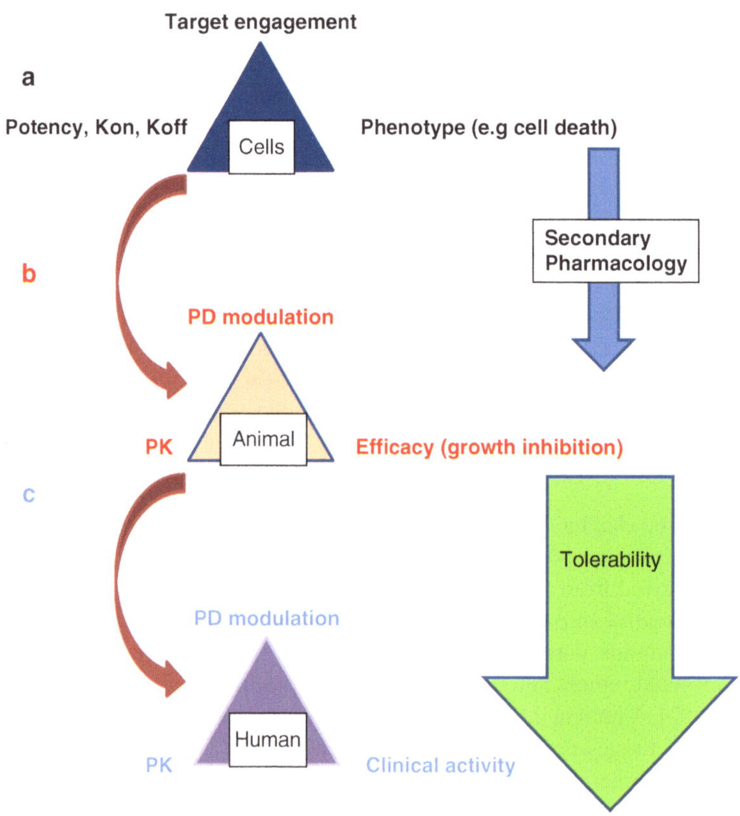

Fig. 3.1 Critical activities from Hit to Lead (**a**) to Lead optimisation (**b**) and candidate selection (**c**)

mechanisms of clearance distribution and absorption is aided by a battery of in vitro tests, including assays in microsomes, hepatocytes, permeability screens, LogP, protein-binding assays, transporter screens, which together support IVIVE (in vitro in vivo evaluations) [46, 94–98]. Even before a compound has been dosed to animals, it is possible to predict the main mechanism of clearance and the resulting concentration-time profiles in animals [99, 100]. If the animal prediction is relatively accurate, it builds confidence in the human prediction. For small molecules metabolised by CYP450 enzymes, pharmacokinetic profiles in man and variability in the population are predicted well. In contrast, the accuracy of the pharmacokinetics of compounds metabolised by aldehyde oxidase or carboxylesterases are more challenging [101–103]. Transport-mediated clearance via the ABC transporters, ABCB1, ABCG2 and ABCC1, is also less accurate than CYP driven metabolism in predicting human pharmacokinetics [104–106], and the compounds that are generated will always suffer drug resistance and efflux from many tumors and cancer stem cells [107–109]. It is therefore preferable for oncology products to be metabolically cleared.

The use of humanised mice models can be of great support in quantification of clearance mechanisms and metabolism of novel agents. For example, engineered mice expressing CYP3A in the liver or gut highlighted the prominence of gut metabolism in the absorption and metabolism of combimetininb [110]. Identification of metabolites serves multiple purposes, including: a check of the potential activity of metabolites; confirmation that no metabolites formed are toxic; and, finally, qualitative and quantitative evaluation of the metabolites formed across species favours selection of the toxicology species where metabolites are closest to those in man. Of note is the fact that metabolites predicted to be more than 10% of parent compound in blood need to be measured in first-in-human studies (ICH guidelines).

Anticancer drugs are mostly administered as tri-therapies and co-administration with steroids, antiemetics or antifungal are frequent. In addition, older patients are often co-medicated for diabetes, high blood pressure or heart disease. It is therefore essential to investigate the potential for drug-drug interaction. The guidelines for what constitutes a risk that needs to be further evaluated in the clinic are different according to the EMA https://www.ema.europa.eu/en/documents/scientific-guideline/guideline-investigation-drug-interactions and FDA Guidelines https://www.fda.gov/drugs/drug-interactions-labeling/drug-development-and-drug-interactions.

Physiologically-based pharmacokinetic models for human prediction are also used for therapeutic antibodies, despite a completely different mechanism of clearance to that of small molecules [111]. In addition, allometric scaling or variants of thereof can be used to predict various pharmacokinetic parameters of small molecules and antibodies [111–113].

Selecting the optimal in-vivo model A challenge in drug discovery is the identification of a suitable model to demonstrate target engagement and resulting efficacy in the in vivo setting. Xenograft models in immunocompromised mice (SCID, NCR nude, NOD) are frequently utilised for PKPD and efficacy studies of non-immune-oncology targets. It is possible to engraft a variety of different tumor types and the experimental turnover is relatively fast compared with other alternatives. However, these models are often criticised for their lack of translation to clinical responses [114].

In vivo studies may also be carried out in patient derived xenografts (PDX). These studies are lower throughput, but are, in general, better predictors of clinical response than simple xenografts derived from cell lines [115, 116]. Alternative in vivo models include genetically engineered mouse models, which validate the effect on the target and the resulting in vivo effect. They can be very useful to test efficacy in models driven by known oncogenic drivers [114, 117]. They are also very useful models in immuno-oncology [115, 118].

For immuno-oncology targets, syngeneic mice serve as appropriate models, provided the immune pathway targeted is similar in mice and humans. Humanised mice models have also been created to mimic the human immune response in mice, including humanisation with PBMC stem cells in blood, liver and thymus. Additional genetic modification of these animals has improved engraftment but these models are still devoid of cytokines and growth factors [119, 120]. Nevertheless, they have been successfully used for the development of CAR-T therapy, NK therapy and PD-1 antibodies [118].

A further complication is that a PD assay developed originally in human cells may not be directly applicable in human tumor xenografts, PDX or GEMM models. For example, antibody-based technologies developed in human cells may be unsuitable in a mouse background, due to interactions of secondary antibody etc, and the assay may need reoptimisation, in the best-case scenario, or complete redevelopment for PD testing in vivo. In some instances, the number of variants of a protein and their structure and regulation can vary across species and careful consideration needs to be given to the potential implications for target engagement, therapeutic effect and potential toxicity.

3.4 Drug Candidate Selection

The selection of a drug candidate presents an important milestone in the drug discovery process. In order to deliver a 'polished' drug candidate optimised for final success in the clinic, a number of criteria that are necessary for success. These are listed in Table 3.2 and are modified from criteria presented by [121]; https://www.ncbi.nlm.nih.gov/books/NBK53196/).

The list of criteria in Table 3.2 for candidate selection in the 'necessary feature' category indicate the minimum properties necessary, with the 'highly desirable' criteria representing features that should be fulfilled before IND submission to the FDA.

Table 3.2 Selection criteria for a drug development candidate to enable IND studies

Necessary features	• Adequate PK (with a validated proximal PD/target engagement biomarker) • Demonstrated in vivo efficacy/activity in ≥2–3 models • Acceptable safety margin (in two species—usually a rat and dog study for 28 days) • Feasibility of GMP manufacture (cost-effective with optimised chemistry synthesis) • Acceptable drug interaction profiles • Definition of therapeutic paradigm – Which disease – Expected clinical impact in context of existing therapies and emerging competition
Highly desirable	• Definition of patient subpopulations with clear genetic, molecular or clinical definitions • Definition of resistance mechanisms • Potential combination strategies • Back up alternative chemical series

3.5 Translating the Drug Development Candidate for IND Submission and First in Human (FIH) Studies

Once the candidate has been selected, a number of parallel yet interdependent activities need to be carried out.

Toxicology evaluation Toxicology studies help to define the starting dose in man, which will impact on the formulation, especially in the case of capsule and tablets. All toxicology studies need to be completed before any regulatory documents, such as IND and protocol, can be finalised. Inability to obtain a sufficiently stable formulation or unacceptable toxicology can derail the project at any point. Full analytical validation of the assays for PK, PD and patient selection must be completed ahead of the clinical trial.

Toxicology is currently carried out in one rodent and one non-rodent species. The choice of the species selected relates to the target biology in the species. If differences exist in the number of isoforms of a target across species, it is preferable to focus on the species closest to man. For given classes of targets, the side effects can be predicted, with knowledge frequently gained from previous preclinical studies (ICH guidelines S7A and B, FDA Guidance for industry M3R2). Compounds with antiproliferative activity often cause gut toxicity and induce myelosuppression. Dogs are extremely prone to emesis which can affect the exposure to drugs, so minipigs can be a good alternative to dogs to test these agents [122–124].

For immune-oncology and biologic agents, humanised mice models are often used alongside cynomolgus monkeys or minipigs [122, 125]. Despite multiple preclinical safety studies, there is always a degree of uncertainty with medicinal products with high human-specificity. Thus, a cautious approach in conduction of FIH trials is always preferable. Under-prediction of toxicity was observed with CD28 superagonist monoclonal antibody TGN1412, as a result of the lack of CD28 expression on the CD4+ effector memory T-cells in primates [126]. For small molecules, it is important to consider the mechanism of clearance and the metabolites produced in the species tested. The evaluation of impurities is also critical in case different batches of compound are used in the toxicology and FIH studies. Additionally, for oral compounds, formulation needs to be considered as it may affect the pharmacokinetic profile of the agent and the resulting toxicity.

It is important to ensure that the duration of the study covers all potential clinical applications as toxicology studies are lengthy and expensive. (https://www.fda.gov/animal-veterinary/guidance-regulations/guidance-industry ICH guidelines S7A and B, FDA Guidance for industry M3R2). In oncology, a 28-day evaluation is usually sufficient for IND application.

Definition of dose and scheduling for FIH studies The pivotal IND-enabling toxicology studies will inform the maximum tolerated dose, will identify the dose-limiting toxicity and establish the NOAEL (No observed adverse effects). From this information, together with the in vivo data from PKPD and therapy studies, it is possible to assess the safety and to evaluate the therapeutic index of the compound. In some instances, the answer may be that there is no predicted therapeutic index and the program will be halted. This was the case with the CDK8/19 project where pleiotropic toxicities not observed in the mice efficacy studies were observed in rat and dogs [127].

The starting dose for FIH studies is an important part of the IND package and fundamentally impacts on speed and success of early clinical trials. Historically, in oncology, for cytotoxic agents, a dose associated with maximal toxicity multiplied by safety margin was used to define the starting dose. As we employ more targeted approaches, we are still using data from preclinical toxicology studies but utilising the NOAEL multiplied by a safety factor. This is combined with in vivo PK/PD and efficacy models to define systemic exposure and correlated with the degree of target engagement and desired efficacy (Fig. 3.1). The extrapolation of doses from animal to human are carried out by allometric scaling, based on body surface, area to define the starting dose (ICH guidelines S7A, S7B, FDA Guidelines for industry M3R2).

Formulation For iv administration, it is necessary for the formulation to maintain the stability of the compound in solution at sufficient concentration to achieve active plasma levels. The infusion rate can modify the profile obtained (Cmax versus exposure), which may offer some versatility pending appropriate solubility. For oral administration, formulation is likely to affect the rate of dissolution in various parts of the gut and therefore the overall absorption profile of the compound. In addition to producing an optimised and reproducible crystalline form of the material, addition of excipients ensures optimal delivery and stability of the end-product. For low molecular weight kinase inhibitors, the low solubility of the salt form has resulted in variable bioavailability in patients [128]. The starting dose can only be established once the toxicology studies have reported, but the projected active doses are often established ahead of time.

Clinically validated biomarker assays The development and validation of robust assays to measure biomarkers of target engagement supports the pharmacological audit trail that drives clinical decisions in first in human studies [58–60, 62, 129].

In solid tumors, the biomarker selected to support preclinical studies is ideally validated for human tumors. Unfortunately, samples are limited by the availability of tumor biopsies and it is important to ensure that paired biopsies are taken: one before treatment and one preferably at peak effect. The use of circulating free DNA in this context is under evaluation and 'liquid biopsies' may provide a less invasive approach.

In order to generate concentration-time-target engagement relationship, surrogate tissues are generally utilised [62]. Identification of the appropriate matrix (blood cells, hair follicles, skin biopsies, plasma) in which to observe biomarker modulation, together with an established PKPD relationship in the preclinical models, will inform clinical decisions, such as scheduling and dose escalation. In haematological malignancies, circulating tumors are available but often limited by the myelosuppressive effect of therapeutics. A variety of techniques are suitable to assess biomarker modulations, including: immunoassays in a variety of formats and platforms; gene expression profiling; flow cytometry; proteomics; and metabolomics [130–132]. In all cases, the level of validation required for clinical assays can be difficult to attain, especially when the technology or the reagents are novel.

In addition, there is an increasing expectation that most agents, particularly where there is a clear patient selection hypothesis, will enter clinical trials with a diagnostic assay at the time of 'first in human' studies. This is particularly the case for drugs that target established drivers of cancer in patient subpopulations, e.g., BRaf-, V600E-mutated melanoma, EGFR-, ALK- and Ras-mutated lung cancer, IDH-mutated AML, and HER2-amplified breast cancer. In addition, excluding patients with certain molecular features, such as Ras mutations for patients undergoing treatment with EGFR antibodies, may be necessary. However, despite the great enthusiasm for personalised/precision medicine (successful in a subgroup of patients), patient selection hypotheses and assays remain elusive for a significant number of new agents. This is true for patients receiving pleiotrophic agents, which target more than one pathway (e.g., multi kinase inhibitors), or target a single pathway with multiple consequences in a cell (e.g., proteosomal inhibitors, IMiD agents, immuno-oncology agents, or agents targeting DNA damage repair pathways). In these cases, multiplex assays or assays based on technologies such as gene expression profile, protein array and immunohistochemistry, can support personalised therapy [130, 133–135].

3.5.1 Modelling and Simulations, Pharmacometrics

Mathematical modelling and simulation can provide a framework to answer important drug development objectives. Earlier in this chapter, the computational analyses that inform druggability assessment of various targets were described [136, 137]. We also mentioned that in silico models can predict permeability of compounds and assist pharmacophore design [45].

Modelling and simulation of data pertaining to pharmacokinetic, pharmacodynamic, and disease progression is often referred to as the pharmacometric analyses. Using a mathematical model to describe the relationship between drug level, effect on the target and the resulting therapeutic effect, allows modelling of the scheduling that can potentially result in the best antitumor activity [136, 138–141]. Using this approach, it was possible to show in preclinical and clinical studies that growth inhibition is observed when EC50 to EC60 of ALK is reached. This was true for two completely different classes of ALK inhibitors [142]. A similar approach utilised with PI3K inhibitors showed that in preclinical models, a minimum of 30% inhibition of AKT phosphorylation is required for antitumor activity in breast cancer models [143].

Using the predicted pharmacokinetic profile in man, it is possible to evaluate the potential efficacious dose once the tumor growth rates have been adjusted. A retrospective analysis of gefitinib and sorafenib using a PK/PD/efficacy model showed that the correct clinical doses of both inhibitors could be predicted from the model established from the preclinical studies, assuming that free steady state concentrations in human and mouse were identical [144]. In addition, a model of resistance was built into the preclinical model that could predict the active doses for sensitive and resistant models [145]. In the field of immune oncology a model of tumor uptake for cytokine-based immunotherapy is now available and can guide development of future agents of this class [146].

Toxicities, such as myelosuppression, which is observed with many cytotoxic agents, can be modelled and compared with target requirements to optimise scheduling [147].

Finally, models can capture and use the predicted PK variability to predict the range of plausible doses. In each case, assumptions are made (especially for the scalability of the PD in human), which need to be considered so that the model can be refined further [148].

3.5.2 Development of a Target Product Profile (TPP)

As part of the IND package or pre-IND meeting with regulatory authorities, a TPP is highly useful though not mandatory (FDA Guidance for Industry https://www.fda.gov/regulatory-information/search-fda-guidance-documents). In addition, a

TPP serves as an important template for defining the ultimate goal of the project and, in this context, will enable definition of the desired therapeutic paradigm and determination of the impact the drug will ultimately have in the context of existing therapies and emerging competition—the ideal version of a claim for the drug label. A TPP should be considered to be a dynamic document, updated as new data emerge and knowledge of the drug is gained. A TPP at the pre-IND stage should include potential indications and usage in defined patient populations, dosage and administration, formulation (with dosage forms and strengths), contraindications, clinical pharmacology, non-clinical toxicology, planned clinical studies, storage, handling and drug stability. Finally, patient information and the consent form for the first in human study should also be included.

3.6 Conclusion

Drug discovery is a risky activity which requires time, resource and a multidisciplinary team with expertise in chemistry, as well as cell, molecular and structural biology, biochemistry, clinical pharmacology, in vivo pharmacology, biomarker development, oncology and Phase 1 trials. Target validation and identification of the correct therapeutic intervention are essential to success. Multiparametric optimisation of selectivity, potency and pharmacokinetics support identification of the clinical development compound. Preclinical models de-risk the project and confer confidence in the rationale for the drug discovery program and the therapeutic paradigm. Modelling and simulations support scheduling and optimal time for tumor analysis in the clinic. In addition, they predict potential drug-drug interactions. Despite all safety precautions and progress in predictive tools, the ultimate test of a novel agent is the clinic. The continuous improvement of models and tools (i.e., organoids, PDX, humanised mice, organs on a chip, pharmacometric analysis [149]) is likely to improve the predictability of our preclinical studies in the future.

Key Expert Opinion Points

- Drug discovery is a multidisciplinary process involving biologists, chemists, pharmacologists, computational scientists and clinicians
- Drug discovery tools are constantly evolving to support all phases of drug discovery/development
- Drug discovery is a dynamic process. It constantly adapts to results from novel basic biology and ongoing projects
- Computational analysis support all aspects of drug discovery and development e.g. target evaluation, in silico analysis, pharmacometric analysis, predictions to man
- Designing the right clinical study must be considered from the onset of the project

References

1. Lambert GK, Duhme-Klair AK, Morgan T, Ramjee MK. The background, discovery and clinical development of BCR-ABL inhibitors. Drug Discov Today. 2013;18:992–1000. https://doi.org/10.1016/j.drudis.2013.06.001.
2. Sun J, et al. A systematic analysis of FDA-approved anticancer drugs. BMC Syst Biol. 2017;11:87. https://doi.org/10.1186/s12918-017-0464-7.
3. Scannell JW, Blanckley A, Boldon H, Warrington B. Diagnosing the decline in pharmaceutical R&D efficiency. Nat Rev Drug Discov. 2012;11:191–200. https://doi.org/10.1038/nrd3681.
4. Coker EA, et al. canSAR: update to the cancer translational research and drug discovery knowledgebase. Nucleic Acids Res. 2019;47:D917–22. https://doi.org/10.1093/nar/gky1129.
5. Begley CG, Ellis LM. Drug development: raise standards for preclinical cancer research. Nature. 2012;483(7391):531–3. https://doi.org/10.1038/483531a.
6. Kaelin WG Jr. Common pitfalls in preclinical cancer target validation. Nat Rev Cancer. 2017;17:425–40. https://doi.org/10.1038/nrc.2017.32.
7. Fisher B, Fisher ER, Redmond C, Brown A. Tumor nuclear grade, estrogen receptor, and progesterone receptor: their value alone or in combination as indicators of outcome following adjuvant therapy for breast cancer. Breast Cancer Res Treat. 1986;7(3):147–60. https://doi.org/10.1007/BF01806245.
8. Johnston SR, Schiavon G. Treatment algorithms for hormone receptor-positive advanced breast cancer: going forward in endocrine therapy-overcoming resistance and introducing new agents. American Society of Clinical Oncology educational book. American Society of Clinical Oncology. Annual Meeting. 2013. https://doi.org/10.1200/EdBook_AM.2013.33.e28.
9. Nabet B, et al. The dTAG system for immediate and target-specific protein degradation. Nat Chem Biol. 2018;14:431–41. https://doi.org/10.1038/s41589-018-0021-8.
10. Blagg J, Workman P. Choose and use your chemical probe wisely to explore cancer biology. Cancer Cell. 2017;32:9–25. https://doi.org/10.1016/j.ccell.2017.06.005.
11. Blagg J, Workman P. Chemical biology approaches to target validation in cancer. Curr Opin Pharmacol. 2014;17:87–100. https://doi.org/10.1016/j.coph.2014.07.007.
12. Workman P, Collins I. Probing the probes: fitness factors for small molecule tools. Chem Biol. 2010;17:561–77. https://doi.org/10.1016/j.chembiol.2010.05.013.
13. Antolin AA, et al. Objective, quantitative, data-driven assessment of chemical probes. Cell Chem Biol. 2018;25:194–205.e195. https://doi.org/10.1016/j.chembiol.2017.11.004.
14. Owens J. Determining druggability. Nat Rev Drug Discov. 2007;6:187.
15. Lipinski CA, Lombardo F, Dominy BW, Feeney PJ. Experimental and computational approaches to estimate solubility and permeability in drug discovery and development settings. Adv Drug Deliv Rev. 2001;46:3–26.
16. An J, Totrov M, Abagyan R. Comprehensive identification of "druggable" protein ligand binding sites. Genome Inform. 2004;15(2):31–41.
17. van Montfort RLM, Workman P. Structure-based drug design: aiming for a perfect fit. Essays Biochem. 2017;61:431–7. https://doi.org/10.1042/ebc20170052.
18. Moffat JG, Rudolph J, Bailey D. Phenotypic screening in cancer drug discovery – past, present and future. Nat Rev Drug Discov. 2014.
19. Collins I, Wang H, Caldwell JJ, Chopra R. Chemical approaches to targeted protein degradation through modulation of the ubiquitin-proteasome pathway. Biochem J. 2017;474:1127–47. https://doi.org/10.1042/bcj20160762.
20. Gollob JA, Wilhelm S, Carter C, Kelley SL. Role of Raf kinase in cancer: therapeutic potential of targeting the Raf/MEK/ERK signal transduction pathway. Semin Oncol. 2006;33:392–406. https://doi.org/10.1053/j.seminoncol.2006.04.002.
21. Das J, Chen P, Norris D, et al. 2-Aminothiazole as a novel kinase inhibitor template. Structure-activity relationship studies toward the discovery of

N-(2-chloro-6-methylphenyl)-2-[[6-[4-(2-hydroxyethyl)-1- piperazinyl)]-2-methyl-4-pyrimidinyl]amino)]-1,3-thiazole-5-carboxamide (dasatinib, BMS-354825) as a potent pan-Src kinase inhibitor. J Med Chem. 2006;49(23):6819–6832. doi:https://doi.org/10.1021/jm060727j
22. Caldwell JJ, et al. Identification of 4-(4-aminopiperidin-1-yl)-7H-pyrrolo[2,3-d]pyrimidines as selective inhibitors of protein kinase B through fragment elaboration. J Med Chem. 2008;51:2147–57. https://doi.org/10.1021/jm701437d.
23. Dillon KJ, Smith GC, Martin NM. A FlashPlate assay for the identification of PARP-1 inhibitors. J Biomol Screen. 2003;8:347–52. https://doi.org/10.1177/1087057103008003013.
24. Popovici-Muller J, et al. Discovery of the first potent inhibitors of mutant IDH1 that lower tumor 2-HG in vivo. ACS Med Chem Lett. 2012;3:850–5. https://doi.org/10.1021/ml300225h.
25. Garcia-Cordero JL, Fan ZH. Sessile droplets for chemical and biological assays. Lab Chip. 2017;17:2150–66. https://doi.org/10.1039/c7lc00366h.
26. Galkin AV, et al. Identification of NVP-TAE684, a potent, selective, and efficacious inhibitor of NPM-ALK. Proc Natl Acad Sci U S A. 2007;104:270–5. https://doi.org/10.1073/pnas.0609412103.
27. Pan S, et al. Discovery of NVP-LDE225, a potent and selective smoothened antagonist. ACS Med Chem Lett. 2010;1:130–4. https://doi.org/10.1021/ml1000307.
28. Mallinger A, et al. Discovery of potent, orally bioavailable, small-molecule inhibitors of WNT signaling from a cell-based pathway screen. J Med Chem. 2015;58:1717–35. https://doi.org/10.1021/jm501436m.
29. Cheeseman MD, et al. Discovery of a chemical probe bisamide (CCT251236): an orally bioavailable efficacious pirin ligand from a heat shock transcription factor 1 (HSF1) phenotypic screen. 2017;60:180–201. https://doi.org/10.1021/acs.jmedchem.6b01055.
30. Arai K, et al. A novel high-throughput 3D screening system for EMT inhibitors: a pilot screening discovered the EMT inhibitory activity of CDK2 inhibitor SU9516. PLoS One. 2016;11:e0162394. https://doi.org/10.1371/journal.pone.0162394.
31. Fernandez-Fuente G, Mollinedo P, Grande L, Vazquez-Barquero A, Fernandez-Luna JL. Culture dimensionality influences the resistance of glioblastoma stem-like cells to multikinase inhibitors. Mol Cancer Ther. 2014;13:1664–72. https://doi.org/10.1158/1535-7163.Mct-13-0854.
32. Kimlin L, Kassis J, Virador V. 3D in vitro tissue models and their potential for drug screening. Expert Opin Drug Discov. 2013;8:1455–66. https://doi.org/10.1517/17460441.2013.852181.
33. Shannan B, et al. Enhancing the evaluation of PI3K inhibitors through 3D melanoma models. Pigment Cell Melanoma Res. 2016;29:317–28. https://doi.org/10.1111/pcmr.12465.
34. LaBarbera DV, Reid BG, Yoo BH. The multicellular tumor spheroid model for high-throughput cancer drug discovery. Expert Opin Drug Discov. 2012;7:819–30. https://doi.org/10.1517/17460441.2012.708334.
35. Carragher N, et al. Concerns, challenges and promises of high-content analysis of 3D cellular models. Nat Rev Drug Discov. 2018;17:606. https://doi.org/10.1038/nrd.2018.99.
36. Ryan SL, et al. Drug discovery approaches utilizing three-dimensional cell culture. Assay Drug Dev Technol. 2016;14:19–28. https://doi.org/10.1089/adt.2015.670.
37. Chi CW, Ahmed AR, Dereli-Korkut Z, Wang S. Microfluidic cell chips for high-throughput drug screening. Bioanalysis. 2016;8:921–37. https://doi.org/10.4155/bio-2016-0028.
38. Hernandez-Perez R, Fan ZH, Garcia-Cordero JL. Evaporation-driven bioassays in suspended droplets. Anal Chem. 2016;88:7312–7. https://doi.org/10.1021/acs.analchem.6b01657.
39. Alsamman K, El-Masry OS. Developmental phases of anticancer screening models. Comb Chem High Throughput Screen. 2017;20:440–50. https://doi.org/10.2174/1386207319666161226142822.
40. Coussens NP, et al. Small-molecule screens: a gateway to cancer therapeutic agents with case studies of food and drug administration-approved drugs. Pharmacol Rev. 2017;69:479–96. https://doi.org/10.1124/pr.117.013755.
41. Collins I, Workman P. New approaches to molecular cancer therapeutics. Nat Chem Biol. 2006;2:689–700. https://doi.org/10.1038/nchembio840.

42. Hoelder S, Clarke PA, Workman P. Discovery of small molecule cancer drugs: successes, challenges and opportunities. Mol Oncol. 2012;6:155–76. https://doi.org/10.1016/j.molonc.2012.02.004.
43. Firth NC, Brown N, Blagg J. Plane of best fit: a novel method to characterize the three-dimensionality of molecules. J Chem Inf Model. 2012;52:2516–25. https://doi.org/10.1021/ci300293f.
44. Langdon SR, Brown N, Blagg J. Scaffold diversity of exemplified medicinal chemistry space. J Chem Inf Model. 2011;51:2174–85. https://doi.org/10.1021/ci2001428.
45. Langdon SR, Westwood IM, van Montfort RL, Brown N, Blagg J. Scaffold-focused virtual screening: prospective application to the discovery of TTK inhibitors. J Chem Inf Model. 2013;53:1100–12. https://doi.org/10.1021/ci400100c.
46. Wang NN, et al. ADME properties evaluation in drug discovery: prediction of Caco-2 cell permeability using a combination of NSGA-II and boosting. J Chem Inf Model. 2016;56:763–73. https://doi.org/10.1021/acs.jcim.5b00642.
47. Wolk O, et al. Segmental-dependent intestinal drug permeability: development and model validation of in-silico predictions guided by in-vivo permeability values. J Pharmaceutical Sci. 2018; https://doi.org/10.1016/j.xphs.2018.07.017.
48. Sánchez-Martín D, Sørensen MD, Lykkemark S, et al. Selection strategies for anticancer antibody discovery: searching off the beaten path. Trends Biotechnol. 2015;33(5):292–301. https://doi.org/10.1016/j.tibtech.2015.02.008.
49. Fransson J, Tornberg UC, Borrebaeck CA, Carlsson R, Frendeus B. Rapid induction of apoptosis in B-cell lymphoma by functionally isolated human antibodies. Int J Cancer. 2006;119:349–58. https://doi.org/10.1002/ijc.21829.
50. Drew AE, et al. Comparison of 2 cell-based phosphoprotein assays to support screening and development of an ALK inhibitor. J Biomol Screen. 2011;16:164–73. https://doi.org/10.1177/1087057110394657.
51. Raynaud FI, et al. Pharmacologic characterization of a potent inhibitor of class I phosphatidylinositide 3-kinases. Cancer Res. 2007;67:5840–50. https://doi.org/10.1158/0008-5472.Can-06-4615.
52. Tan DS, et al. Biomarker-driven early clinical trials in oncology: a paradigm shift in drug development. Cancer J. 2009;15:406–20. https://doi.org/10.1097/PPO.0b013e3181bd0445.
53. Lynch TJ, et al. Activating mutations in the epidermal growth factor receptor underlying responsiveness of non-small-cell lung cancer to gefitinib. N Engl J Med. 2004;350:2129–39. https://doi.org/10.1056/NEJMoa040938.
54. Raynaud FI, et al. Biological properties of potent inhibitors of class I phosphatidylinositide 3-kinases: from PI-103 through PI-540, PI-620 to the oral agent GDC-0941. Mol Cancer Ther. 2009;8:1725–38. https://doi.org/10.1158/1535-7163.mct-08-1200.
55. Sarker D, et al. First-in-human phase I study of pictilisib (GDC-0941), a potent pan-class I phosphatidylinositol-3-kinase (PI3K) inhibitor, in patients with advanced solid tumors. Clinical Cancer Res. 2015;21:77–86. https://doi.org/10.1158/1078-0432.ccr-14-0947.
56. Yap TA, et al. Preclinical pharmacology, antitumor activity, and development of pharmacodynamic markers for the novel, potent AKT inhibitor CCT128930. Mol Cancer Ther. 2011a;10:360–71. https://doi.org/10.1158/1535-7163.Mct-10-0760.
57. Yap TA, et al. First-in-man clinical trial of the oral pan-AKT inhibitor MK-2206 in patients with advanced solid tumors. J Clin Oncol. 2011b;29:4688–95. https://doi.org/10.1200/jco.2011.35.5263.
58. Banerji U, Workman P. Critical parameters in targeted drug development: the pharmacological audit trail. Semin Oncol. 2016;43:436–45. https://doi.org/10.1053/j.seminoncol.2016.06.001.
59. Workman P. Using biomarkers in drug development. Clin Adv Hematol Oncol. 2006;4:736–9.
60. Sarker D, Workman P. Pharmacodynamic biomarkers for molecular cancer therapeutics. Adv Cancer Res. 2007;96:213–68. https://doi.org/10.1016/s0065-230x(06)96008-4.
61. Yap TA, et al. Interrogating two schedules of the AKT inhibitor MK-2206 in patients with advanced solid tumors incorporating novel pharmacodynamic and functional imaging biomarkers. Clinical Cancer Res. 2014;20:5672–85. https://doi.org/10.1158/1078-0432.Ccr-14-0868.

62. Yap TA, Sandhu SK, Workman P, de Bono JS. Envisioning the future of early anticancer drug development. Nat Rev Cancer. 2010;10:514–23. https://doi.org/10.1038/nrc2870.
63. Faisal A, et al. Characterisation of CCT271850, a selective, oral and potent MPS1 inhibitor, used to directly measure in vivo MPS1 inhibition vs therapeutic efficacy. Br J Cancer. 2017;116:1166–76. https://doi.org/10.1038/bjc.2017.75.
64. Moore AS, et al. Selective FLT3 inhibition of FLT3-ITD+ acute myeloid leukaemia resulting in secondary D835Y mutation: a model for emerging clinical resistance patterns. Leukemia. 2012;26:1462–70. https://doi.org/10.1038/leu.2012.52.
65. Yang W, et al. Genomics of drug sensitivity in cancer (GDSC): a resource for therapeutic biomarker discovery in cancer cells. Nucleic Acids Res. 2013;41:D955–61. https://doi.org/10.1093/nar/gks1111.
66. Pawlak M, Carragher NO. Reverse Phase Protein Arrays elucidate mechanisms-of-action and phenotypic response in 2D and 3D models. Drug Discov Today Technol. 2017;23:7–16. https://doi.org/10.1016/j.ddtec.2017.05.002.
67. Zhao X, Modur V, Carayannopoulos LN, Laterza OF. Biomarkers in pharmaceutical research. Clin Chem. 2015;61:1343–53. https://doi.org/10.1373/clinchem.2014.231712.
68. Bowes J, et al. Reducing safety-related drug attrition: the use of in vitro pharmacological profiling. Nat Rev Drug Discov. 2012;11:909–22. https://doi.org/10.1038/nrd3845.
69. Lynch JJ III, Van Vleet TR, Mittelstadt SW, Blomme EAG. Potential functional and pathological side effects related to off-target pharmacological activity. J Pharmacol Toxicol Methods. 2017;87:108–26. https://doi.org/10.1016/j.vascn.2017.02.020.
70. Anon. ICHS7A Safety pharmacology studies for human phamaceuticals. Federal register 66. 2001.
71. Anon. ICH harmonised tripartite guideline S7B Safety pharmacology assesment of the potential for delayed ventricular repolarisation by human pharmaceuticals. 2005.
72. Clemons PA, et al. Quantifying structure and performance diversity for sets of small molecules comprising small-molecule screening collections. Proc Natl Acad Sci U S A. 2011;108:6817–22. https://doi.org/10.1073/pnas.1015024108.
73. Schreiber SL, et al. Towards patient-based cancer therapeutics. Nat Biotechnol. 2010;28:904–6. https://doi.org/10.1038/nbt0910-904.
74. Covell DG, Huang R, Wallqvist A. Anticancer medicines in development: assessment of bioactivity profiles within the National Cancer Institute anticancer screening data. Mol Cancer Therap. 2007;6:2261–70.
75. Park ES, Rabinovsky R, Carey M, Hennessy BT, Agarwal R, Liu W, Ju Z, Deng W, Lu Y, Woo HG, Kim SB, Lee JS, Garraway LA, Weinstein JN, Mills GB, Lee JS, Davies MA. Integrative analysis of proteomic signatures, mutations, and drug responsiveness in the NCI 60 cancer cell lines set. Mol Cancer Therap. 2010;9:257–67.
76. Gurden MD, et al. Naturally occurring mutations in the MPS1 gene predispose cells to kinase inhibitor drug resistance. Cancer Res. 2015;75:3340–54. https://doi.org/10.1158/0008-5472.Can-14-3272.
77. Yamaoka T, Ohba M, Ohmori T. Molecular-targeted therapies for epidermal growth factor receptor and its resistance mechanisms. Int J Mol Sci. 2017;18. https://doi.org/10.3390/ijms18112420.
78. Madoux F, et al. A 1536-Well 3D viability assay to assess the cytotoxic effect of drugs on spheroids. SLAS Discov Advancing Life Sci R&D. 2017;22:516–24. https://doi.org/10.1177/2472555216686308.
79. Artegiani B, Clevers H. Use and application of 3D-organoid technology. Hum Mol Genet. 2018;27:R99–107. https://doi.org/10.1093/hmg/ddy187.
80. Drost J, Clevers H. Organoids in cancer research. Nat Rev Cancer. 2018;18:407–18. https://doi.org/10.1038/s41568-018-0007-6.
81. Nagle PW, Plukker JTM, Muijs CT, van Luijk P, Coppes RP. Patient-derived tumor organoids for prediction of cancer treatment response. Sem Cancer Biol. 2018. https://doi.org/10.1016/j.semcancer.2018.06.005.
82. Vlachogiannis G, et al. Patient-derived organoids model treatment response of metastatic gastrointestinal cancers. Science. 2018;359:920–6. https://doi.org/10.1126/science.aao2774.

83. Bein A, et al. Microfluidic organ-on-a-chip models of human intestine. Cell Mol Gastroenterol Hepatol. 2018;5:659–68. https://doi.org/10.1016/j.jcmgh.2017.12.010.
84. Karolak A, Markov DA, McCawley LJ, Rejniak KA. Towards personalized computational oncology: from spatial models of tumour spheroids, to organoids, to tissues. J Roy Soc Interf. 2018;15. https://doi.org/10.1098/rsif.2017.0703.
85. Caballero D, et al. Organ-on-chip models of cancer metastasis for future personalized medicine: from chip to the patient. Biomaterials. 2017;149:98–115. https://doi.org/10.1016/j.biomaterials.2017.10.005.
86. Hassell BA, et al. Human organ chip models recapitulate orthotopic lung cancer growth, therapeutic responses, and tumor dormancy in vitro. Cell Rep. 2018;23:3698. https://doi.org/10.1016/j.celrep.2018.06.028.
87. Beckwitt CH, et al. Liver 'organ on a chip'. Exp Cell Res. 2018;363:15–25. https://doi.org/10.1016/j.yexcr.2017.12.023.
88. Wang YI, et al. Self-contained, low-cost Body-on-a-Chip systems for drug development. Exp Biol Med (Maywood, NJ). 2017;242:1701–13. https://doi.org/10.1177/1535370217694101.
89. Wu J, et al. Lab-on-a-chip platforms for detection of cardiovascular disease and cancer biomarkers. Sensors (Basel). 2017;17. https://doi.org/10.3390/s17122934.
90. Ishida S. Organs-on-a-chip: current applications and consideration points for in vitro ADME-Tox studies. Drug Metab Pharmacokinet. 2018;33:49–54. https://doi.org/10.1016/j.dmpk.2018.01.003.
91. Biselli E, et al. Organs on chip approach: a tool to evaluate cancer-immune cells interactions. Sci Rep. 2017;7:12737. https://doi.org/10.1038/s41598-017-13070-3.
92. Mertz DR, Ahmed T, Takayama S. Engineering cell heterogeneity into organs-on-a-chip. Lab Chip. 2018;18:2378–95. https://doi.org/10.1039/c8lc00413g.
93. Kola I, Landis J. Can the pharmaceutical industry reduce attrition rates? Nat Rev Drug Discov. 2004;3:711–5. https://doi.org/10.1038/nrd1470.
94. Obach RS. Nonspecific binding to microsomes: impact on scale-up of in vitro intrinsic clearance to hepatic clearance as assessed through examination of warfarin, imipramine, and propranolol. Drug Metab Disposition Biol Fate Chem. 1997;25:1359–69.
95. Obach RS, et al. The prediction of human pharmacokinetic parameters from preclinical and in vitro metabolism data. J Pharmacol Exp Ther. 1997;283:46–58.
96. Obach RS, Zhang QY, Dunbar D, Kaminsky LS. Metabolic characterization of the major human small intestinal cytochrome p450s. Drug Metab Disposition Biol Fate Chem. 2001;29:347–52.
97. Cho HJ, Kim JE, Kim DD, Yoon IS. In vitro-in vivo extrapolation (IVIVE) for predicting human intestinal absorption and first-pass elimination of drugs: principles and applications. Drug Dev Ind Pharm. 2014;40:989–98. https://doi.org/10.3109/03639045.2013.831439.
98. Kratochwil NA, et al. Metabolic profiling of human long-term liver models and hepatic clearance predictions from in vitro data using nonlinear mixed-effects modeling. AAPS J. 2017;19:534–50. https://doi.org/10.1208/s12248-016-0019-7.
99. Varma MV, Steyn SJ, Allerton C, El-Kattan AF. Predicting clearance mechanism in drug discovery: extended clearance classification system (ECCS). Pharm Res. 2015;32:3785–802. https://doi.org/10.1007/s11095-015-1749-4.
100. El-Kattan AF, Varma MVS. Navigating transporter sciences in pharmacokinetics characterization using the extended clearance classification system. Drug Metab Disposition Biol Fate Chem. 2018;46:729–39. https://doi.org/10.1124/dmd.117.080044.
101. Terao M, et al. Structure and function of mammalian aldehyde oxidases. Arch Toxicol. 2016;90:753–80. https://doi.org/10.1007/s00204-016-1683-1.
102. Argikar UA, Potter PM, Hutzler JM, Marathe PH. Challenges and opportunities with non-CYP enzymes aldehyde oxidase, carboxylesterase, and UDP-glucuronosyltransferase: focus on reaction phenotyping and prediction of human clearance. AAPS J. 2016;18:1391–405. https://doi.org/10.1208/s12248-016-9962-6.
103. Zhou L, Zhong DF, Chen XY. Research advances in non-P450-mediated drug oxidative metabolism. Yao xue xue bao/Acta Pharmaceutica Sinica. 2017;52:8–18.

104. Lee SC, Arya V, Yang X, Volpe DA, Zhang L. Evaluation of transporters in drug development: current status and contemporary issues. Adv Drug Deliv Rev. 2017;116:100–18. https://doi.org/10.1016/j.addr.2017.07.020.
105. Feng B, Varma MV, Costales C, Zhang H, Tremaine L. In vitro and in vivo approaches to characterize transporter-mediated disposition in drug discovery. Expert Opin Drug Discov. 2014;9:873–90. https://doi.org/10.1517/17460441.2014.922540.
106. Li R, Barton HA, Varma MV. Prediction of pharmacokinetics and drug-drug interactions when hepatic transporters are involved. Clin Pharmacokinet. 2014;53:659–78. https://doi.org/10.1007/s40262-014-0156-z.
107. Jiang ZS, Sun YZ, Wang SM, Ruan JS. Epithelial-mesenchymal transition: potential regulator of ABC transporters in tumor progression. J Cancer. 2017;8:2319–27. https://doi.org/10.7150/jca.19079.
108. Begicevic RR, Falasca M. ABC transporters in cancer stem cells: beyond chemoresistance. Int J Mol Sci. 2017;18. https://doi.org/10.3390/ijms18112362.
109. Ceballos MP, et al. ABC transporters: regulation and association with multidrug resistance in hepatocellular carcinoma and colorectal carcinoma. Curr Med Chem. 2018; https://doi.org/10.2174/0929867325666180105103637.
110. Choo EF, et al. Use of transgenic mouse models to understand the oral disposition and drug-drug interaction potential of cobimetinib, a MEK inhibitor. Drug Metab Disposition Biol Fate Chem. 2015;43:864–9. https://doi.org/10.1124/dmd.115.063743.
111. Ferl GZ, Theil FP, Wong H. Physiologically based pharmacokinetic models of small molecules and therapeutic antibodies: a mini-review on fundamental concepts and applications. Biopharm Drug Dispos. 2016;37:75–92. https://doi.org/10.1002/bdd.1994.
112. Ling J, Zhou H, Jiao Q, Davis HM. Interspecies scaling of therapeutic monoclonal antibodies: initial look. J Clin Pharmacol. 2009;49:1382–402. https://doi.org/10.1177/0091270009337134.
113. Oitate M, et al. Prediction of human plasma concentration-time profiles of monoclonal antibodies from monkey data by a species-invariant time method. Drug Metab Pharmacokinet. 2012;27:354–9.
114. Rossanese O, et al. The pharmacological audit trail: use of tumor models to adress critical issues in preclinical development of anticancer agents. Drug Discov Today. 2016;21:23–9.
115. Pauli C, et al. Personalized in vitro and in vivo cancer models to guide precision medicine. Cancer Discov. 2017;7:462–77. https://doi.org/10.1158/2159-8290.Cd-16-1154.
116. Williams JA. Using PDX for preclinical cancer drug discovery: the evolving field. J Clin Med. 2018;7. https://doi.org/10.3390/jcm7030041.
117. Singh M, Murriel CL, Johnson L. Genetically engineered mouse models: closing the gap between preclinical data and trial outcomes. Cancer Res. 2012;72:2695–700. https://doi.org/10.1158/0008-5472.Can-11-2786.
118. Li QX, Feuer G, Ouyang X, An X. Experimental animal modeling for immuno-oncology. Pharmacol Ther. 2017;173:34–46. https://doi.org/10.1016/j.pharmthera.2017.02.002.
119. De La Rochere P, et al. Humanized mice for the study of immuno-oncology. Trends Immunol. 2018;39:748–63. https://doi.org/10.1016/j.it.2018.07.001.
120. Ibarrola-Villava M, Cervantes A, Bardelli A. Preclinical models for precision oncology. Biochim Biophys Acta. 2018; https://doi.org/10.1016/j.bbcan.2018.06.004.
121. Strovel J, Sittampalam S, Coussens NP, et al. Early drug discovery and development guidelines: For academic researchers, collaborators, and start-up companies. In: Sittampalam GS, Grossman A, Brimacombe K, et al., editors. Assay guidance manual. Bethesda, MD: Eli Lilly & Company and the National Center for Advancing Translational Sciences; 2004. Updated 2012, 2016.
122. Stricker-Krongrad A, et al. Miniature swine breeds in toxicology and drug safety assessments: what to expect during clinical and pathology evaluations. Toxicol Pathol. 2016;44:421–7. https://doi.org/10.1177/0192623315613337.
123. Svendsen O. The minipig in toxicology. Exp Toxicol Pathol. 2006;57:335–9. https://doi.org/10.1016/j.etp.2006.03.003.

124. Vamathevan JJ, et al. Minipig and beagle animal model genomes aid species selection in pharmaceutical discovery and development. Toxicol Appl Pharmacol. 2013;270:149–57. https://doi.org/10.1016/j.taap.2013.04.007.
125. Brennan FR, et al. Current strategies in the non-clinical safety assessment of biologics: new targets, new molecules, new challenges. Regul Toxicol Pharmacol. 2018;98:98–107. https://doi.org/10.1016/j.yrtph.2018.07.009.
126. Pallardy M, Hunig T. Primate testing of TGN1412: right target, wrong cell. Br J Pharmacol. 2010;161:509–11. https://doi.org/10.1111/j.1476-5381.2010.00925.x.
127. Clarke PA, et al. Assessing the mechanism and therapeutic potential of modulators of the human mediator complex-associated protein kinases. eLife 2016;5. https://doi.org/10.7554/eLife.20722.
128. Herbrink M, Schellens JH, Beijnen JH, Nuijen B. Inherent formulation issues of kinase inhibitors. J Control Rel. 2016;239:118–27. https://doi.org/10.1016/j.jconrel.2016.08.036.
129. Cummings J, Raynaud F, Jones L, Sugar R, Dive C. Fit-for-purpose biomarker method validation for application in clinical trials of anticancer drugs. Br J Cancer. 2010;103:1313–7. https://doi.org/10.1038/sj.bjc.6605910.
130. Chae YK, et al. Challenges and future of biomarker tests in the era of precision oncology: can we rely on immunohistochemistry (IHC) or fluorescence in situ hybridization (FISH) to select the optimal patients for matched therapy? Oncotarget. 2017;8:100863–98. https://doi.org/10.18632/oncotarget.19809.
131. VanMeter A, et al. Reverse-phase protein microarrays: application to biomarker discovery and translational medicine. Expert Rev Mol Diagn. 2007;7:625–33. https://doi.org/10.1586/14737159.7.5.625.
132. Yuan J, et al. Novel technologies and emerging biomarkers for personalized cancer immunotherapy. J Immunother Cancer. 2016;4:3. https://doi.org/10.1186/s40425-016-0107-3.
133. Gulley JL, et al. Immunotherapy biomarkers 2016: overcoming the barriers. J Immunother Cancer. 2017;5:29. https://doi.org/10.1186/s40425-017-0225-6.
134. Infante JR, et al. Safety, pharmacokinetic, pharmacodynamic, and efficacy data for the oral MEK inhibitor trametinib: a phase 1 dose-escalation trial. Lancet Oncol. 2012;13:773–81. https://doi.org/10.1016/s1470-2045(12)70270-x.
135. Iorio F, et al. A landscape of pharmacogenomic interactions in cancer. Cell. 2016;166:740–54. https://doi.org/10.1016/j.cell.2016.06.017.
136. Benson N, van der Graaf PH, Peletier LA. Use of mathematics to guide target selection in systems pharmacology; application to receptor tyrosine kinase (RTK) pathways. Eur J Pharm Sci. 2017;109:S140–8. https://doi.org/10.1016/j.ejps.2017.05.049.
137. Sato K, Sato K. Recent progress in the development of microfluidic vascular models. Anal Sci. 2018;34:755–64. https://doi.org/10.2116/analsci.17R006.
138. Chen KG, et al. Pluripotent stem cell platforms for drug discovery. Trends Mol Med. 2018; https://doi.org/10.1016/j.molmed.2018.06.009.
139. Chen Y, et al. Predicting antitumor effect of deoxypodophyllotoxin in NCI-H460 tumor-bearing mice on the basis of in vitro pharmacodynamics and a physiologically based pharmacokinetic-pharmacodynamic model. Drug Metab Disposition Biol Fate Chem. 2018;46:897–907. https://doi.org/10.1124/dmd.117.079830.
140. Snowden TJ, van der Graaf PH, Tindall MJ. Model reduction in mathematical pharmacology: integration, reduction and linking of PBPK and systems biology models. J Pharmacokinet Pharmacodyn. 2018;45:537–55. https://doi.org/10.1007/s10928-018-9584-y.
141. van der Graaf PH, Benson N. The role of quantitative systems pharmacology in the design of first-in-human trials. Clin Pharmacol Therap. 2018; https://doi.org/10.1002/cpt.1145.
142. Yamazaki S, et al. Mechanistic understanding of translational pharmacokinetic-pharmacodynamic relationships in nonclinical tumor models: a case study of orally available novel inhibitors of anaplastic lymphoma kinase. Drug Metab Disposition Biol Fate Chem. 2015;43:54–62. https://doi.org/10.1124/dmd.114.061143.
143. Salphati L, et al. Pharmacokinetic-pharmacodynamic modeling of tumor growth inhibition and biomarker modulation by the novel phosphatidylinositol 3-kinase inhibitor GDC-0941.

Drug Metab Disposition Biol Fate Chem. 2010;38:1436–42. https://doi.org/10.1124/dmd.110.032912.

144. Eigenmann MJ, Frances N, Hoffmann G, Lave T, Walz AC. Combining nonclinical experiments with translational PKPD modeling to differentiate erlotinib and gefitinib. Mol Cancer Ther. 2016;15:3110–9. https://doi.org/10.1158/1535-7163.Mct-16-0076.
145. Eigenmann MJ, Frances N, Lave T, Walz AC. PKPD modeling of acquired resistance to anti-cancer drug treatment. J Pharmacokinet Pharmacodyn. 2017;44:617–30. https://doi.org/10.1007/s10928-017-9553-x.
146. Ribba B, et al. Prediction of the optimal dosing regimen using a mathematical model of tumor uptake for immunocytokine-based cancer immunotherapy. Clin Cancer Res. 2018;24:3325–33. https://doi.org/10.1158/1078-0432.Ccr-17-2953.
147. Mould DR, Walz AC, Lave T, Gibbs JP, Frame B. Developing exposure/response models for anticancer drug treatment: special considerations. CPT Pharmacomet Syst Pharmacol. 2015;4:e00016. https://doi.org/10.1002/psp4.16.
148. Bender BC, Schindler E, Friberg LE. Population pharmacokinetic-pharmacodynamic modelling in oncology: a tool for predicting clinical response. Br J Clin Pharmacol. 2013;79:56–71. https://doi.org/10.1111/bcp.12258.
149. Ribba B, et al. Methodologies for quantitative systems pharmacology (QSP) models: design and estimation. CPT Pharmacomet Syst Pharmacol. 2017;6:496–8. https://doi.org/10.1002/psp4.12206.

Chapter 4
Practicalities of Setting Up a Phase I Clinical Trial Unit Within an Academic Center

David S. Hong, Kathrina L. Marcelo-Lewis, and Patricia LoRusso

Abstract Over 1100 cancer drugs are in development representing an increase in effort and progress in cancer drug discovery. The starting point of clinical development is Phase 1 clinical trials and the need for dedicated Phase I units have emerged as forefront necessity even in academic centers. Early phase oncology clinical trial units within an academic center allow for the conduct of clinical research at the highest standards combined with unique opportunities for intellectual development and research collaborations. We outline here some of the practical elements of a robust early drug development unit.

Keywords Phase 1 unit · Early phase oncology trials · Academic center · Drug development · Human research

Key Points

- Early phase oncology clinical trial units within an academic center fosters the conduct of clinical research at the highest standards.
- Significant considerations must be made about the infrastructure necessary for the formal creation of a dedicated early phase clinical trial unit.

D. S. Hong (✉)
Department of Investigational Cancer Therapeutics, University of Texas-MD Anderson Cancer Center, Houston, TX, USA
e-mail: dshong@mdanderson.org

K. L. Marcelo-Lewis
Department of Thoracic/Head and Neck Medical Oncology, University of Texas-MD Anderson Cancer Center, Houston, TX, USA
e-mail: klmarcelo@mdanderson.org

P. LoRusso
Section of Medical Oncology, Department of Internal Medicine, Yale School of Medicine, New Haven, CT, USA
e-mail: patricia.lorusso@yale.edu

T. A. Yap et al. (eds.), *Phase I Oncology Drug Development*,
https://doi.org/10.1007/978-3-030-47682-3_4

- Among the minimum requirements for a robust early drug development unit within an academic center are: organizational structure, dedicated facilities, cores and space, institutional human research infrastructure, personnel and services, and standard operating procedures.

As of May 2018, over 1100 cancer drugs have been reported to be in development in the United States alone, all of which are either in clinical trials or awaiting FDA review (REF: PhRMA report 2018). This represents a clear increase in effort and progress in cancer drug discovery, with more targeted approaches being developed, including genomically-matched therapies or treatments that harness the capabilities of the immune system, as well as even combinations thereof. With the shifting landscape of drug design and development, the need for dedicated Phase I units in academic centers that would facilitate efficient development and implementation of clinical trials has never been more front and center.

Setting up an early phase oncology clinical trial unit within an academic center allows for the conduct of clinical research at the highest standards, in part due to the accessibility of existing research infrastructures and programs, facilities, as well as state-of-the-art resources and equipment within such institutions. Unique opportunities for intellectual development and research collaborations are also naturally fostered, which may then translate into healthcare innovations that could eventually be integrated into clinical practice.

This chapter provides a guide on the necessary structure and components that would allow for the formal creation of a dedicated early phase clinical trial unit in any academic center.

4.1 Organizational Structure

Most academic oncology centers in the western world, whether a cancer center or oncology unit within a university hospital setting, are tumor histology-focused. In fact, early therapeutics programs are often embedded within a specific tumor histology department. An advantage of such embedded units is that there is more synchrony relative to transitioning to phase 2 tumor-specific trials and expansions. Although most phase 1 trials are histology-independent, embedded units can also work across tumor types to collaborate and enroll other histologies, especially in smaller institutions.

Stand-alone units have emerged because of the need for expertise in the early development of new molecules for cancer discovery. We could argue that a dedicated unit allows for the development of expertise for all staff and processes in order to better serve the sponsor, clinical trial and most importantly, the patient (Fig. 4.1). Dedicated units have emerged in several academic centers, such as Royal Marsden Hospital, University of Texas MD Anderson Cancer Center, Princess Margaret Cancer Centre, and Yale Cancer Center.

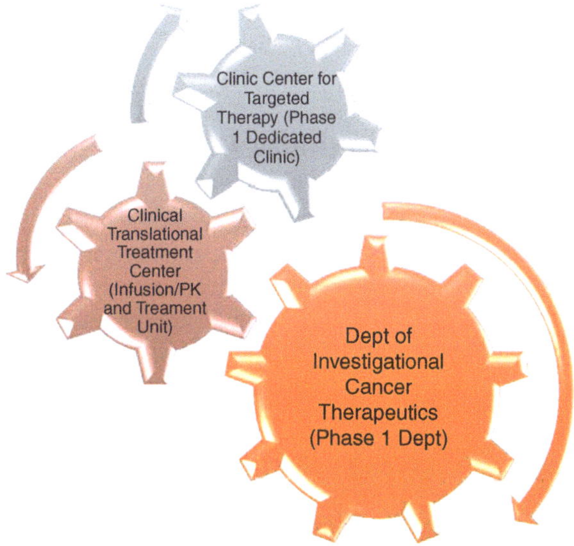

Fig. 4.1 Overall organizational structure

Regardless of whether a unit is stand-alone or embedded within a tumor histology context, it is key for any early therapeutics program to have access to the full resources of the university or cancer center, thus creating a unique opportunity for research collaborations. Frequent meetings of researchers in various scientific disciplines with clinical team members can spark new collaborations and push the edge of exploration in new directions. It is of paramount importance to foster translational research by providing outstanding facilities with state-of-the-art equipment and, most critically, by bringing together in daily interchange the best and brightest minds.

All early therapeutics personnel and functional cores optimally should report directly to a Program Director, who would, in turn, report directly to the Cancer Center Director. Interaction with the Cancer Center administration, clinical trials office (CTO), and other functions should be on a liaison basis for policy and procedure coordination but not in a direct reporting relationship. An early therapeutics Senior Leadership Council should be formed, consisting of the Program Director, the early therapeutics Associate Directors and Executive Director, and the Core Service Managers. The Senior Leadership Council should have a monthly standing meeting as well as ad hoc meetings. A regular weekly meeting should be scheduled for review and discussion of all patients, studies, slot assignments and general business.

It is critical that the organizational and management structure outlined be in place for either an embedded or stand-alone unit. Commitment to personnel growth is essential since this increases their long-term commitment and thus increases the expertise of the team. In addition, commitment to facilities and processes are likewise needed in order to present a cohesive case to sponsors that study commitments can be handled efficiently and effectively and to convince them that transferring currently open studies will be beneficial.

4.2 Dedicated Facilities, Cores and Space

Any early phase Clinical Therapeutics Center ideally should include a dedicated clinic, documentation and electronic health records (EHR), treatment unit, pharmacokinetics, laboratory, investigational pharmacy preparation facility, patient records storage, study supply storage, conference facility linked to off-site locations by full AV capacity, and sufficient offices/workspace for all staff as well as visiting monitors. This arrangement allows the unification of all early therapeutics clinical trials activities, and brings into close proximity all necessary core clinical research functions, which will increase efficiency and quality assurance with management coordination.

Clinic An outpatient Clinic dedicated to early phase trials with varied therapeutic areas of interest is optimal to provide a central resource not only for oncologists throughout the academic institution or even the community that are in search of clinical trials for patients with advanced cancer, but also for patients and their families themselves. Adequate space for exam rooms, physician and advanced practice provider work areas, and nursing work areas are necessary, as well as areas for patient screening/consenting and storage of patient records.

Documentation and Electronic Health Records (EHR) EHR systems have been employed in most academic centers with varied success. Access to the medical records is crucial for the monitoring of trials. Ideally, the EHR will allow for easy access to source documentation. All regulatory documents, such as the Form FDA 1572 (Statement of Investigator), training documentation, and other study-related source documentation also need to be in an easily accessed format, whether paper or electronic. Per 21 CFR 21.62, records are required to be kept a minimum of two (2) years either after the date a marketing application is approved for a drug for the indication for which it is being investigated, or after the study is discontinued and FDA is notified that no application is to be filed or if the application is not approved. The sponsor and/or FDA should also send a written confirmation granting permission to destroy the records. Institutional requirements may specify a longer record retention period.

Treatment Unit A treatment unit where investigational therapeutic agents will be administered to patients, having a sufficient number of beds to accommodate the anticipated volume of patients enrolled in phase I clinical trials, is also integral to early stage clinical trial units. Here, patients will receive intensive, time-sensitive monitoring from clinical nursing staff who are experienced in recognizing treatment-emergent adverse events. Nurses should also coordinate and communicate with patients' treating physicians. Pharmacokinetic and pharmacodynamic studies are often intertwined with study drug or regimen administration, therefore EKG and laboratory services are ideally integrated with the treatment unit, or at least in close coordination with the nursing staff. The laboratory unit should be able to provide phlebotomy services by certified technicians and technologists, prompt specimen processing, on-site storage, tracking and shipment. A sample documentation/tracking system that collects collection, testing, storage, and shipment information for every patient sample collected per protocol is essential, especially for data monitoring purposes. Lastly, 24-hour availability per day may be required per study protocol, hence sufficient staffing should be considered to support extended weekday and weekend hours of treatment unit operation, as needed.

With the advent of complex cellular therapies that require intensive monitoring for cytokine release syndrome (CRS) and neurotoxicity from cellular therapies, dedicated inpatient units that Foundation for the Accreditation of Cellular Therapy (F.A.C.T) certified with trained nurses who can identify the signs and symptoms of CRS are essential. In addition, other immunotherapies such as bispecific immunotherapy antibodies can also lead to significant CRS and often require inpatient monitoring.

Investigational Pharmacy An Investigational Pharmacy responsible for managing all investigational drugs used at any academic center is an essential component of an early phase clinical trial unit. Among its operational responsibilities include drug acquisition, inventory control and investigational drug accountability, as well as "provision of drug information of investigational agents and protocols for health care professionals both within and outside the institution". The Investigational Pharmacy staff should also ensure pharmacy compliance with protocol requirements. All equipment used in the pharmacy must be appropriately calibrated, and the site must also take the appropriate measures, such as keeping a limited supply of the investigational product on hand, locked, and in a temperature-controlled room to ensure security.

Imaging Core and Interventional Radiology support A centralized platform for quantitative image analysis for clinical and translational oncology research that provides independent tumor measurements according to the response assessment criteria (RECIST 1.1, irRECIST, PERCIST, RANO, etc.) as required per protocol is an advantage for any Early Phase Clinical Trial Unit. An Imaging Core acts as a comprehensive computational and communication resource for image-based analytics, and provides services such as image acquisition consulting, quality control, and standardization of tumor measurement and result reporting.

In addition, Phase 1 trials increasingly require biopsies to correlate the pharmacodynamic markers included in modern early drug development studies. Also, an increasing number of new therapies include direct tumor injections which also requires experienced Interventional radiology colleagues who understand the nuances and complexities of research tumor biopsies and injections. Ideally, faculty imbedded in the phase 1 unit eliminates miscommunication. If however, organizational structure does not allow for this, clear SOPs about communication to the interventional radiology colleague about biopsy selection, sample acquisition, and tumor injection techniques are necessary.

Molecular Profiling Core In the past few decades, tremendous advances in cancer therapy have been made possible by targeted therapy and genomic testing. Personalized cancer therapy, an approach that utilizes molecular diagnostics to its full extent to inform therapeutics in patient care, has become a cornerstone for oncology drug development so as to improve patient outcomes. Access to molecular testing is therefore critical for all cancer patients, but even more so for those that will be seen and treated in clinical trial centers. A Molecular Profiling Core that tests patient biopsies (solid/tissue or liquid/blood) for aberrations in actionable genes and gene products allows for the proper screening of patients and selection of appropriate targeted therapies. A Molecular Profiling Core also supports and fosters preclinical and translational research efforts that are driven by better characterization of tumors and their microenvironment, along with the integration of such molecular data with clinical information on patient diagnosis, response, adverse events, and the like.

4.3 Institutional Human Research Infrastructure

Institutional Review Board (IRB) The main purpose of an IRB, an administrative committee that protects human subjects' rights and welfare should they decide to participate in clinical trials under the oversight of the academic institution, is to provide an independent review of research protocols and activities that fall within its jurisdiction, as specified by federal regulations and institutional policy. IRBs should be registered with the Office for Human Research Protections (OHRP) and are associated with the Federal-wide Assurance Document FWA-363. Human research subject involvement will only be permitted if the IRB has reviewed and approved the research protocol, and if informed consent has been appropriately obtained as required by 45 CFR 46.116. Several IRBs may be established depending on the volume and scope of the studies, and ideally each study will be assigned to a home IRB for review (initial or continuing) until termination.

Federal regulations also require each IRB to be composed of at least five (5) members, each with varying backgrounds and professions, and should be composed of male and female members. At minimum, there should be one member of the community who represents the perspective of research participants, a member with a science background and another with a non-science background, and one who is not affiliated with the academic institution.

Internal Protocol Review Committee An Internal Protocol Review Committee is responsible for evaluating the science behind all research activities requiring a clinical protocol, as well as overseeing the scientific research incorporated within such protocols. This includes those that originated from private pharmaceutical and biotechnology companies, cooperative groups, studies sponsored by the National Cancer Institute (NCI), protocols initiated by investigators or physician-scientists within the Institute, and all others that require a written protocol for review by the

IRB. An assessment of the scientific merit of each protocol's specific aims, background, rationale, pharmaceutical information, and methods, including biostatistical analyses and radiologic and pathologic procedures, should be made by the committee members to preserve the standards of clinical investigations within the academic center.

Investigational New Drug (IND) Office An academic setting provides fertile ground for clinical research initiatives, including investigator-initiated studies (IITs). The FDA holds investigators responsible to the same standards as industry sponsors, and the responsibilities, liabilities, and funding required to support such studies can be overwhelming. The IND Office is a central office that serves to assume responsibility for, and take the obligation of, IND sponsorship off of investigators within the academic institution for investigator-initiated studies. In this manner, investigators are provided regulatory and monitoring support while ensuring compliance with sponsor and federal regulatory requirements. Ideally, this office should assist investigators and provide oversight on the following areas: Regulatory Affairs, Monitoring Services, and Medical Affairs/Safety.

The amount of monitoring required is significant for IITs, especially if the trial is recruiting at multiple institutions. Not only is it important that the PI confirms timely data entry, but must also assure accuracy of data starting with eligibility confirmation through all data required to be collected through patient coming off trial, and often through death if the trial is a Phase 2 or Phase 3 study with overall survival as an endpoint. Having dedicated monitors that can review the data in a timely fashion and meet on a regular basis with the trial PI and review data, is important. This helps to assure all relevant data is collected to help assure fulfillment of the trial objectives. Personnel need to be available who have the experience and knowledge to maintain and submit relevant regulatory documents, beyond the IND, to the FDA and/or sponsors, as well as central IRB if one is used for multi-institutional trials, assures compliance. This would include such things as amendments to the protocol, updated Investigator Brochures, relevant patient safety information, etc.

4.4 Personnel and Services

The most important piece in the success of an early drug development unit is the people who lead, serve, and run the organization day to day. For viable growth, it is important that new personnel be added sufficiently in advance of new studies opening to allow necessary training to competently handle all studies. Projected study openings should be adjusted yearly and new staff added as required in advance based upon agreed-upon study ratios (Fig. 4.2).

The **ratio of personnel to studies** depend on the design of studies, since studies with multiple arms or open enrollment to expansion cohorts have high accrual per study. Trials that require a higher number of patient visits, long treatments, more tests and procedures require more time from personnel and reduce the number of

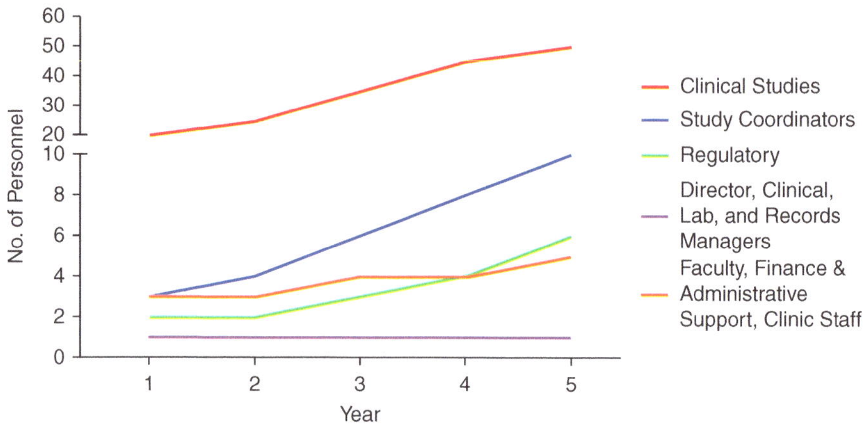

Fig. 4.2 Staffing requirements in an early phase clinical trial unit. The number of essential clinical trial personnel, such as study coordinators and regulatory staff, should grow sufficiently in advance of new studies opening so studies are handled competently and patient safety is not sacrificed. Projected study openings should be adjusted yearly and new staff added as required in advance based upon agreed-upon study ratios

studies each can handle. Since the design of early therapeutics studies are becoming more complex, the patients' status can change dramatically and quickly, which can impact support services, additional visits and procedures, and clinicians and treatment unit staff.

A. **Faculty.** Dedicated faculty who have expertise in early drug are necessary in the development of a competitive unit. Ideally, the faculty should be medical oncology- or medical and hematological malignancy-trained. Faculty need to have experience and expertise in running complex early trials with an understanding of pharmacokinetic principles, and pharmacodynamic and molecular endpoints. They should also have a grasp of varying trial designs, both early and late, and need a strong working understanding of, at minimum, standard and Bayesian statistical designs. Understanding of adverse event (AE) reporting and all standard reporting requirements such as SAEs, deviations, and violations are also essential for running any early trial. Perhaps most importantly, the faculty need strong leadership, management, and organizational skills since their role in leading these complex trials primarily centers on managing their research teams of clinical, data, regulatory, and financial coordinators.

B. **Clinical Study Nurses/Coordinators.** Early phase studies tend to be more complicated than later phase trials. Patients/subjects also tend to experience more AEs and/or serious adverse events (SAE) than average. Clinical study nurses/coordinators are therefore essential not only to provide advanced patient care services but also for operational management of clinical trials. They are responsible for ensuring that patient visits and activities are scheduled in accordance to what is indicated in the IRB-approved protocol, reconciling performed assessments and following up on patient-related issues. In this manner, they closely coordinate quality control of clinical research studies to avoid missing protocol-specific assessments. It is important that they interact closely with other clinical study team members so daily patient data are captured. In addition, they serve as the point of contact for all external and internal agencies. Study coordinators should be trained to understand and adhere to ICH-GCP, FDA, and institutional policies and procedures related to the conduct of clinical trials, since they ultimately serve a large part in providing collaborative oversight by documenting patient care, maintaining patient safety, and coordinating with the rest of the multidisciplinary team to achieve the objectives of the phase I trials.

C. **Clinical Data Coordinators.** Data coordinators, working closely with study coordinators or research nurses, are responsible for the accurate and timely capture of subject information in various research data system applications. Data coordinators should perform source document verification of protocol compliance and drug accountability prior to research data capture to ensure consistency between protocol database and source documentation. Their knowledge of various disease states is important in determining the appropriate clinical information to report, as well as their ability to thoroughly review information within treatment records, clinical evaluations, diagnostic test results, records of surgery, and pathology information. As with other study team members, data coordinators should be trained to understand and adhere to ICH-GCP, FDA, and institutional policies and procedures related to the conduct of clinical trials.

D. **Advanced Practice Providers.** Primarily in the United States, Advanced Practice Providers (APPs), which include both Advanced Practice Nurses and Physician Assistants, are vital to the operations of any early phase clinical trial unit, especially for clinic operations. They are responsible for seeing patients enrolled in trials in clinic. Hence, APPs should be well versed with study work-ups and with common AEs that are associated with specific classes of investigational drugs, as well as those associated with FDA-approved oncology drugs. They provide prompt detection of other unusual treatment-emergent and -associated AEs, and also provide immediate medical support to patients.

E. **Treatment Unit Nursing Staff**. The nursing staff in an early phase clinical trial unit should also display familiarity with the conduct of phase I trials, especially with the administration of investigational therapeutics and the required treatment-related and timepoint-specific assessments such as vitals, EKGs, and blood draws. Therefore, the treatment unit nurses work in close coordination with the Investigational Pharmacy staff for study drug administration, and with the laboratory staff for treatment-related procedures. As with any medical support providers, the treatment unit nursing staff should also be familiar with common AEs associated with both investigational drugs and FDA-approved oncology drugs, and should be prompt both in detecting unusual AEs and also in providing the appropriate medical attention and response.

F. **Laboratory staff.** Laboratory staff specialize in patient specimen collection, processing, and storage for analysis in the laboratory. Attention to detail is critical for the laboratory staff especially during the accurate labeling of all samples and entering sample data into a database in accordance with prescribed procedures. Likewise, it is important that samples are processed according to protocol requirements, transferred to appropriate containers, and stored at the specified temperature to ensure sample integrity. Laboratory staff may also be trained to perform EKGs for patients on protocol.

G. **Regulatory Staff.** Working closely with the entire research team, the Regulatory Staff provides support to Clinical Trial Units by serving as the primary contact with external sponsors to ensure compliance with local and federal regulatory requirements. They act on behalf of the principal investigators beginning from submission of the protocol and other study-related documents all the way to study close-out to obtain approval from regulatory review bodies such as the Institutional Review Board (IRB), National Cancer Institute (NCI), and the Food and Drug Administration (FDA). Regulatory Coordinators assist in developing protocols and informed consent forms, amend existing investigator-initiated protocols, and assist in ensuring quality control of research design.

H. **Finance Staff.** The Finance or Business Operations team supports Clinical Trial Units by assessing the financial components of clinical trials and issuing appropriate recommendations, from initial negotiations to eventual trial close-out. Having a Finance staff integrated within a Clinical Trial Unit allows them to work closely with the Principal Investigators, trial unit Director, Managers, and leadership team throughout the lifetime of any clinical trial. During the pre-award stage, the Finance team functions to develop budgets for clinical trial costs, perform coverage analysis, provide expertise in contract negotiations, and facilitate contract routing and approvals, among others. They also serve to ensure compliance to grants and contracts, invoice sponsors for billable services and associated collections, generate financial reports, and prevent cost overruns and address them if they ever happen during the post-award stage.

4.5 Standard Operating Procedures (SOPs)

Development of a defined set of phase I standard operating procedures (SOPs) that apply to all operations, center participants and processes should be in place. Below is a list of some of the essential topics that SOPs should cover:

- Reporting of AEs, SAEs, continuing reviews, other compliance issues
- Physicians including coverage, team meeting participation and study acceptance
- Advance Practice Providers, including their responsibilities, research activity and schedule

- Training manuals for clinical research coordinators/research nurses/data coordinators
- Study management
- Study acceptance & Portfolio management
- Study closure and maintenance of documents
- Internal Review Committees
- Publications and Authorship
- Finance
- Coverage and scheduling
- Patient intake and clinics
- Investigational Pharmacy
- Drug administration
- Pharmacokinetics
- Tissue and blood handling
- Inpatient and outpatient clinic policies

4.6 Study Portfolio

A balanced study portfolio is important to include a diversity of novel compounds, targets, sponsors, and study designs to provide sufficient and appropriate patient assignments to studies and open slots. This balance should be the result of multiple variables and study assessment factors. Ideally the portfolio should meet the needs of the patient population seen at the institution. Other considerations include the expertise of the unit faculty and their familiarity with the class of molecules, disease subtypes needed to be enrolled, or molecular subtypes. In starting a Phase 1 unit, the number of studies that need to be activated depends on the number of experienced principle investigators and research nurses/coordinators on hand.

A standard process of determining which studies should be accepted and prioritized should be in place. Proposed studies should be evaluated based on the interest of the team in the target and compound, current study portfolio, considering anticipated study openings or closings, compelling scientific questions to be answered, access to potential further interesting studies based on outcome of proposed study, sponsor relationships, master contracts and other relevant factors. Any of the early therapeutics physicians/faculty should be able to bring forward a proposal to the Senior Leadership Council for review and discussion of the study fit with the Center portfolio needs.

Letters of Intent (LOIs), grant projects, Investigator Initiated (IIT) studies, etc. should become a significant portion of the Early Therapeutics Portfolio to push forward concepts, protocols and treatments that allow for ideas and concepts outside industry strategies. Junior faculty and fellows should be mentored and encouraged to bring forward proposals. Study Principal Investigators should be determined by a variety of factors including: relationship with the sponsor, which investigator brought the study forward, previous experience with the compound and/or target, balance of study responsibilities and mentoring of junior faculty.

4.7 Protocol Review and Activation Process

To attract the best clinical trials of the most promising compounds (first in human, first in class, best in class), it is critical to commit to strict standards for the time it takes to open new studies. Ideally, the activation process should occur as quickly as possible without compromising a thoughtful and thorough review of the protocol for feasibility and safety. On average, activation of studies should take 12 weeks from receipt of protocol through all internal and IRB reviews, receipt of written approvals to site initiation visit (SIV), and study opening. Progress through protocol review, including all component committees, should be transparent and seamless so that the entire timeline from receipt to SIV falls within the 12-week metric. Processes such as scientific review, budget and contracting should be done, whenever possible, in parallel.

All internal study review committee (scientific and other) processes from the time of protocol submission to written receipt approval from all committees must be completed within a 4–6 week metric. Budgeting and contracting processes for each study must proceed in parallel with all internal and IRB review committee processes and must be completed by the time of IRB approval with no extension of the overall timeline metric of 12 weeks from receipt of protocol to SIV. Budgets should be competitive with local and national standards. Service charges may require negotiation. Budgeting and contract negotiations are often the slow link in any activation process. Creation of budgets are complex and require understanding of research costs vs. standard of care costs. Institutional clinical research finance staff and processes that understand these complexities, create and negotiate a budget rapidly, is key to any activation process.

Finally, whenever feasible, the potential first subject in (FSI) will be identified at the team meeting prior to the SIV so that FSI can be consented and screened within 1 week of SIV.

Interacting with sponsors and tumor focused departments:

Sponsors such as mid/small biotech and large pharma are the key customers of any phase 1 unit. Increasingly, Clinical Research Organizations (CROs), on behalf of sponsors, determine sites for any clinical trial. Ideally any phase 1 unit will have several investigators with deep relationships with biotech, large pharma, and CROs. Selection of a site depends on several key factors: experience and knowledge of the principal investigator, staffing, patient volume, inpatient capability, time to activation, cost, and importantly previous trial performance. Many sponsors and CROs maintain large databases to track these metrics on sites. This poses a challenge to an academic site that is beginning a phase 1 unit with no previous relationships or track record. Nationally recognized faculty at an academic site who may not have a phase 1 focus but have deep connections with a sponsor may help to bridge this gap and help build the portfolio of a phase 1 unit just starting. Sponsors and CROs will seek sites out that can deliver on quick activation of trials, patient enrollment, and data quality. Hence, it is paramount that the phase 1 unit leadership build an infrastructure to deliver.

As shared in the introduction, stand alone phase I units are the exception. If an academic site decides to build a stand alone phase 1 unit clear boundaries, rules of engagement, and collaboration need to be written down and agreed upon. Phase 1 trials have evolved where seamless studies have become an increasingly common trial design. Phase 1 trials, rapidly after dose escalation, transition to multi-arm basket trials or phase 2 studies that can include several different tumor types. Clear boundaries of which studies will go to a tumor specific PI or a phase 1 PI, whether the phase I PI remains the overarching PI when the trial transitions to expansion, where the patients will be treated and followed, are but some of the points that will need to be agreed upon. Finally, the currency of academia-authorship needs to be clearly agreed upon before acceptance of the trial.

4.8 Conclusion

As a renaissance of new oncology drugs emerge onto the screen of drug development, there has been a need to rapidly transition new molecules from the preclinical to the clinical space. As a result, phase 1 units have taken center stage. Academic centers face competition from alternative clinical trial sites and the need to develop focused phase 1 units in the academic setting is a new challenge for administrators. As shared in this chapter, significant investment in space, staff, and SOPs are necessary to guarantee success.

Key Expert Opinion Points

- There are advantages to having an academic dedicated phase 1 unit: a focused and dedicated unit to the development of new drugs in oncology.
- Organizational structure and resources are the bedrock to success.
- Clear SOPs must be laid out before creating a unit.
- Staff and Faculty who are dedicated are ultimately will decide whether the unit will succeed and developing staff and junior faculty is paramount.

Chapter 5
Novel Trial Designs for Early Phase Clinical Trials

Chia-Chi Lin

Abstract Oncology phase I trials consist of the dose escalation part and the dose expansion part. The former traditionally uses the "3+3" design, which takes lots of patients, takes a long time, and may expose a substantial proportion of patients to low (and ineffective) doses. Therefore the novel designs such as the accelerated titration design, the continual reassessment method, the escalation with overdose control were implemented in some phase I trials. The latter nowadays serves multiple purposes to confirm the safety profile, to characterize the pharmodynamics/pharmacokinetics, and to define the objective response rates in certain tumor/molecular types (seamless design).

Keywords Dose limiting toxicity · Maximum tolerated dose · Optimal biologic dose · Pharmacokinetics · Pharmacodynamics · Accelerated titration design Continual reassessment method · Seamless design

Key Points

- The tradition (3+3) design of the dose escalation part leads to many apparent drawbacks.
- The novel designs of the dose escalation part theoretically could solve those problems.
- The optimal biologic (immunologic) dose has been proposed to replace the maximum tolerated dose.
- The dose expansion part has become more complex in the modern oncology phase I trials.
- There were several oncology agents developed by trials using the seamless design.

C.-C. Lin (✉)
Department of Oncology, National Taiwan University Hospital, Taipei, Taiwan

Graduate Institute of Clinical Medicine, National Taiwan University College of Medicine, Taipei, Taiwan
e-mail: cclin1@ntu.edu.tw

T. A. Yap et al. (eds.), *Phase I Oncology Drug Development*,
https://doi.org/10.1007/978-3-030-47682-3_5

5.1 Introduction

The objective of a phase I trial is to determine the appropriate dosage of an agent or combination to be taken into further study and to provide initial pharmacologic and pharmacokinetic studies. It is generally assumed, at this stage of testing, that increased dose is associated with increased chance of clinical efficacy. Therefore, the phase I trial is designed as a dose-escalation study to determine the maximum tolerated dose (MTD), that is, the maximum dose associated with an acceptable level of dose-limiting toxicity (DLT—usually defined to be grade 3 or above toxicity, except for grade 3 neutropenia unaccompanied by either fever or infection). This MTD is then taken into further testing. Since evaluation of efficacy is generally not the objective of a phase I trial, it is not necessary to restrict to a patient population homogeneous with respect to disease, or even to restrict to patients with measurable disease (for which tumor response is determinable). It is important, however, to exclude patients with impaired organ function, who may therefore be more prone to serious toxicity. The fundamental conflict in phase I trials is between escalating too fast, so as to expose patients to excessive toxicity, and escalating too slow, so as to deny patients the opportunity to be treated at potentially efficacious dose levels.

Phase I clinical trials in oncology have been conducted using a modified Fibonacci "3+3" design whereby between three and six patients are accrued per dose level and no more than one of up to six patients experience a DLT prior to proceeding to the next step. Dose escalations increments are approximately 100%, 67%, 50%, 40%, and 33% thereafter. The purpose is to allow more aggressive dose escalation for the initial levels, which are expected to be sufficiently remote from the MTD for this to be safe. If the mice LD_{10} (lethal dose in 1/10th of a rodent species tested pre-clinically) accurately predicted the human MTD, only 5–6 such dose escalations would be necessary to complete this traditional phase I design. Unfortunately, this is often not the case [1].

The statistical operating characteristics of this approach are as follows. If at least two of three patients treated at a particular dose show DLT, we can conclude with 90% confidence that the true probability of DLT at that dose is greater than 20%. In other words, as we see in Table 5.1, unless the true probability of DLT at that dose is at least 20%, the probability of at least two out of three patients exhibiting DLT is less than 10%. On the other hand, if 0 of 3 patients show DLT, we can conclude with 90% confidence that the true probability of DLT is less than 55%. Again, as we see in Table 5.1, unless the true probability of DLT is less than 55%, the probability of 0 out of 3 patients exhibiting DLT is less than 10%. In the interest of efficiency, we accept either of these situations as sufficient to halt or continue escalation after treating only three patients at the current level. Allowing for expansion to six patients in case one of the initial three show DLT, the dose escalation rule gives 91% probability that dose escalation will not halt at doses associated with DLT probability less than 10%, and it gives 92% probability that escalation will not proceed beyond doses associated with DLT probability in excess of 60% (Table 5.1). The process of approaching

Table 5.1 Probabilities of halting or continuing dose escalation for various probabilities of DLT associated with the dose level, for the standard phase I trial design

True probability of DLT for dose level	0.05	0.1	0.2	0.3	0.4	0.5	0.6	0.7
Probability of halting dose escalation after accruing either three or six patients (≥2 DLT)	0.03	0.09	0.29	0.51	0.69	0.83	0.92	0.97
Probability of continuing escalation after only three patients (0 DLT)	0.86	0.73	0.51	0.34	0.22	0.13	0.06	0.03
Probability of halting escalation after only three patients (≥2 DLT)	0.01	0.03	0.10	0.22	0.35	0.50	0.65	0.78

the MTD from below, in successive steps, further protects against defining an MTD associated with excessive toxicity. Table 5.1 plus simulations show that, for a wide variety of dose-toxicity curves, the probability is approximately 85–90% that the defined MTD will be associated with DLT probability of approximately 10–45%.

The primary criticisms of the standard phase I design [2–5] are:

(1) It does not target a particular probability of DLT to be associated with the MTD, and, in practice, the DLT rate associated with the defined MTD will be somewhat dependent on the DLT rates of the various dose levels. This issue could be solved by the modified toxicity probability interval design [6].
(2) With standard designs many patients are treated at doses well below the biologically active level, minimizing the opportunity for antitumor response.
(3) The dose escalation is unnecessarily slow, leading to treatment of excessive numbers of patients at dose levels less likely to be efficacious.
(4) Traditional designs provide little information about inter-patient variability, cumulative toxicity or the steepness of the dose-toxicity relationships.

Despite much criticism for being overly cautious, the modified Fibonacci approach remains the most widely used methodology for dose escalation in phase I trials [7, 8]. The trend seems to change in the era of more modern phase I trials of targeted therapy [9].

5.2 Accelerated Titration Design

The accelerated titration design was proposed with the shortcomings of the modified Fibonacci approach in mind and have slowly been incorporated into some phase I dose escalation designs. The premise behind the accelerated titration design was to achieve the MTD using fewer patients without undue toxicity to the participating subjects [3].

The concept of one patient per dose level initially was originally described by Storer [5]. The accelerated titration scheme including those described by Simon et al. [3] utilizes one patient per dose level and dose escalate until a DLT is achieved or until grade 2 toxicities are experienced by two separate patients. There were three separate accelerated dose escalation schemes (Design 1 being the traditional modified Fibonacci "3+3" approach). (1) Design 2: one patient per dose level till DLT or two patients experiencing grade 2 toxicities during course 1. Dose escalation increments were according to usual modified Fibonacci schemes; (2) Design 3: dose escalation increments 100%, otherwise similar to Design 2; and (3) Design 4: DLT during any course causes design to revert to modified Fibonacci design, otherwise similar to Design 3. Additionally, two intra-patient dose escalation schema were described. (1) Option A: no intra-patient dose escalation allowed, and de-escalation if grade 3 or worse toxicity encountered; and (2) Option B: intra-patient dose escalation allowed if grade 0–1 at previous course, no change if grade 2, and de-escalation if grade 3 or worse. With all these designs, in the setting of toxicities described above, they would revert to a modified Fibonacci dose escalation scheme (i.e. Design 1) with the advent of DLTs or two patients with grade 2 toxicities. Many phase I trials had employed this design. For example, onalespib (AT11387, heat shock protein 90 [HSP90] inhibitor) [10].

5.3 Pharmacologically Guided Dose Escalation Design (PGDE)

Collins et al. [11, 12] proposed using the area under the curve (AUC) for the concentration versus time curve as an aid to decision making in phase I trials. The rationale was to achieve an LD_{10}, or the equivalent (e.g., STD_{10} [severely toxic dose in 10% animals]) observed in mice (or another species). This approach had some shortcomings in that it could only be used in those situations where a sensitive assay for the new agent was available clinically and where interspecies differences for the drug did not exist. It was not a good approach in the case of anti-metabolites which tend to have somewhat less predictable pharmacokinetics. It also required that pharamacokinetic analyses were performed in real-time. CI-958, a DNA intercalator, was studied in the phase I setting using this approach [13]. Despite having many attractive features, a pure version of this design is not routinely used in new drug development. On the other hand, pharmacokinetic outcomes are routinely used as one of many factors that serve as decision points in dose escalation decisions.

5.4 Modified Continual Reassessment Method (mCRM)

The continual reassessment method is an adaptive design first introduced by O'Quigley et al. [4] in 1990. It is felt by its proponents to be superior to the traditional modified Fibonacci approach because it learns from new information that is encountered during the course of the trial to make dose escalation decisions. Several modifications were suggested to the original design proposed by O'Quigley et al. [4] and these have generally been referred to as modified continual reassessment method (mCRM). The general idea behind the mCRM is that a dose-toxicity curve is generated using a priori assumptions about the dose-toxicity relationship of the anti-cancer agent in question. As new data is generated with dose escalations and subsequent patients, the curve is "refitted" to incorporate this new information according to Bayes' theorem. This aspect of the mCRM makes it a dynamic dose escalation scheme whereas the modified Fibonacci is a static scheme where all dose levels are chosen a priori using a starting dose and appropriate increments. O'Quigley et al. [4] proposed that when the sample size reached a preset limit of 20–25, the MTD can be calculated from the final state of the dose-toxicity model. Numerous anti-cancer agents have been developed using this methodology. These include pemetrexed (LY232514, an antimetabolite) [14], and DX-8951f (exatecan mesylate, topoisomerase I inhibitor) [15]. The most prominent barriers to implementation of a model-based design such as mCRM were lack of suitable training, principal investigators' preference for rule-based designs, and limited resources for study design [16].

5.5 Escalation with Overdose Control (EWOC)

The escalation with overdose control (EWOC) trial design is an adaptive design which takes into account inter-patient variability due to known or presumed factors such as renal function, hepatic function, and age [17, 18]. Much like the mCRM, EWOC assimilates new information into decision making with the caveat that they emphasize an inter-patient variability as well. The importance of inter-patient variability is probably best illustrated from the impact of renal function on appropriate dosing of carboplatin [19]. EWOC was successfully employed in the development of PNU-214936 (a murine Fab fragment of 5T4 fused to a mutated superantigen of staphylococcal enterotoxin A) [20] and ribociclib (LEE011, CDK4/6 inhibitor) [21]. EWOC, like mCRM, needs extensive statistical support and this drawback has limited its practical application to no more than a handful of phase I trials.

5.6 Dose Escalation for Targeted Therapy and Immunotherapy

Certain types of therapeutics are not expected to be toxic in the dose range used. Some targeted therapies and immunotherapies are of this type [22, 23]. Conventional phase I designs are not suitable for such drugs because there is no interest in the MTD. Nevertheless, there may be uncertainty about the appropriate dose to use for clinical development. Resolving this uncertainty may not be possible, however, in the context of small 3–6 patient per cohort studies used for chemotherapy. Much larger studies may be required, depending on the specific objectives.

5.7 Pharmacokinetics Design

A pharmacokinetics based design generally can be accomplished with a limited number of subjects. One determines a target serum concentration based on preclinical or ex-vivo studies. For molecularly targeted drugs, the target concentration is chosen to maximally inhibit the target. The phase I trial then includes n patients for each of several dose levels. The serum concentration of the active metabolite is measured and the dose chosen that best achieves the target concentration. The target concentration is often a steady state level or a concentration integrated over time.

5.8 Optimum Biologic Dose (OBD)

One may define biological activity based on inhibition of a molecular target or based on an immunogenic response, and attempt to identify the smallest dose that is biologically active. Trying to characterize the shape of the dose-biological response relationship or finding an optimum biologic dose (OBD) is a more ambitious objective than a two dose comparison of biological response rates. It is rarely practical in a phase I study unless there is an accurate quantitative assay of biological response with little intra-patient or inter-patient variability in assay results.

Trials utilizing biological response endpoints are also complicated by issues of assay adequacy and access to biological tissues. Because of the difficulties of accessing tumor tissue, some studies have used normal tissue in which the molecular target is highly expressed. Thus, one strategy for phase I trials of targeted therapies is to compare dose levels with regard to biological response in accessible normal tissue using an optimized highly reproducible assay. The use of normal tissue may serve to reduce inter-patient variability. One example to use surrogate normal tissue to define OBD is everolimus (RAD001, mTOR inhibitor) [24].

If use of normal tissue for assessing biological response is not acceptable or if a highly reproducible assay is not available, trying to characterize an OBD is probably not feasible. In such cases it would probably be better to optimize the dose level utilizing clinical response as the endpoint. It would probably take more patients and more time to characterize the OBD than to compare dose levels with regard to clinical response. Such studies can either use tumor shrinkage or time to progressive disease as the clinical endpoint. The studies are best conducted as randomized trials but the type I error level does not need to be set stringently at the conventional 5% level.

5.9 Cohort Expansion

Phase I trial designs increasingly go beyond their former focus on safety and aim to identify the most-promising agents by adding cohort expansion before moving to phase II trials [25, 26]. Patient eligibility criteria for cohort expansion are often narrow and focus on specific tumor types, molecular characteristics (basket design), or both. Cohort expansions have various objectives: confirming that a safe level of drug exposure has been established; obtaining preliminary evidence of efficacy; and identifying specific patient subgroups that might derive particular benefits from the investigational treatment. Cohort expansions enable investigators to identify drugs that work best for specific patient populations in the context of a single trial, rather than using separate phase I trials and multiple phase II trials in specific patient populations. There remain many important questions. Are cohort expansions efficient, and to what extent do they help clinicians decide which drugs to take forward for further testing?

Current cohort expansions typically add an additional number of patients (usually $\geq$12) who are all treated at the established MTD. Use of such cohorts can reduce the uncertainty in estimating the MTD, which is especially relevant in trials of combination regimens involving targeted agents [27]. Experimenting with multiple doses to better evaluate the dose-response curve is also a rational approach [28]. Other trial designs can address certain questions, such as factors contributing to differing levels of treatment tolerance, or whether variations in tolerance correspond with differences in efficacy [28].

5.10 Seamless Design

The premise for phase I trials of targeted therapy is different from that of chemotherapy. For targeted therapies, toxicity and efficacy do not necessarily increase monotonically with increasing dose levels, but likely plateau after they reach maximal toxicity or efficacy. Hoering et al. [29] proposed a seamless phase I-II trial design to assess both toxicity and efficacy to find the best dose as well as a good dose [30]. Although consolidation and rapid accrual may yield efficiencies, widespread use of seamless first-in-human trials without careful consideration of objectives, statistical analysis plans, or trial oversight raises concerns. There are many phase I trials using seamless design. For example, pembrolizumab [31], atezolizumab [32], durvalumab [33], and avelumab [34].

Key Expert Opinion Points

- Novel dose escalation designs could prevent the phase I trial from enrolling lots of patients, taking a long time, and exposing a substantial proportion of patients to low (and effective dose).
- Novel dose escalation designs to determine the maximum tolerated dose include the accelerated titration design, the continual reassessment method, and the escalation with overdose control.

- If there is no MTD, the optimal biologic dose could be determined by other endpoints such as pharmacokinetics and pharmacodynamics.
- The dose expansion cohorts serve many purposes in the modern oncology phase I trials to become the so-called seamless design.
- The designs of the dose expansion cohorts should be based on the sound statistics.

References

1. Newell DR. Pharmacologically based phase I trials in cancer chemotherapy. Hematol Oncol Clin North Am. 1994;8:257–75.
2. Goodman SN, Zahurak ML, Piantadosi S. Some practical improvements in the continual reassessment method for phase I studies. Stat Med. 1995;14:1149–61.
3. Simon R, Freidlin B, Rubinstein L, et al. Accelerated titration designs for phase I clinical trials in oncology. J Natl Cancer Inst. 1997;89:1138–47.
4. O'Quigley J, Pepe M, Fisher L. Continual reassessment method: a practical design for phase 1 clinical trials in cancer. Biometrics. 1990;46:33–48.
5. Storer BE. Design and analysis of phase I clinical trials. Biometrics. 1989;45:925–37.
6. Ji Y, Wang SJ. Modified toxicity probability interval design: a safer and more reliable method than the 3 + 3 design for practical phase I trials. J Clin Oncol. 2013;31:1785–91.
7. Rogatko A, Schoeneck D, Jonas W, et al. Translation of innovative designs into phase I trials. J Clin Oncol. 2007;25:4982–6.
8. Le Tourneau C, Lee JJ, Siu LL. Dose escalation methods in phase I cancer clinical trials. J Natl Cancer Inst. 2009;101:708–20.
9. Le Tourneau C, Gan HK, Razak AR, Paoletti X. Efficiency of new dose escalation designs in dose-finding phase I trials of molecularly targeted agents. PLoS One. 2012;7:e51039.
10. Do K, Speranza G, Chang LC, et al. Phase I study of the heat shock protein 90 (Hsp90) inhibitor onalespib (AT13387) administered on a daily for 2 consecutive days per week dosing schedule in patients with advanced solid tumors. Invest New Drugs. 2015;33:921–30.
11. Collins JM, Zaharko DS, Dedrick RL, Chabner BA. Potential roles for preclinical pharmacology in phase I clinical trials. Cancer Treat Rep. 1986;70:73–80.
12. Collins JM, Grieshaber CK, Chabner BA. Pharmacologically guided phase I clinical trials based upon preclinical drug development. J Natl Cancer Inst. 1990;82:1321–6.
13. Dees EC, Whitfield LR, Grove WR, et al. A phase I and pharmacologic evaluation of the DNA intercalator CI-958 in patients with advanced solid tumors. Clin Cancer Res. 2000;6:3885–94.
14. Rinaldi DA, Burris HA, Dorr FA, et al. Initial phase I evaluation of the novel thymidylate synthase inhibitor, LY231514, using the modified continual reassessment method for dose escalation. J Clin Oncol. 1995;13:2842–50.
15. Rowinsky EK, Johnson TR, Geyer CE Jr, et al. DX-8951f, a hexacyclic camptothecin analog, on a daily-times-five schedule: a phase I and pharmacokinetic study in patients with advanced solid malignancies. J Clin Oncol. 2000;18:3151–63.
16. Love SB, Brown S, Weir CJ, et al. Embracing model-based designs for dose-finding trials. Br J Cancer. 2017;117:332–9.
17. Babb J, Rogatko A, Zacks S. Cancer phase I clinical trials: efficient dose escalation with overdose control. Stat Med. 1998;17:1103–20.
18. Tighiouart M, Rogatko A, Babb JS. Flexible Bayesian methods for cancer phase I clinical trials. Dose escalation with overdose control. Stat Med. 2005;24:2183–96.
19. Harland SJ, Newell DR, Siddik ZH, et al. Pharmacokinetics of cis-diammine-1,1-cyclobutane dicarboxylate platinum(II) in patients with normal and impaired renal function. Cancer Res. 1984;44:1693–7.

20. Cheng JD, Babb JS, Langer C, et al. Individualized patient dosing in phase I clinical trials: the role of escalation with overdose control in PNU-214936. J Clin Oncol. 2004;22:602–9.
21. Infante JR, Cassier PA, Gerecitano JF, et al. A phase I study of the cyclin-dependent kinase 4/6 inhibitor ribociclib (LEE011) in patients with advanced solid tumors and lymphomas. Clin Cancer Res. 2016;22:5696–705.
22. Tosi D, Laghzali Y, Vinches M, et al. Clinical development strategies and outcomes in first-in-human trials of monoclonal antibodies. J Clin Oncol. 2015;33:2158–65.
23. Viala M, Vinches M, Alexandre M, et al. Strategies for clinical development of monoclonal antibodies beyond first-in-human trials: tested doses and rationale for dose selection. Br J Cancer. 2018;118:679–97.
24. Tanaka C, O'Reilly T, Kovarik JM, et al. Identifying optimal biologic doses of everolimus (RAD001) in patients with cancer based on the modeling of preclinical and clinical pharmacokinetic and pharmacodynamic data. J Clin Oncol. 2008;26:1596–602.
25. Manji A, Brana I, Amir E, et al. Evolution of clinical trial design in early drug development: systematic review of expansion cohort use in single-agent phase I cancer trials. J Clin Oncol. 2013;31:4260–7.
26. Dahlberg SE, Shapiro GI, Clark JW, Johnson BE. Evaluation of statistical designs in phase I expansion cohorts: the Dana-Farber/Harvard Cancer Center experience. J Natl Cancer Inst. 2014;106
27. Cannistra SA. Challenges and pitfalls of combining targeted agents in phase I studies. J Clin Oncol. 2008;26:3665–7.
28. Iasonos A, O'Quigley J. Dose expansion cohorts in Phase I trials. Stat Biopharm Res. 2016;8:161–70.
29. Hoering A, LeBlanc M, Crowley J. Seamless phase I-II trial design for assessing toxicity and efficacy for targeted agents. Clin Cancer Res. 2011;17:640–6.
30. Hobbs BP, Barata PC, Kanjanapan Y, et al. Seamless designs: current practice and considerations for early-phase drug development in oncology. J Natl Cancer Inst. 2018.
31. Kang SP, Gergich K, Lubiniecki GM, et al. Pembrolizumab KEYNOTE-001: an adaptive study leading to accelerated approval for two indications and a companion diagnostic. Ann Oncol. 2017;28:1388–98.
32. Herbst RS, Soria JC, Kowanetz M, et al. Predictive correlates of response to the anti-PD-L1 antibody MPDL3280A in cancer patients. Nature. 2014;515:563–7.
33. Massard C, Gordon MS, Sharma S, et al. Safety and efficacy of durvalumab (MEDI4736), an anti-programmed cell death ligand-1 immune checkpoint inhibitor, in patients with advanced urothelial bladder cancer. J Clin Oncol. 2016;34:3119–25.
34. Heery CR, O'Sullivan-Coyne G, Madan RA, et al. Avelumab for metastatic or locally advanced previously treated solid tumours (JAVELIN Solid Tumor): a phase 1a, multicohort, dose-escalation trial. Lancet Oncol. 2017;18:587–98.

Chapter 6
Examining Performance of Phase I Designs: 3+3 Versus Bayesian Optimal Interval (BOIN)

Kenneth R. Hess and Bryan M. Fellman

Abstract In Phase I oncology trials, the primary goal is to assess dose limiting toxicities (DLT) and estimate the maximum tolerated dose (MTD). The classical 3+3 design is still used in the vast majority of studies. In this chapter, we review the 3+3 design and the new Bayesian Optimal Interval (BOIN) design. BOIN is easy to implement, similar to the 3+3, using a simple table to guide dose escalation/de-escalation. As opposed to the 3+3 design, BOIN can target a DLT rate well above or below the usual 25–33% target. We explain how computer simulations can be used to evaluate phase I designs and present results comparing the designs under a large number of true dose-toxicity scenarios. We show that BOIN has better performance than 3+3. BOIN selects the true MTD at a much higher rate and treats a higher percentage of patients at the MTD. BOIN allocates fewer patients to low toxicity doses. Unlike older Bayesian designs (e.g., modified continual reassessment method), BOIN does not require a statistician to be available during the trial. Readily-available, free software makes BOIN simple to implement. We recommend the use of BOIN over the 3+3 design.

Keywords 3+3 · Bayesian optimal interval · Statistical properties and performance Novel phase I design

Key Points

1. A key goal of phase I oncology trials is to estimate the maximum tolerated dose (MTD)
2. The vast majority of phase I oncology trials use the simple 3+3 design
3. The Bayesian Optimal Interval (BOIN) design is one of a new class of model-assisted designs

---

K. R. Hess (✉) · B. M. Fellman
Department of Biostatistics, UT MD Anderson Cancer Center, Houston, TX, USA
e-mail: khess@mdanderson.org; bmfellman@mdanderson.org

T. A. Yap et al. (eds.), *Phase I Oncology Drug Development*,
https://doi.org/10.1007/978-3-030-47682-3_6

4. BOIN has superior statistical properties as shown by numerous computer simulation studies
5. Free BOIN software is available on a wide range of platforms.

6.1 Introduction

The key goals of a phase I dose-escalation study in oncology are to assess the types, severities and incidences of dose-limiting toxicities (DLTs) and to estimate the maximum tolerated dose (MTD) of experimental therapy. In designing a phase I study, the following must be specified: the patient population, the types of toxicities of interest, the route and schedule of administration of the experimental therapy, and a set of possible doses to be studied (see Chap. 1). We assume that the probability of DLT increases with dose (Fig. 6.1).

In a typical phase I dose-escalation study, at a given dose-level, small cohorts of patients are treated and DLT outcomes are observed. Based on the DLT outcomes the dose is escalated, de-escalated or retained at the current level. This process is repeated until either the maximum dose level is studied or the MTD is reached.

An ideal phase I study design is intuitive both to clinical investigators and statisticians, painless to implement and has good statistical properties including reliably and accurately estimating the MTD.

Fig. 6.1 Example toxicity-dose curve

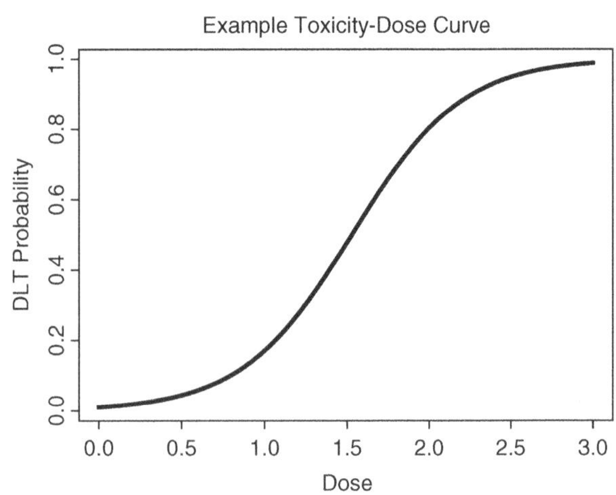

6.2 Classic 3+3 Dose Escalation Design

Historically, the 3+3 design has been used in the vast majority of oncology studies. This design treats patients in cohorts of 3 following a strict set of rules (Fig. 6.2). At a given dose level, the dose for the next cohort is esclated if 0 of 3 patients experience DLT, the dose is retained if 1 of 3 patients experience DLT, and the dose is de-escalated if >1 of 3 patients experience DLT. The maximum number of patients for the 3+3 design is six times the number of dose levels. However, if no DLTs are encountered, the expected number of patients is three times the number of dose levels plus three additional patients to have six treated at the MTD. So, for 5 dose levels, the maximum number of patients would be 30 and if no DLTs are observed, the expected number of patients would be 18.

For example, a 3+3 design would proceed (given hypothetical DLT results) as:

- Step 1: 3 patients are treated at dose level 1 and 0 experience DLT;
- Step 2: 3 patients are treated at dose level 2 and 0 experience DLT;
- Step 3: 3 patients are treated at dose level 3 and 1 patient develops DLT;
- Step 4: 3 more patients are treated at dose level 3 and 0 of these patients experience DLT (so 1/6 patients experience DLT at dose level 3);
- Step 5: 3 patients are treated at dose level 4 and 1 patient develops DLT;

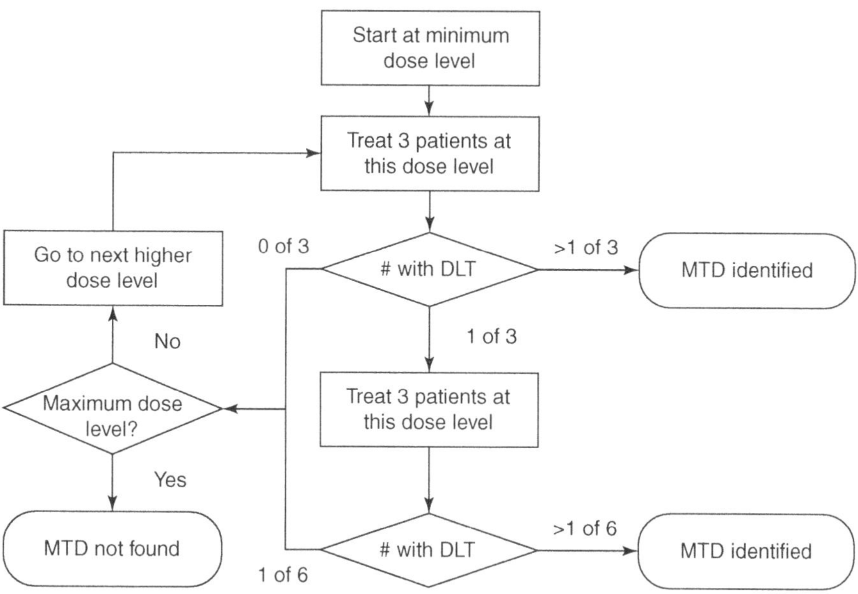

Fig. 6.2 3+3 Flow Diagram

- Step 6: 3 more patients are treated at dose level 4 and 1 of these patients experiences DLT (so 2/6 patients experience DLT at dose level 4);
- Step 7: stop dose escalation and establish dose level 3 as the MTD. Thus a total of 18 patients were treated and the DLT rate at the MTD was 1/6 = 17%.

6.3 Newer Designs: Bayesian Statistics Applied to Dose Escalation Designs

Over the years, statisticians have developed several dose escalation designs with superior statistical properties compared to the 3+3 design [1]. Designs have also been developed specifically for targeted and immunotherapy ([2]; see more in Chap. 10).

They are typically model-based or model-assisted. A model-based design like the modified Continual Reassessment Method (mCRM) establishes a statistical model that relates DLT probability to dose level. Other more recent designs are termed model-assisted because, while they are based on probability models, updating the model parameters based on accruing data is not necessary. The decision rule for dose escalation and de-escalation can be predetermined and included in the trial protocol. This greatly simplifies their implementation and means that a statistician does not need to be available to update the model during the trial. The BOIN design described below is an example of such a design.

BOIN Design The Bayesian Optimal Interval, or BOIN design [3] is a model-assisted Bayesian design which is straight-forward to implement and has superior performance to the 3+3 design [1]. The BOIN design is very flexible in that any DLT rate can be used as the target rate for estimating the MTD; any reasonable cohort size (e.g., 1, 2, 3, 4) can be used; and the maximum number of patients to be studied can be pre-specified. The design is easy to implement because the underlying probability model and the design parameters are used to generate *a priori,* a single table that guides dose finding. This table is easily generated using freely available software which can also be used to estimate the statistical properties of the design for a wide range of hypothetical dose-toxicity scenarios using computer simulations.

The goal of the BOIN design [4] is to minimize decision errors of escalating (or deescalating) the dose when the current dose actually is above (or below) the MTD. The design creates three distinct probability regions for the observed DLT rate: "escalate", "retain" and "de-escalate" (Fig. 6.3). The boundaries between regions are derived to satisfy statistical optimization properties. The boundaries for the oft-chosen 30% target toxicity rate are 0.236 and 0.358 [3]. Thus, the probability regions are: *escalate* = 0 to 0.236, *retain* (i.e., stay at current dose level): 0.237 to 0.357, and *de-escalate* = 0.358 to 1. The design monitors which probability region the observed DLT rate of the current dose level falls and makes decisions accordingly (Fig. 6.4). For example, if the observed DLT rate at the current dose (e.g., 1/6 = 0.167) is less than 0.236, the design escalates the dose; if the observed DLT rate at the current dose (e.g., 3/6 = 0.5) is greater than 0.358, the design de-escalates the dose. BOIN allows for the maximum number of patients to be specified as well as the maximum number of patients to be treated at any given dose level.

An example of a BOIN dose-finding decision table is shown in Table 6.1 (design parameters: target DLT rate = 30%, maximum number of patients treated at single dose = 15, cohort size = 3). For example, if 3 patients have been treated at a given dose level, the decisions are to escalate if 0 patients experience DLT, stay at current dose (i.e., retain) if 1 patient experiences DLT (determined by process of elimination because other options are explicitly ruled out); de-escalate if 2 or more patients experience DLT; and to eliminate the dose level from future consideration if all 3 of the patients experience DLT.

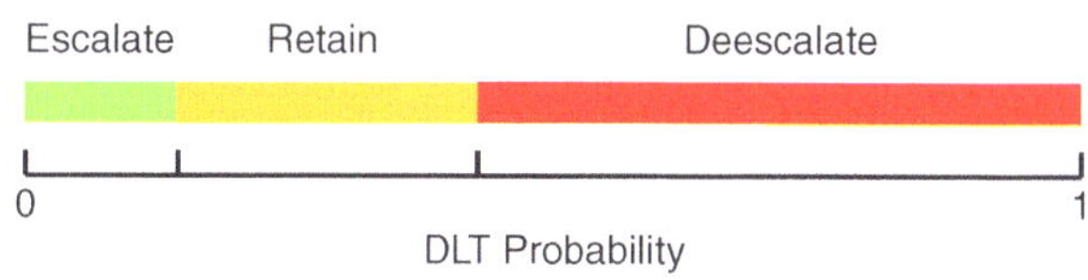

Fig. 6.3 Three distinct probability regions for the observed DLT rate

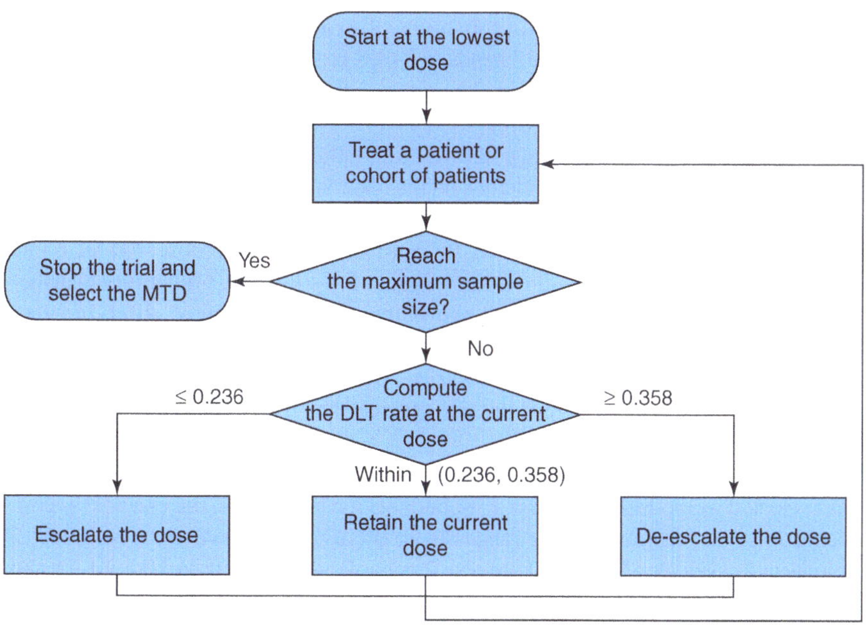

Fig. 6.4 BOIN Flow Diagram

Table 6.1 Dose escalation/de-escalation rule for the BOIN design

	The number of patients treated **at the current dose**														
Actions	1	2	3	4	5	6	7	8	9	10	11	12	13	14	15
Escalate if # of DLT ≤	0	0	0	0	1	1	1	1	2	2	2	2	3	3	3
De-escalate if # of DLT ≥	1	1	2	2	2	3	3	3	4	4	4	5	5	6	6
Eliminate if # of DLT ≥	NA	NA	3	3	4	4	5	5	5	6	6	7	7	8	8

6.4 Making Decisions with Small Cohorts: The Role of Random Variation in DLT Results

Because only a relatively small number of patients are typically studied at a given dose level in a phase I study, it is important to understand the effect of random variation on the observed DLT results. DLT events are binary (yes/no) in nature (i.e., did patient experience DLT during pre-specified observation period). Binary events can be viewed as coin flips (i.e., two well-defined, mutually exclusively outcomes). Observing the number of patients experiencing DLTs out three patients total is analogous to observing the number heads in 3 coin flips. With 3 flips, there are 4 possibilities: 0, 1, 2, or 3 heads. If we assume that the number of heads follows the binomial distribution, then we can compute the probability of observing 0, 1, 2, or 3 heads in 3 flips if we know the true probability of getting a head on a given flip of the coin.

Figure 6.5 shows the probability distribution for a 0.5 probability of heads. It shows that even though the true probability of heads is 50%, the probability of observing zero heads in 3 flips or 3 heads in 3 flips is 12.5%. Of course the probability of observing 1 head in 3 flips or 2 heads in 1 flip is much higher at 27.5%. So given the small number of flips, while there is a 75% chance of observing either 1/3 or 2/3 heads, there is a 25% chance of observing either 0/3 or 3/3 heads. The lesson for phase I trials is that basing decisions on the observed DLT outcomes of 3 patients is fraught with uncertainty. If the true DLT rate at a given dose level is 0.5, and we treat 3 patients at this level, there is a 25% probability that the observed DLT rate will be extreme (0/3 = 0% or 3/3 = 100%). Figure 6.6 shows the probability distribution for a 0.1 probability of heads. It shows that the probability of observing zero heads in 3 flips is 72.9%, probability of 1 head is 24.3%, the probability of 2 heads is 2.7% and the probability of 3 heads is 0.1%. So in the phase I setting, even though the true DLT rate is 0.1, there is a 27% chance that the observed DLT rate will be >0.1.

We can also think of the precision in our estimation of the DLT rate at the dose level selected as the MTD. If 1/6 = 17% patients develops DLT, the exact 95% confidence interval for this estimate ranges from 0% to 64%. However, if we treat 12 patients at the selected MTD and observe 2 patients with DLT, then 2/12 = 17% and the exact 95% confidence interval extends from 2% to 48% and if we treat 24 patients and observe 4 patients with DLT, then 4/24 = 17% with an exact 95% confidence interval extending from 5% to 37%. Clearly the estimate based on 24

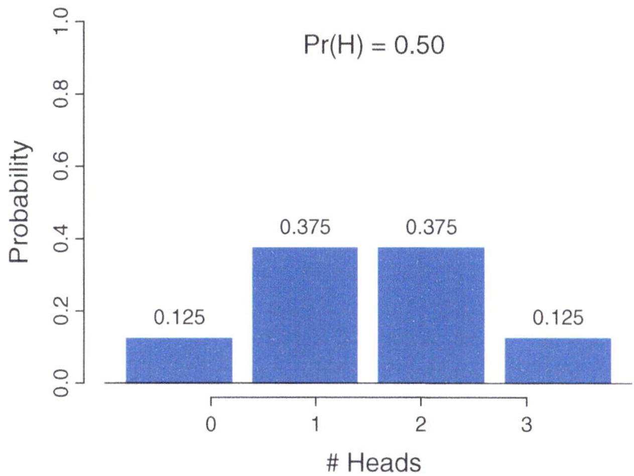

Fig. 6.5 Probability of 0–3 heads in 3 flips

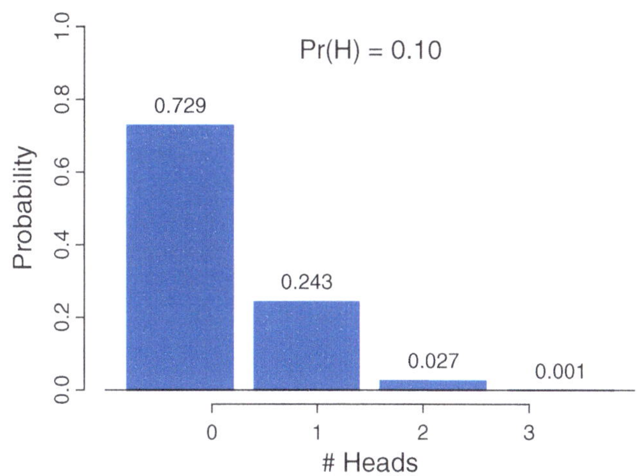

Fig. 6.6 Probability of 0-3 heads in 3 flips

patients has much more precision (i.e., less uncertainty). Knowing that the observed data at the presumed MTD are consistent with a range of DLT rates from 5% to 37% is much more informative than one that ranges from 0% to 64%.

6.5 Simulating Trial Conduct to Assess Design Performance

In order to assess the statistical properties of how a phase I dose-finding method performs, investigators design computer simulations. Given a number of dose levels, they specify a series of scenarios of true DLT rates at each dose level (i.e., dose-toxicity relationships). Given a cohort size (typically 3 patients), the idea is to generate random data to represent the number of patients experiencing DLTs given the cohort size and true DLT rate (e.g., 3 patients total with DLT rate = 0.5 might yield 2 patients with DLT). The computer uses a random number generator to randomly select a number representing the number of patients experiencing DLT given the cohort size and true DLT rate and assuming the results follow the binomial distribution. A computer program implementing the dose-finding method (e.g., 3+3 or BOIN) is used to determine for each set of generated data how the method would act in terms of escalating, de-escalating, or retaining the dose level. The simulation continues for a given trial until the MTD is found, the maximum number of allowable patients is treated at the highest dose level or, in the case of BOIN, the maximum total number of patients is reached. This process is repeated many, many times (typically 10,000) and the results averaged over these simulations.

Generally a wide range of scenarios is specified to "stress test" the design to show how it operates under a wide range of scenarios, including ones where the true DLT rates are very low for all dose levels (well below the targeted DLT rate); ones were the targeted DLT rate is associated with the lowest dose level; ones were the targeted DLT rate is associated with a middle dose level; ones were the targeted DLT rate is associated with the highest dose level; and ones were all dose levels have high true DLT rates (well above the targeted DLT rate).

Various performance metrics are reported as "operating characteristics" of a phase I design. These are the statistical properties of the design that demonstrate how it performs over a wide range of hypothetical dose-toxicity scenarios. These metrics include: the probability of selecting the dose level with DLT rate closest to the target as the MTD; the percentage of patients treated at the dose level with DLT rate closest to the target as the MTD; percentage of patients treated at dose levels with DLT rates well above the target; and the percentage of patients treated at dose levels with DLT rates well below the target.

6.5.1 Example Simulation

Table 6.2 shows results from a very limited simulation study of the 3+3 design with 3 dose levels with true DLT rates of 0.10, 0.25 (target), and 0.45. For each simulated cohort, random data are generated using the true DLT rates. In the first experiment, first cohort, 0 simulated patients experience DLT and the dose is escalated to level 2. In the second cohort of 3 patients now being treated at dose level 2, 1 patient develops DLT so 3 more patients are treated at this dose level. In the third cohort of 3 patients (2nd cohort at dose level 2), 1 patient develops DLT (for a total of 2/6 DLTs at dose level 2). Given the rules of 3+3 design this means that we conclude that dose level 2 exceeds the MTD and that dose level 1 is chosen as the MTD. For the 6 experiments (simulated trials) shown, dose level 1 is selected as the MTD 2 times (33%) while dose level 2 (with target DLT rate of 25%) is selected as the MTD 3 times (50%), dose level 3 is selected 0 times (0%), and no dose is selected 1 time (17%).

6.5.2 BOIN Versus 3+3 Comparison, Example Simulation

For the second experiment in Table 6.2 and Fig. 6.7 illustrates the results graphically for both 3+3 and BOIN. For 3+3 (Fig. 6.7, top), in the first cohort of 3 patients, 0 patients experience DLT and the dose is escalated to level 2. In the second cohort of 3 patients now being treated at dose level 2, 1 patient develops DLT so 3 more patients are treated at this dose level. In the third cohort of 3 patients (2nd cohort at dose level 2), 0 patients develops DLT (for a total of 1/6 DLTs at dose level 2). Given the rules of 3+3 design this means that we escalate to dose level 3. In the fourth cohort of 3 patients, 2 patients develop DLT and we conclude that dose level 3 exceeds the MTD and that dose level 2 is chosen as the MTD. The DLT rate at the selected MTD is 1/6 = 17% with 95% exact confidence interval from 0% to 64%.

For BOIN (Fig. 6.7, bottom), following the decision rules shown in Table 6.1, the path is the same as for 3+3 (for ease of comparison we are using the same random data for the first 4 cohorts). After cohort #4, Table 6.1 indicates we should de-escalate from dose level 3 to dose level 2. For cohort #5 (now the third cohort treated at dose level 2), 0 patients develop DLT and Table 6.1 indicates we should escalate back to dose level 3. For cohort #5, (now the second cohort treated at dose level 3), 2 patients develop DLT and Table 6.1 indicates we should de-escalate back to dose level 2 (and eliminate dose level 3 from future consideration). For cohort #6, (now the fourth cohort treated at dose level 2), 1 patient develops DLT and Table 6.1 indicates we should stay at dose level 2. For cohort #7 (now the fifth cohort treated at dose level 2), 2 patients experience DLT and Table 6.1 indicates we should remain at dose level 2. However, we have treated 15 patients at dose level 2 which is the maximum allowed. Dose level 2 is chosen as the MTD and the corresponding DLT

Table 6.2 Six simulated 3+3 trials with true DLT rates of 10%, 25%, 45%

EXP #	Results	MTD	# Pts
1	0/3, 1/3 +1/3	1	9
2	0/3, 1/3 + 0/3, 2/3	2	12
3	0/3, 3/3	1	6
4	2/3	Exceeded	3
5	1/3 + 0/3, 0/3, 2/3	2	12
6	0/3, 0/3, 1/3 + 2/3	2	12

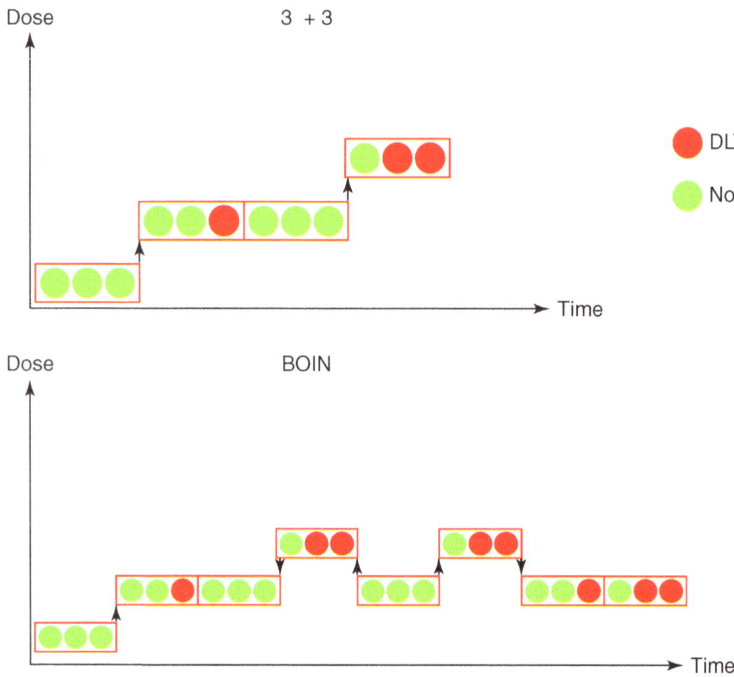

Fig. 6.7 Graphical illustration of phase I trial conduct

rate = 4/15 = 27% with exact 95% confidence interval from 8% to 55%. Thus, the BOIN estimate of the DLT rate at the MTD is both more accurate (i.e., closer to the target of 25%) and more precise (narrower confidence interval) than that from 3+3. Key differences between the 3+3 and BOIN designs are the ability of BOIN to visit a dose level multiple times, the ability of BOIN to treat more than 6 patients at a dose level and the ability of BOIN to repeatedly escalate and de-escalate across dose levels. By doing so, BOIN allows us to collect more information to learn the true DLT rate of a dose and adaptively corrects incorrect decisions possibly made at earlier stages of the trial caused by the random variation of small amounts of data described previously.

6.5.3 BOIN Versus 3+3 Comparison, Simulations

An increasingly common approach to computer simulations for phase I studies is to generate a large number of dose-toxicity scenarios using an algorithm that creates a wide range of scenarios such that the DLT probabilities are an non-decreasing function of dose level [1]. Based on 10,000 generated scenarios with 2000 trials simulated trials each, we can compare the performance of the 3+3 design and the BOIN design (assuming 6 dose levels, a DLT target of 25%, and a maximum sample size

Table 6.3 Comparison of simulation results for 3+3 and BOIN designs

	3+3	BOIN
Probability of correctly selecting MTD	33%	49%
Proportion of patients treated at MTD	26%	31%
Probability of selecting doses with DLT rate ≥ 33%	8%	12%
Proportion of patients treated at doses with DLT rate ≥ 33%	10%	14%
% of selecting doses with DLT rate ≤ 16%	40%	25%
% of patients treated at doses with DLT rate ≤ 16%	45%	42%

Note: These metrics are more completely defined in [1]

for 36 patients for BOIN, Table 6.3) using the data from simulations reported in Zhou et al. [1]. The probability of correctly selecting the target dose level (i.e., dose level with DLT rate closest to target) is 33% for 3+3 compared to 49% for BOIN. The proportion of patients treated at the target dose level is 26% for 3+3 and 31% for BOIN. The probability of selecting as the MTD doses with DLT rate ≤16% is 40% for 3+3 and 25% for BOIN. Thus, importantly, BOIN is more likely to correctly select the MTD (49% vs 33%) and less likely to select as the MTD doses with low DLT rates (25% vs 40%).

6.6 Expansion Cohorts

Increasingly, phase I studies include expansion cohorts to confirm safety and develop preliminary efficacy data for patients treated at the MTD. Multiple cohorts with different molecular defects or different histologies are sometimes specified. Expansion cohorts typically include 10–30 patients. The number of patients included is usually not given statistical justification but can be specified to achieve a given level of precision in estimation. E.g., to have 95% confidence interval with half-width not more than 0.2 for a targeted proportion of 0.3, requires at least 21 patients while targeting a 0.15 half-width would require at least 36 patients.

Because the toxicity data for patients treated at the MTD at the time the expansion phase begins is generally limited (often based on just 6 patients), it is prudent to monitor toxicity in the expansion phase. For the 3+3 design, we can add Bayesian monitoring rules [5] based on the beta distribution which stop enrollment if the probability of excessive toxicity exceeds some pre-specified threshold. Such rules are superior to deterministic rules such as stopping enrollment if DLT rate in the expansion cohort exceeds some threshold (e.g., 0.30) because their statistical properties can be calibrated by changing the threshold. Also, when excessive toxicity is observed in the expansion phase after 3+3, it is often not clear how to proceed. Since 6 is a very small sample, as more patients are treated at the MTD in an expansion cohort, the additional toxicity data may easily contradict the earlier conclusion that the selected dose is the MTD. For example, what should we do if the first three patients in an expansion cohort all have toxicity? Should we stop the trial according to Bayesian monitoring rule or de-escalate? If we de-escalate, what sort of rule or algorithm should be applied to choose a dose? On the other hand, if the toxicity rate in the cohort expansion is very low, should we escalate the dose? If so, what sort of rule or algorithm should be applied to choose a dose? The point is that the idea of treating a fixed expansion cohort at a chosen MTD may seem sensible, but in practice can be very problematic. BOIN does not have this issue as it allows dose escalation/de-escalation continuously in light of accruing data. With the BOIN design, the expansion toxicity can be monitored using an expanded decision table like the one used for dose escalation. This allows the dose level declared to be the MTD to be updated based on accruing toxicity data.

6.7 Conclusion/Discussion

The classical 3+3 design is simple in concept and implementation and transparent during trial conduct. However, this design suffers from poor statistical properties. The BOIN design is somewhat complicated in concept due to its statistical underpinnings but is easy to implement and has clearly superior statistical properties compared to the 3+3 design. The BOIN design is also considerably more flexible than the 3+3 design. The target DLT rate for the MTD can be set at any value. Extensions for the BOIN design have been developed for drug combination studies [6] and for phase I studies with prolonged observation periods [7]. Free software can be downloaded to develop BOIN designs and compute operating characteristics. A web-based version, a desktop version, and versions for R and Stata are available for download. The web-based and desktop versions also provide templates of text describing the design giving necessary parameters and tables of decision rules and operating characteristics. These templates can be inserted into appropriate sections in phase I protocols. The web links for the software are provided at the end of the chapter.

Key Expert Opinion Points

1. The 3+3 design in phase I oncology studies should be replaced by newer designs with better statistical properties
2. Phase I designs with better statistical properties have been available for decades but have not been widely used
3. This is partly related to the difficulty in creating and implementing model-based designs
4. Another difficulty is that the comparisons between designs are based on results of computer simulations which many clinical trialists find inaccessible
5. BOIN is easy to implement; very flexible; has superior statistical properties and is widely available as free software in several platforms.

Acknowledgements Authors would like to thank Ying Yuan, PhD for advice; Heng Zhou, PhD for assistance with computer simulations; Rachel Hess for assistance with graphics and editing;

and the clinical investigators in the Phase I program at MDACC for their continued collegial collaboration.

References

1. Zhou H, Yuan Y, Nie L. Accuracy, safety, and reliability of novel phase I trial designs. Clin Cancer Res. 2018;24:4357–64.
2. Zhou Y, Lee JJ, Yuan Y. A utility-based Bayesian optimal interval (U-BOIN) phase I/II design to identify the optimal biological dose for targeted and immune therapies. Statistics in Medicine. 2019;38(28):5299–316.
3. Yuan Y, Hess KR, Hilsenbeck SG, Gilbert MR. Bayesian optimal interval design: a simple and well-performing design for phase I oncology trials. Clin Cancer Res. 2016;22:4291–301.
4. Liu S, Yuan Y. Bayesian optimal interval designs for phase I clinical trials. Appl Stat. 2015;64:507–23.
5. Thall PF, Simon RM, Estey EH. Bayesian sequential monitoring designs for single-arm clinical trials with multiple outcomes. Stat Med. 1995;14:357–79.
6. Lin R, Yin G. Bayesian optimal interval designs for dose finding in drug-combination trials. Stat Methods Med Res. 2017;26:2155–67.
7. Yuan Y, Lin R, Li D, Nie L, Warren KE. Time-to-event Bayesian optimal interval design to accelerate phase I trials. Clin Cancer Res. 2018;24:4921–30.

Web Links

Web-based version: http://www.trialdesign.org/one-page-shell.html#BOIN
Desktop version: https://biostatistics.mdanderson.org/SoftwareDownload/SingleSoftware.aspx?Software_Id=99
R version: https://cran.r-project.org/web/packages/BOIN/index.html
Stata version: https://www.stata-journal.com/article.html?article=st0372

Chapter 7
Considerations for the Attribution and Management of Toxicities in Phase I Clinical Trials

Pedro C. Barata and David S. Hong

Abstract The process of describing the association of adverse events with investigational drugs in clinical research is known as symptom attribution. The focus of attribution varies and in early phases of drug development, the use of attribution data is predominantly used for safety assessment and ensure patient protection. The current symptom attribution process is often not easy and has a number of limitations and challenges. In this review, we review the current status of attribution in the context of early-phase studies, highlight some of the limitations and challenges, and expand on future directions and the number of actions that may improve the efficiency of the attribution process in clinical research. This review includes the discussions, challenges and recommendations from the consensus-building workshop on toxicity attribution (Silver Springs 2017) to develop guidance for improving attribution of adverse events in Oncology.

Keywords Symptom attribution · Early-phase studies · Adverse events · Phase I trials · Clinical research · Patient reported outcomes · Drug development

Key Points

- In the early stages of drug development, the focus of attribution is predominantly for safety assessment of the patients included in the phase I trials;
- Misattribution, insufficient baseline information, trial logistics and cost/time, lack of education and lack of communication are among the several challenges and inefficiencies of the attribution process;

P. C. Barata
Department of Internal Medicine, Section of Hematology and Oncology, Tulane University, New Orleans, LA, USA
e-mail: pbarata@tulane.edu

D. S. Hong (✉)
Department of Investigational Cancer Therapeutics, University of Texas MD Anderson Cancer Center, Houston, TX, USA
e-mail: dshong@mdanderson.org

T. A. Yap et al. (eds.), *Phase I Oncology Drug Development*,
https://doi.org/10.1007/978-3-030-47682-3_7

- Optimization of the attribution process may require the revision of the 5-tier system; the incorporation of baseline data that includes patient-reported outcomes, as well as long-term data on low-grade adverse events; and elimination of uninformed safety reports;
- There is an increase dialogue between from industry, academia and regulatory agencies, with an intent to achieve a better harmonization and synchronization of the attribution process in clinical trials.

7.1 Introduction

In clinical research, attribution is the determination of whether a clinical event is related to the investigational treatment under study, or non-treatment causes, such as the underlying disease, or comorbidities [1]. The term "attribution" is most likely to be used in the area of clinical trials, while it is also referred to as "relatedness to study treatment" in published reports [2] or as "causality" in certain regulatory contexts.

About three decades ago (1983), an uniform and objective tool to report treatment-related adverse events was developed and named Common Terminology Criteria for Adverse Events (CTCAE) [3]. A few years later, CTCAE started the process of AE collection and reporting based on a set of five nominal categories of attribution to study drug: "definite," "probable," "possible," "unlikely," and "unrelated" [4]. The CTCAE has since been updated several times as new therapies come available and the current CTCAE version 5, with new AE terms, has recently been published [5].

The focus of attribution differs during the different phases of drug development. In early-stage development, the use of attribution data is for safety assessment to ensure patient protection. Endpoints such as maximum tolerated dose (MTD) and dose-limiting toxicities (DLTs) are carefully defined and these data is then used to characterize the new drug's safety profile and to determine the adverse drug reactions [6, 7].

In later stages of development, the safety profile of an investigational drug is usually completed with key toxicities of special interest and less attention is paid to mild and expected adverse events.

From a regulatory perspective, premarket toxicity attribution is a requirement in ongoing clinical trials (concerned primarily with the safety of the participating patients and dose finding); and regulatory use of attribution data in the evaluation of new drugs and indications, i.e. New Drug Application (NDA), US Food and Drug Administration (FDA); Marketing Authorization Application (MAA), European Medicines Agency (EMA). Safety evaluation is a core component of the risk-benefit assessment.

There are different causality reporting requirements between the FDA and EMA, [8] with the most important distinction being that the FDA ultimately requires sponsors to make the causality determination for an AE, while according to EMA's ICH

E2A, AE causality is determined by either the investigator or the sponsor [8]. FDA requirements mandate that for serious adverse events (SAEs), attributions have to be made by the PI and the PI must report to the sponsor, regardless of attribution. The sponsor is required to expedite reporting of the SAE to the FDA if the SAE is serious, unexpected, suspected, regardless of attribution/causality. Either the investigator or the sponsor can make the determination that an AE is serious. However, in practice in the US, sponsors rarely change the causality assessment provided by the investigator. At the site, all SAEs have to be reported to the sponsor by the site investigator, regardless of whether the SAE is considered drug-related or not (21 CFR 312.64). Investigators must also include a causality assessment (21 CFR 312.64). All treatment-emergent AEs should be reported as per the clinical protocol. The site PI has ultimate responsibility for attributions at the site. There are periodic safety conference calls during trial among sponsor and site investigators to assess toxicity.

Regarding trials sponsored by NCI-CTEP, a source document called the Comprehensive Adverse Events and Potential Risks (CAEPR), is provided and serves as a guide to the investigator and is a way of determining what toxicities have been seen with a specific drug. CAEPR is a single source document containing reported and/or potential AEs associated with an agent. CAEPR utilizes CTCAE terminology and hierarchy. CTEP examines various items to develop a CAEPR, including the investigators brochure, any animal data, safety communications, and publications.

7.2 Current Status of Symptom Attribution: Challenges and Inefficiencies

Accurate attribution of toxicities to an experimental drug versus confounding factors, such as concomitant chemotherapy or patient comorbidities itself is not always clear. An event may be incorrectly attributed to other causes when it is related with the investigational drug (type A error) or may be attributed to the experimental therapy by the investigator when in fact it is related to other causes (type B) [2, 9]. Consequently, type A errors can result in more patients being exposed to potentially toxic levels of the investigational drug, with a negative impact on their quality of life and survival. On the other hand, type B errors lead to an early termination of clinical trials due to a predefined sub-therapeutic dosing for further investigation. These errors are known to significantly impact the MTD estimation, and consequently, accuracy, safety, sample size and/or duration. Furthermore, the magnitude of impact of these errors seems to be related with the trial design used, as data suggest that the standard "3+3" dose escalation schema is particular sensitive to type B errors [9, 10].

Misattribution also results in substantial implications to sponsors due to the underestimation of the MTD due to dose-limiting toxicities that are erroneously attributed. Downstream consequences of misattribution include not being able to demonstrate clinical benefit/appropriate efficacy signals in later studies, and inaccurate safety profiling of the study drug within the label. The end-result of misattribution is that the safety and treatment experience information that patients receive is not necessarily reflective of their experience.

Often, phase I studies allow enrollment of patients with various cancers with different biology and treatment strategies. Attribution of AEs is particularly challenging in patients with advanced disease who may have gone through multiple prior treatments (including chemotherapy, radiation, hormonal therapy, targeted agents, hospitalizations). They may often also be older adults with multiple comorbidities and concomitant medications [8].

Multiagent combinations of oncologic drugs are often times tested in early phase trials. Sometimes, two or more novel compounds are evaluated in combination with each other, and the safety profile for either of the novel drugs being tested in combination may not be available. Also, although some of the individual drugs being tested may not have direct drug-drug interactions, they may have functional interactions, and one has to decipher if these two different oncology compounds are augmenting, either synergistically or significantly additively with each other even in terms of AEs, making attributions in combination drug trials particularly challenging.

For compliance purposes, extensive amount of data on AEs are reported and collected, representing an extensive burden for researchers, research sites and the FDA [11, 12]. The process of reporting adverse events (AEs) in the regulatory process is acknowledged to be flawed and inefficient, producing much information that is of little benefit to the regulatory process and is ultimately uninformative [8]. A recent study revealed that FDA's office of Hematology and Oncology Products received on average 17,686 expedited safety reports each year between January 1, 2006 and December 31, 2014 [13]. An audit of 160 randomly selected expedited safety reports submitted to the FDA Office of Hematology and Oncology Products, revealed that only 14% of these reports were informative and met all three criteria for expedited IND safety reports of detailing serious, unexpected, and suspected adverse reactions [13]. These inefficiencies add to cost, time, and the involvement of investigators effort, perhaps limiting the number of agents that can advance through the clinical trial trajectory.

Several studies have documented that AEs collection represent one of the most burdensome steps during the clinical research process, as they often include useless information and represent a major consuming of the overall time and resources required for the conduct of a clinical trial [14–17]. In a retrospective analysis of 26 trials coordinated by the North-Central Cancer Treatment Cooperative Group, only 3% of CTCAE grade 3 or higher were noted; the majority of them had no significant impact on clinical practice [18]. In addition, 72% of data would be eliminated if only maximum severity per patient and per type were considered. In another study evaluating the relevance of collection of safety data for supplemental approval, none of the concomitant medication records contributed to labeling changes for supplemental indications [16].

Typically, clinical trials report the incidence of the AEs irrespective of the timing and frequency of adverse events. Baseline AEs collection is often insufficient or absent, as well as the low-grade but persistent, chronic AEs that may continue to affect patients after they discontinue study. In reality, the number of targeted therapies, small molecules and monoclonal antibodies evaluated in early-phase trials have been increasing, which are often associated with low-grade durable AEs, but only uncovered with longer follow up [19]. However, useful information about duration, frequency and timing of toxicities is usually not captured nor reported [20].

Once the AE data are collected, there seems to be a lack of optimal communication between the different players in drug development, including regulators, researchers, and sponsors/Contract Research Organizations (CROs). Often, the CRO requirements and what the FDA requires and what sites are audited for by auditors, are very different and inconsistent. The overall communication of AE data between sponsors and FDA continues to be suboptimal as sponsors still report serious adverse events independent of drug exposure, manifestations of the underlying disease, or that are study endpoints not related with the investigational drug. These generally uninformative reports drain resources for the FDA, researchers and institutional review boards, and divert them from other important activities [21].

On the other hand, investigators are not reporting high-quality or complete information in safety reports, and there is still lack of specific training on how to assign attribution [22]. Even though several guidelines integrating symptom management recommendations already exist [23, 24], compliance is not mandatory and is still suboptimal [25, 26]. In addition, educational programs in clinical research do not prepare attendees on how to properly report serious AEs in an accurate manner.

In fact, selective reporting of clinical trial results is a well-documented issue. Positive studies are more likely to be published than those with non-significant or negative results, and AEs are reported inconsistently in a significant proportion of the trials. In addition, publications usually report fewer serious AEs compared with the public database ClinicalTrials.gov [27, 28]. Reasons for this suboptimal level of AE reporting include the use of studies with poor capture of toxicities, space restriction imposed by medical journals and intentional concealing of unfavorable data [29, 30]. Moreover, results from individual trials are now being reported in multiple forms, including regulatory documents, clinical study reports (CSRs), registries, publications, scientific meetings and presentations, as well as patient level data portals, and other databases [20]. Table 7.1 summarizes the current opportunities for the optimization of the symptom attribution process in clinical trials.

Table 7.1 Challenges and inefficiencies with symptom attribution

Misattribution due to confounding factors (prior therapies, comorbidities, multiagent studies)
Insufficient baseline information
Trial logistics, cost and time
Lack of education on attribution
Lack of communication between regulators, investigators and sponsors
Inconsistent publication of safety reports

7.3 Next Steps for Optimization of Attribution Assessment and Efficiency

The optimization of the attribution process is a priority in the drug development process and a number of meetings have been promoted between the different players, including the FDA, academic institutions and pharmaceutical companies [31, 32]. In fact, there is a published white paper summarizing the consensus-building workshop held on toxicity attribution (Silver Springs 2017) to develop guidance for improving attribution of adverse events [33]. Interestingly, among these different meetings, there are similar actions suggested to improve the efficiency of the attribution process. One possibility would be to reduce the current 5-tier system by eliminating the "possible" and "probably related" categories that are often difficult to interpret [6]. Two- and 3-tier systems have been proposed, as well as arguments in favor of both; this change could alleviate burden and is more concordant to investigator assessments on a daily basis [6]. Sample wording for the 2-tier system is: "more likely related to study drug (than other causes)" vs. "more likely related to other causes (than study drug)". Sample wording for the 3-tier system is "more likely related to study drug," "equally likely related to study drug and other causes," or "more likely related to other causes".

Regardless of whether a 3- or 2-tiered system is recommended, clear communication based on investigators current knowledge to convey a probability assessment rather than the ultimate "true" attribution is needed. This could increase the quality of attribution by reducing the proportion of attributions to the drug that are made just in order to be on the "safe side".

As mentioned before, baseline scores and pretrial data are extremely important because they help in attribution by providing an individual control thus, helping to establish if a patient's symptom is worsening or improving. This baseline data could also include patient-reported outcomes (PROs), as well as objective information such as laboratory levels, comorbidities and current medications. Although symptom attribution is the responsibility of the investigators, the inclusion of PROs especially for symptomatic toxicities best reported by the patients (such as pain, fatigue, nausea or neuropathy) could be extremely helpful [31, 34].

By the same token, long-term data, including low-grade AEs, are very important to be captured from patients who had previous cancer treatments as they inform the researchers about potential chronic toxicity complications. The example of radiation therapy trials where long-term AEs were assessed [35, 36] may be generalized and used in other clinical studies investigating new therapies.

PROs are a systematic capture of the patient perspective and are increasingly being included in cancer clinical trials [37]. There is a broad number of different instruments to collect health-related quality of life, but they were largely developed in an older therapeutics area, are static instruments, and have different measures to include the same questions irrespective of disease stage or current therapy. This is particularly true in the era of targeted therapies.

As a consequence of a renewed effort to incorporate valuable information from patients, the FDA's Office of Hematology and Oncology Products has developed the systemic assessment of symptomatic adverse events reported by patients as a way to objectively describe the safety and tolerance of an investigational drug [34, 38, 39]. The National Cancer Institute's PRO version of the CTCAE (PRO-CTCAE) was subsequently created and provides a standard but flexible method to assess symptomatic AEs from the perspective of patients, and complement safety and tolerability data across clinical trials [40, 41]. As patient experience is being incorporated more often in clinical studies, standardizing this process will foster systemic and consistent data collection as part of drug development and improve our knowledge about how to integrate patient's data as part of a treatment risk/benefit assessment [42].

On the other hand, it is frequently not possible to attribute a specific AE to an individual drug when testing a combination regimen in phase I studies. Thus, attribution in combinatorial studies should be focused on the combination regimen rather than to individual drugs, alleviating the unnecessary burden to investigators.

In order to improve the quality of safety reporting, the FDA published the 2010 Final Rule elucidating the requirements for expedited IND safety reporting [43, 44]. These guidelines were intended to reduce the number of uninformative reports generated by trial sponsors, so as to ease the detection of true safety signals and improve the overall quality of safety data. However, extensive data have shown problems and limitations in the current attribution process and the extent of the toxicity burden is unknown [1, 7, 11, 45]. For investigators already involved in clinical research, their engagement on teleconference call meetings with sponsors is highly recommended as expertise is cumulative over clinical trials. In addition, a minimum requirement to join safety calls may be employed, as this may have major implications for the attribution process and MTD definition. There must also be attention paid to developing better content to provide training in attribution (for example, using case-studies from prior trials to train on AE attribution).

With the change in the goals and conduct of early-phase trials including the increasing use of seamless designs, there has been a shift towards multi-institutional studies and centralized study management by CROs instead of research centers. To adapt to this shift, junior faculty, fellows and trainees may need additional training in all aspects of drug development and also more years of experience to become truly independent with opportunities to advance their academic careers [46]. Similarly, continuous efforts to improving communication between multi-center studies should be made, to better interpret AEs in the context of clinically-relevant information and greater understanding the available non-clinical data [47]. Recognizing the instrumental value that experienced researchers offer to early-phase studies, the quality and experience of a clinical research center and their investigators shall continue to be the major selection criteria, rather than their ability to enroll patients in trials.

Finally, there has been a crescent number of meetings and discussions between the different players from industry, academia and regulatory agencies, intended to achieve a better harmonization and synchronization of attribution [8]. This communication is key to improving consistency and compliance, and common recommendations may be the results of those discussions.

Key Expert Opinion Points

1. In the early phases of drug development, symptom attribution focuses mainly on patient's safety and impact important endpoints that include the maximum tolerated dose and dose-limiting toxicities, defining the investigational drug safety profile.
2. The current symptom attribution process is not simple or straight forward. Inaccuracies are frequent given the number of possible confounding factors. While a significant amount of resources and time is spent on data collection and trial logistics, there are inefficiencies associated with uninformative data collection, misattribution and lack of effective communication.
3. Optimizing the symptom attribution process is considered a priority among the different players in the drug development process. The number of meetings to discuss opportunities to discuss this topic and to enhance the overall efficiency and quality of symptom attribution has increased in last few years. Communication improvement, collection of baseline and long term data, Patient-Reported Outcomes while minimizing collection of non-informative reports are some of are some of the right steps being taken in that direction.

References

1. Cleeland CS, Allen JD, Roberts SA, et al. Reducing the toxicity of cancer therapy: recognizing needs, taking action. Nat Rev Clin Oncol. 2012;9(8):471–8.
2. Le-Rademacher J, Hillman SL, Meyers J, Loprinzi CL, Limburg PJ, Mandrekar SJ. Statistical controversies in clinical research: value of adverse events relatedness to study treatment: analyses of data from randomized double-blind placebo-controlled clinical trials. Ann Oncol. 2017;28(6):1183–90.
3. Trotti A, Colevas AD, Setser A, et al. CTCAE v3.0: development of a comprehensive grading system for the adverse effects of cancer treatment. Semin Radiat Oncol. 2003;13(3):176–81.
4. Committee IS. ICH harmonised tripartite guideline. Clinical safety data management: definitions and standards for expedited reporting E2A. Step 4 version. Paper presented at International Conference on Harmonisation of Technical Requirements for Registration of Pharmaceuticals for Human Use; 1994.
5. Institute NC. Common terminology criteria for adverse events (CTCAE). 2018.; www.ctep.cancer.gov. Accessed February 2018.
6. Eaton A, Iasonos A, Gounder MM, et al. Toxicity attribution in phase I trials: evaluating the effect of dose on the frequency of related and unrelated toxicities. Clin Cancer Res. 2016;22(3):553–9.
7. Sharma MR, Ratain MJ. Taking a measured approach to toxicity data in phase I oncology clinical trials. Clin Cancer Res. 2016;22(3):527–9.
8. Levit LA, Perez RP, Smith DC, Schilsky RL, Hayes DF, Vose JM. Streamlining adverse events reporting in oncology: an American Society of Clinical Oncology research statement. J Clin Oncol. 2018;36(6):617–23.

9. Iasonos A, Gounder M, Spriggs DR, et al. The impact of non-drug-related toxicities on the estimation of the maximum tolerated dose in phase I trials. Clin Cancer Res. 2012;18(19):5179–87.
10. Zohar S, O'Quigley J. Sensitivity of dose-finding studies to observation errors. Contemp Clin Trials. 2009;30(6):523–30.
11. Perez R, Archdeacon P, Roach N, et al. Sponsors' and investigative staffs' perceptions of the current investigational new drug safety reporting process in oncology trials. Clin Trials. 2017;14(3):225–33.
12. U.S. Department of Health and Human Services, Food and Drug Administration. Guidance for industry and investigators safety reporting requirements for INDs and BA/BE Studies; 2010.
13. Jarow JP, Casak S, Chuk M, Ehrlich LA, Khozin S. The majority of expedited investigational new drug safety reports are uninformative. Clin Cancer Res. 2016;22(9):2111–3.
14. Steensma DP, Kantarjian HM. Impact of cancer research bureaucracy on innovation, costs, and patient care. J Clin Oncol. 2014;32(5):376–8.
15. Sargent DJ, George SL. Clinical trials data collection: when less is more. J Clin Oncol. 2010;28(34):5019–21.
16. Kaiser LD, Melemed AS, Preston AJ, et al. Optimizing collection of adverse event data in cancer clinical trials supporting supplemental indications. J Clin Oncol. 2010;28(34):5046–53.
17. Roche K, Paul N, Smuck B, et al. Factors affecting workload of cancer clinical trials: results of a multicenter study of the National Cancer Institute of Canada Clinical Trials Group. J Clin Oncol. 2002;20(2):545–56.
18. Mahoney MR, Sargent DJ, O'Connell MJ, Goldberg RM, Schaefer P, Buckner JC. Dealing with a deluge of data: an assessment of adverse event data on North Central Cancer Treatment Group trials. J Clin Oncol. 2005;23(36):9275–81.
19. Drye LT, Casper AS, Sternberg AL, Holbrook JT, Jenkins G, Meinert CL. The transitioning from trials to extended follow-up studies. Clin Trials (London, Engl). 2014;11(6):635–47.
20. Lineberry N, Berlin JA, Mansi B, et al. Recommendations to improve adverse event reporting in clinical trial publications: a joint pharmaceutical industry/journal editor perspective. BMJ. 2016;355 https://doi.org/10.1136/bmj.i5078.
21. Food and Drug Administration. Best practices for communication between IND Sponsors and FDA during drug development guidance for industry and review staff 2018; www.fda.gov/. Accessed February 2018.
22. Crepin S, Villeneuve C, Merle L. Quality of serious adverse events reporting to academic sponsors of clinical trials: far from optimal. Pharmacoepidemiol Drug Saf. 2016;25(6):719–24.
23. Albizu-Rivera A, Portman DG, Thirlwell S, Codada SN, Donovan KA. Implementation of NCCN palliative care guidelines by member institutions. Support Care Cancer. 2016;24(2):929–32.
24. Dillmon M, Goldberg JM, Ramalingam SS, Mayer RJ, Loehrer P, Van Poznak C. Clinical practice guidelines for cancer care: utilization and expectations of the practicing oncologist. J Oncol Pract. 2012;8(6):350–3. 352 p following 353.
25. Hakonsen GD, Strelec P, Campbell D, Hudson S, Loennechen T. Adherence to medication guideline criteria in cancer pain management. J Pain Symptom Manag. 2009;37(6):1006–18.
26. Mahe I, Puget H, Buzzi JC, et al. Adherence to treatment guidelines for cancer-associated thrombosis: a French hospital-based cohort study. Support Care Cancer. 2016;24(8):3369–77.
27. Hartung D, Zarin DA, Guise J-M, McDonagh M, Paynter R, Helfand M. Reporting discrepancies between the ClinicalTrials.gov results database and peer reviewed publications. Ann Intern Med. 2014;160(7):477–83.
28. Song F, Parekh S, Hooper L, et al. Dissemination and publication of research findings: an updated review of related biases. Health Technol Assess. 2010;14(8):iii, ix–xi, 1–193.
29. Pitrou I, Boutron I, Ahmad N, Ravaud P. Reporting of safety results in published reports of randomized controlled trials. Arch Intern Med. 2009;169(19):1756–61.
30. Ioannidis JP. Adverse events in randomized trials: neglected, restricted, distorted, and silenced. Arch Intern Med. 2009;169(19):1737–9.

31. Cleeland CS, Sloan JA, Cella D, et al. Recommendations for including multiple symptoms as endpoints in cancer clinical trials: a report from the ASCPRO (Assessing the symptoms of cancer using patient-reported outcomes) multisymptom task force. Cancer. 2013;119(2):411–20.
32. Barsevick AM, Cleeland CS, Manning DC, et al. ASCPRO recommendations for the assessment of fatigue as an outcome in clinical trials. J Pain Symptom Manag. 2010;39(6):1086–99.
33. George GC, Barata PC, Campbell A, et al. Improving attribution of adverse events in oncology clinical trials. Cancer Treat Rev. 2019;76:33–40. https://doi.org/10.1016/j.ctrv.2019.04.004.
34. Dueck AC, Mendoza TR, Mitchell SA, et al. Validity and reliability of the US National Cancer Institute's patient-reported outcomes version of the common terminology criteria for adverse events (PRO-CTCAE). JAMA Oncol. 2015;1(8):1051–9.
35. Whelan TJ, Pignol J-P, Levine MN, et al. Long-term results of hypofractionated radiation therapy for breast cancer. N Engl J Med. 2010;362(6):513–20.
36. Ducassou A, Gambart M, Munzer C, et al. Long-term side effects of radiotherapy for pediatric localized neuroblastoma: results from clinical trials NB90 and NB94. Strahlenther Onkol. 2015;191(7):604–12.
37. Kluetz PG, Chingos DT, Basch EM, Mitchell SA. Patient-reported outcomes in cancer clinical trials: measuring symptomatic adverse events with the National Cancer Institute's patient-reported outcomes version of the common terminology criteria for adverse events (PRO-CTCAE). Am Soc Clin Oncol Educ Book. 2016;35:67–73.
38. Trask PC, Dueck AC, Piault E, Campbell A. Patient-reported outcomes version of the common terminology criteria for adverse events: methods for item selection in industry-sponsored oncology clinical trials. Clin Trials. 2018; https://doi.org/10.1177/1740774518799985.
39. Hay JL, Atkinson TM, Reeve BB, et al. Cognitive interviewing of the US National Cancer Institute's patient-reported outcomes version of the common terminology criteria for adverse events (PRO-CTCAE). Qual Life Res. 2014;23(1):257–69.
40. Basch E, Pugh SL, Dueck AC, et al. Feasibility of patient reporting of symptomatic adverse events via the patient-reported outcomes version of the common terminology criteria for adverse events (PRO-CTCAE) in a Chemoradiotherapy Cooperative Group Multicenter Clinical Trial. Int J Radiat Oncol Biol Phys. 2017;98(2):409–18.
41. Kim J, Singh H, Ayalew K, et al. Use of PRO measures to inform tolerability in oncology trials: implications for clinical review, IND safety reporting, and clinical site inspections. Clin Cancer Res. 2018;24(8):1780–4.
42. Kluetz PG, O'Connor DJ, Soltys K. Incorporating the patient experience into regulatory decision making in the USA, Europe, and Canada. Lancet Oncol. 2018;19(5):e267–74.
43. Food Drug Administration. Investigational new drug safety reporting requirements for human drug and biological products and safety reporting requirements for bioavailability and bioequivalence studies in humans. Final rule. Federal Reg. 2010;75(188):59935.
44. Behrman Sherman R, Woodcock J, Norden J, Grandinetti C, Temple RJ. New FDA regulation to improve safety reporting in clinical trials. N Engl J Med. 2011;365(1):3–5.
45. Shimizu T, Saijo N. Common toxicity criteria: version 2.0, an improved reference for grading the adverse reaction of cancer treatment. Nihon Rinsho. 2003;61(6):937–42.
46. Wong KM, Capasso A, Eckhardt SG. The changing landscape of phase I trials in oncology. Nat Rev Clin Oncol. 2016;13(2):106–17.
47. Pietanza MC, Basch EM, Lash A, et al. Harnessing technology to improve clinical trials: study of real-time informatics to collect data, toxicities, image response assessments, and patient-reported outcomes in a phase II clinical trial. J Clin Oncol. 2013;31(16):2004–9.

Chapter 8
Strategies for Incorporating Pharmacokinetic Studies into Oncology Phase I Trials

Lingzhi Wang, Wan Qin Chong, Pei Shi Ong, and Boon Cher Goh

Abstract The ultimate goal of therapeutics is to ensure that the appropriate treatment is administered to the individual patient at the most appropriate dose for optimal effects. In drug development, clinical trials are conducted in 3 broad phases (Phase I, II and III) before registration for a new drug is granted. In Phase I clinical trials, the primary objectives are to define safety and tolerability of a new treatment and to establish the recommended dose/s for efficacy studies. Clinical pharmacokinetics (PK) is an invaluable tool that can help with achieving this goal, when applied early and throughout the clinical drug development phases. In this chapter, the following topics will be covered:

1. Selected PK concepts specific to clinical drug development of oncology drugs.
2. Practical issues in designing PK studies in Phase I trials.
3. Application of PK in specific situations and drug interactions.

L. Wang (✉)
Cancer Science Institute of Singapore, Singapore, Singapore

Department of Pharmacology, Yong Loo Lin School of Medicine, Singapore, Singapore
e-mail: csiwl@nus.edu.sg

W. Q. Chong
Department of Haematology-Oncology, National University Hospital, Singapore, Singapore
e-mail: wan_qin_chong@nuhs.edu.sg

P. S. Ong
Faculty of Science, Department of Pharmacy, National University of Singapore, Singapore, Singapore
e-mail: phcops@nus.edu.sg

B. C. Goh
Cancer Science Institute of Singapore, Singapore, Singapore

Department of Pharmacology, Yong Loo Lin School of Medicine, Singapore, Singapore

Department of Haematology-Oncology, National University Hospital, Singapore, Singapore
e-mail: phcgbc@nus.edu.sg

T. A. Yap et al. (eds.), *Phase I Oncology Drug Development*,
https://doi.org/10.1007/978-3-030-47682-3_8

Keywords Pharmacokinetic studies · Oncology drugs · Phase 1 trials · Special populations

Key Points

- Pharmacokinetic analysis is a valuable tool to understand and guide early development of investigational new drugs
- The design and conduct of PK studies requires careful thought and planning
- Drugs have considerable propensity for PK issues in real world use, and in such situations, understanding the influence of drugs, food, pharmacogenetics, renal or liver function on PK of a new drug is essential to prepare for its eventual use in the clinic.

8.1 Selected PK Concepts Specific to Clinical Drug Development of Oncology Drugs

8.1.1 Introduction to Pharmacokinetic Concepts

PK refers to the study of the time course of drug absorption, distribution, metabolism and excretion after drug administration. It essentially refers to what the body does to the drug. Pharmacodynamics (PD) on the other hand, is the study of the effects of a drug on the body. It essentially means what the drug does to the body which encompasses both on target and off-target effects. Both PK and PD are important disciplines within clinical pharmacology, where the basic premise is that free drug concentration at the target tissue of action will determine the magnitude and the duration of drug response. This is in turn manifested clinically as observed effects or measurable effects, which include the intended therapeutic effects of the drug and its off-target adverse effects. Unlike drug exposure at fixed concentrations in cell line models, in patients, systemic drug concentrations vary as they undergo processes of absorption (A), distribution (D), metabolism (M) and excretion (E), which are processes that determine the clinical PK of a drug.

In oncology, orally administered small molecule chemotherapeutic agents will be subjected to absorption processes including dissolution, ionisation, active transport and gastric emptying. This is followed by drug metabolism at the intestinal lining and liver before reaching the systemic circulation. For these drugs, a high hepatic drug metabolism prior to reaching the systemic circulation, also known as high first pass effect, will in turn reduce their respective bioavailabilities in the systemic circulation. In general, drugs that are well absorbed and have low hepatic first pass will give rise to higher plasma concentrations or have higher bioavailabilities following oral consumption compared to those that are poorly absorbed or have high hepatic first pass effect. Regardless, there is always a lag time between drug administration and the appearance of the drug in the blood for an orally administrated drug due to the absorption and first pass metabolic processes. In repeated administration, accumulation occurs when the drug is administered before the previous dose is completely eliminated. The amount of drug in the body will then progressively rise to reach a plateau due to saturation of membrane transporters. On the contrary, high hepatic drug metabolism prior to reaching the systemic circulation, also known as the high first pass effect, contributes to the reduced bioavailability of orally administrated chemotherapeutic drugs.

Within the plasma, a small amount of administered drug remains as free molecules while majority are bound to plasma proteins especially for more lipophilic drugs. In the end, both bound and unbound drugs are carried to various parts of the body via the circulatory system. Those that are lipophilic are partitioned largely into fat tissues, resulting in large apparent volumes of distribution. At the tumor site, free drug molecules are transported into tumor cells where they exert their PD effects. Unbound free drug molecules that are water soluble may either be filtered in the renal glomeruli and excreted, or secreted at the renal tubules while those that are more lipophilic are metabolised, largely in the liver. Within the liver, phase 1 enzymes metabolise these drugs through the processes of oxidation, reduction or carboxylation, while phase 2 enzymes conjugate a moiety to make the phase 1 metabolites more water soluble for subsequent drug elimination. It has been observed that some metabolites retain PD activity, albeit at a different potency to the parent molecule. Due to these ADME processes, plasma concentrations of drugs at any point after administration is thus the summation of processes of absorption and distribution, metabolism and elimination from the body.

8.1.1.1 Interindividual Variability

In a given population, it has been observed that different individuals when given the same dose of drug exhibit different drug effects. This is attributed to differences in the PK processes between them that in turn result in different PK parameters such as drug clearance (CL), half-life ($t_{1/2}$), area under the concentration-time curve (AUC). This interindividual variability in PK results in higher exposure in some individuals, and lower exposure in others and hence the differences in drug effects among different members of a population. For oncology drugs, this poses as a significant challenge for precision dosing to achieve consistency in drug effects in different patients. This is because the therapeutic window, which is the range of drug concentrations required to achieve the intended therapeutic effect without unacceptable toxicity is narrow for most chemotherapeutic agents. In other words, the desired target concentrations are close to that associated with toxic effects. Fortunately, these adverse events are most frequently due to PD effects exerted by the drug binding to its other targets and are dose dependent, rather than due to unpredictable, idiosyncratic effects. Nonetheless, the high interindividual variability in drug response can act as a significant conundrum to development of chemotherapeutic drugs in the clinic as they are often dosed at close to the highest clinically tolerable dose in the hope of getting optimal benefit.

8.1.1.2 Plasma Protein Binding

Another crucial factor potentially affecting the effect of an anticancer drug is its protein binding capacity which is variable between different anticancer drugs. Plasma proteins that can bind chemotherapeutic agents include albumin, alpha-1-acid glycoprotein (α_1AGp), globulins and lipoprotein. α1AGp is a crucial plasma protein involved in the binding and transport of many drugs, especially basic compounds. This also applies to chemotherapeutic agents whereby for example, docetaxel is 98% bound to α_1AGp, leading to potential risk for those with lower protein binding [1–3]. This protein binding process is reversible and the free drug fraction is relatively constant for a given drug in a given patient. This is an important parameter for some oncology drugs with extremely high protein binding as it could result in a big difference in free drug (unbound fraction) concentration since it is this form of the drug that is active and can cross the membrane to reach targeted sites. Hence, there has been increasing interest in the measurement of plasma free drug, and the most commonly used approaches for determination of plasma free drug concentration include ultrafiltration and equilibrium dialysis before actual drug concentration analysis. For the former, the drug containing plasma samples are filtered through a very small pore size membrane filter by centrifugation at 37 °C. The unbound fraction may be calculated as the ratio of the free drug concentration in the filtrate over the total drug concentration in the plasma. For the latter, free drug is separated from the bound drug in the plasma by utilizing a dialysis chamber divided by a semipermeable membrane which allows the transfer of the free drug but not the drug bound to proteins.

8.1.1.3 Clearance, Volume of Distribution and Half-Life

Clearance (CL), a commonly used parameter in clinical PK, links the rate of elimination with plasma concentration of a drug. It is defined as the volume of plasma that is completely cleared of the drug in a unit of time. As most drugs are mainly cleared from liver or renal routes, the summation of CL via all these routes of CL is therefore the total CL of the drug. For an intravenously administered drug, the CL derived reflects the whole administered dose assuming full bioavailability via this route of administration. For orally administered agents, the parameter derived is called apparent oral CL (CL/F), which takes into account the reduced bioavailability of the drug due to drug absorption efficiency and first pass elimination. This parameter is calculated from an oral PK experiment by dividing the actual dose administered by the AUC attributable to the dose given. An understanding of the factors of interindividual variability of a drug such as body size estimates, liver function, renal function, can be obtained by studying their effects on drug clearance. In drugs administered continuously, at steady state, rate of elimination will be balanced by the rate of dosing. Since CL relates the drug concentration to rate of elimination, CL will determine the maintenance dose to be administered to maintain therapeutic concentration. This parameter is in turn related to drug exposure and dose. Since drug exposure is related to its PD effect, the effect of a drug can thus be adjusted by changing the administered dose. Depending on the main routes of CL of drugs, careful selection of agents is prudent in patients with impairment of either liver or renal function (see below, special populations).

Volume of distribution (Vd) of a drug is the apparent volume of fluid into which a drug distributes on the basis of the amount of drug in the body and the measured concentration in the plasma or serum. Since the drug is not equally distributed to all parts of the body, Vd does not represent a real volume, such that it is often known as the apparent Vd. Vd may be affected by many factors, such as physicochemical property of the drug, tissue characteristics, protein binding and co-administered drugs, etc. Hence, the Vd of a drug affects the difference between peak and trough concentrations at steady state or maximum concentrations for single intravenous bolus dosing. The Vd can be used to determine the loading dose needed to achieve a certain concentration.

Half-life ($t_{1/2}$) is the time required for the concentration or amount of drug in the body to be reduced by one-half when a drug follows linear PK (dose and concentration independent PK, also called first-order kinetics). In fact, $t_{1/2}$ which can be calculated using CL and Vd and is a hybrid parameter that takes into account drug CL as well as its Vd. Although CL can be easily related to the elimination capacity of a specific organ such as the liver and kidney, it is not easy to have a precise judgement on how fast a drug is removed from the body based on CL. The elimination $t_{1/2}$ is better suited for this because after 5 half-lives, approximately 97% of the drug has been eliminated from the body. Hence, understanding $t_{1/2}$ is particularly important when determining dosing intervals for chronically-administered drugs, such as various kinase inhibitors, as dosing adjustments may impact a drug's systemic exposure and changes in plasma concentrations.

8.1.1.4 Dose-Proportionality

In drug development, it is essential to determine if the disposition of a new drug is linear (dose-proportional) or nonlinear. Linear PK is also known as dose-independent and concentration-independent PK because the PK parameters ($t_{1/2}$, CL, Vd) are constant and do not change with a change in drug dose. These drugs are said to have first-order kinetics. Examples of drugs that follow linear kinetics include most small molecule drugs and chemotherapeutic agents whereby drug metabolism is the main pathway of drug disposition. In addition, for these drugs, the change in drug dose results in a proportional alteration in the drug concentrations in both the systemic circulation and tumor tissue. Owning to the difficulty in direct measurement of drug concentration in tumor tissues, plasma drug concentration is thus used as a surrogate marker for tumor drug concentration in studies investigating dose proportionality and PK of investigational oncology drugs assuming kinetic homogeneity.

Conversely, drugs with nonlinear PK exhibit distinct PK properties at different plasma concentrations. Nonlinear PK is also known as dose-dependent or concentration-dependent PK whereby one or more ADME PK processes parameters (such as $t_{1/2}$, CL, Vd) are dose-dependent. They do not follow first-order kinetics whereby doubling of drug dose will result in doubling of plasma drug concentration. Rather, an increase in dose will result in a disproportional increase in plasma concentration. These drugs are therefore more difficult to use in clinics especially when the drug therapeutic window is narrow. Examples of oncology drugs with non-linear PK include high dose methothrexate and monoclonal antibodies widely used recently in the treatment of cancer. The latter are not typically metabolised.

In general, based on FDA guidelines, a drug in development does not need to be dose proportional or exhibit first-order kinetics. However, dose proportionality of investigational new drugs—where an increase in the administered dose is accompanied by a proportional increase in a measure of drug exposure, such as AUC or maximum plasma drug concentration (Cmax)—will greatly help clinicians have better control over their safety and toxicity when used clinically. Of note, it should be highlighted that the use of different formulations of the same drug can also impact its dose proportionality. For instance, the PK of cremophor-formulated paclitaxel is non-linear following short (<6 h) infusions, whereas that of long (24 h) infusions is linear [4]. Reformulating paclitaxel as Abraxane, where paclitaxel is available as an albumin-bound nanoparticle also results in dose-proportionality in patients.

A few approaches are available for the evaluation of dose proportionality. The most commonly used method is known as the power model approach (physiologie.envt.fr/wp.../04/Dose_linearity_and_dose_proportionality.ppt). In this model, an empirical relationship between AUC and dose is established based on the following equation:

$$Ln(AUC) = a + \beta Ln(Dose) + \epsilon \tag{8.1}$$

Here, β also known as the slope, is a measure of the proportionality between Dose and AUC. If $\beta = 0$, it implies that the response is independent from the dose. If beta = 1, dose proportionality can be declared. Investigational new drugs that are dose proportional are therefore attractive candidates for further development as precision dosing to ensure that the right drug dose is given to individual patients to maximize therapeutic benefit and minimise risk.

8.2 Practical Issues in Designing PK Studies for Phase I Trials

8.2.1 Pharmacokinetics, Bioanalytical Method Development and Validation in Phase I Clinical Trials

A Phase I trial involves the initial introduction of an investigational new drug into humans. These studies are typically closely monitored and are designed in cohorts of patients with gradual escalation of doses. The purpose of such a study design is to minimise potential exposure to serious toxicity and yet maximise the chances of antitumor response. Patients are started at a safe starting dose according to preclinical animal studies and each dosing cohort is kept small during the dose escalation phase according to a dose escalation schema that is typically either model-based or algorithm-based. From these studies, the metabolism and pharmacologic actions of the drug in humans and side effects associated with increasing drug doses are evaluated. Such studies may also provide early evidence on the antitumor activity of the investigational new drugs.

Importantly, sufficient information about the drug's PK property and PD effects should be obtained during these studies. This is because the early assessment of PK parameters at initial doses of a first-in-human study would be highly informative about the estimation of bioavailability, and the AUC compared with the intended target AUC in animal models. This in turn provides an estimation of the dose ranges that would achieve target modulation, assuming PK linearity. Conversely, the investigation of PD effects of the drug will provide information on target and pathway inhibition. This is particularly relevant to targeted drug therapy in oncology whereby the PD biomarkers will act as surrogates of target engagement. More importantly, such PD biomarker endpoints should be interpreted in the light of PK results of the drug to provide a more thorough understanding of its mechanism of action in relation to systemic drug levels. From all this gathered information, the investigator should also be able to determine if the dosing regimen is appropriate, and to assess the relevance of active metabolites to the PD effects of the drug. Such PK and PD data accumulated during the early phases of clinical drug development, when iteratively integrated into population PK and PD models, will also provide valuable insights into patient variables that influence drug effect. It in turn aids in choosing doses and dose intervals for subsequent Phase II studies (FDA Good Review Practice: Clinical Review of Investigational New Drug Applications).

In first in human (FIH) studies of oncology drugs, the key objectives are to investigate the safety, tolerability, PK and PD of these drugs in humans. Importantly, PK data from FIH phase I trials of these new investigational drugs in oncology are essential for the following: (i) to discern whether a given dose and schedule provides a potentially effective level of systemic exposure to the drug by comparison with biologically relevant concentrations or exposure that inhibits the target, (ii) to monitor the magnitude of intra-patient and inter-patient variability which is critical in understanding interindividual PK/PD variability, (iii) to assess whether changes in drug disposition or metabolism are related to the development of toxicity or the lack of efficacy, and (iv) to predict or monitor drug-drug interactions, with the ultimate goal of optimizing clinical outcomes [5]. With this information, early PK studies in a phase I trial may provide essential guidance for the development of investigational oncology drugs. For example, PK data from a FIH study may reveal unfavourable pharmacology which would lead to discontinuation of development, or reformulation. This is exemplified by vemurafenib (PLX4032), the first structurally designed small molecule inhibitor of BRAF V600E [6]. In the initial phase I study of vemurafenib using a crystalline formulation, a modest bioavailability of vemurafenib using this preparation was revealed. This led to the replacement of this formulation by a microprecipitated bulk powder, which yielded a tenfold increase in bioavailability.

Another important aspect in the conduct of Phase I trials is the development and analytical validation of suitable analytical methods that will facilitate PK analysis of the investigational oncology drugs. These assays must fulfil all the requirements enumerated in FDA regulations. The parameters and acceptance criteria based on the latest bioanalytical validation guidance updated in May 2018 can be found at https://www.fda.gov/downloads/Drugs/Guidances/ucm070107.pdf. Of note, for the determination of small-molecule oncology drugs, nearly all analytical methods used in the past decade utilised chromatographic assays (CCs) such as LC-MS/MS and GC-MS etc. In contrast, ligand-binding assays (LBAs) are used for large molecules, such as antibodies. For the former, method development involves optimization of procedures and conditions involved with extraction and quantification of the analytes. This however is not necessary for large molecule investigational oncology drugs. Nonetheless, for both types of investigational oncology drugs, several key elements such as the use of suitable reference standards, construction of calibration curves, the use of suitable quality control samples, as well as their recovery, the stability of the analyte in the assay matrix and method selectivity, specificity, sensitivity, precision and accuracy, should all be considered in the development and validation of their bioanalytical methods as summarised in Table 8.1.

Overall, oncology drug development is a process with a high attrition rate with only 5% of drugs evaluated in Phase I eventually registered. In the past, poor PK was one of the most common causes of early termination of a drug in development. However, with an improved understanding of clinical PK, together with its incorporation into Phase I studies, such PK issues have been mitigated. At present, drug ineffectiveness is the key cause of unsuccessful oncology drug approval.

8.2.2 Pointers for PK Sampling When Conducting a Phase I Oncology Trial

The basic PK parameters such as elimination rate constant (Kel), Cmax, AUC and CL of the investigational small molecule anticancer drugs obtained from initial PK studies during phase I trials will provide information on the dose proportionality and accumulation ratio of the investigational drugs at steady state.

- In order to obtain accurate information on these parameters, the use of an appropriate PK sampling schedule is crucial. In designing the sampling schedule, considerations would be whether there have been prior human PK data of the drug studied, or whether previous drugs with similar chemical properties are available to guide the choice of the sampling following single- and multiple-dose administration. This will in turn allow for a thorough evaluation of the exposure-response relationships across multiple dose levels. Thus, a well-designed sampling schedule should define the full time-course of drug concentrations (and

Table 8.1 Key elements of bioanalytical methods

Reference standards	A reference standard is a chemical substance of known purity and identity which is used to prepare calibration standards and quality controls. Three types of reference standards are usually used: (1) certified (e.g., USP compendial standards), (2) commercially supplied, and (3) custom-synthesized.
Calibration curve	The calibration curve—also known as the standard curve—is the relationship between the instrument response and the calibration standards within the intended quantitation range.
Quality control samples (QCs)	Calibrators, or calibration standards, refer to a biological matrix to which a known amount of analyte has been added. Calibration standards are used to construct calibration curves from which the concentrations of analytes in QC samples and PK samples are determined.
Selectivity and specificity	Selectivity is the extent to which the method can determine a particular compound in the analyzed matrices without interference from matrix components. Specificity is the ability of the method to assess, unequivocally, the analyte in the presence of other components that are expected to be present (e.g., impurities, degradation products, matrix components, etc.).
Sensitivity	Sensitivity is defined as the lowest analyte concentration in the matrix that can be measured with acceptable accuracy and precision (i.e., LLOQ).
Accuracy and precision	Accuracy is the degree of closeness of the determined value to the nominal or known true value under prescribed conditions. Accuracy is also sometimes termed trueness. Precision is the closeness of agreement (i.e., degree of scatter) among a series of measurements obtained from multiple sampling of the same homogenous sample under the prescribed conditions.
Recovery	Recovery refers to the extraction efficiency of an analytical process, reported as a percentage of the known amount of an analyte carried through the sample extraction and processing steps of the method.
Stability of the analyte in the matrix	Stability is a measure of the intactness an analyte (lack of degradation) in a given matrix under specific storage and use conditions relative to the starting material for given time intervals.

its metabolites) following a given dose, and all inflection points of the PK curve should be adequately sampled. Ideally, at least 3 time points are required for each of the different kinetic phases of drug absorption (for extravascular drug administration), distribution and elimination. Typically, 10–15 time points including baseline at predose should be adopted for each dose group in an intensive PK study as part of Phase I trials since this is conducted in only a small number of study subjects in a 3+3 dose escalation design. The sampling scheme should not be too sparse as this can potentially risk a biased estimate of Cmax and AUC values which in turn affects further evaluation of dose-proportionality during dose escalation studies, drug interaction studies and investigations of the effects of food on the drug's PK parameters. Apart from this, the actual time the PK samples are taken with respect to the dosing should also be recorded to ensure precise PK analysis and derivation of accurate PK parameters, such as AUC, kel, Cmax, CL and Vd.

8.3 Application of PK to Understand and Rationalize Drug Development for Special Situations

Apart from the usefulness of PK in aiding dose determination for subsequent clinical studies, PK can also be used to investigate the effects of food on the bioavailability of an investigational new drug, to study drug-drug interactions between the drug in development and currently approved drugs, as well as to provide a better understanding on the changes in PK parameters of the investigational new drug in special patient populations. All of these applications are discussed in the succeeding section of this book chapter.

8.3.1 Food Effect Studies

Food can affect the bioavailability of orally administered drugs by various means, such as delaying gastric emptying, stimulating bile flow, changing the gastrointestinal pH and physically or chemically interacting with the drug. Food-effect bioavailability (BA) studies should be conducted early in the clinical development for all new chemical entities to determine the effect food has on their absorption and PK. Conversely, fed bioequivalence (BE) studies are conducted for abbreviated new drug applications to demonstrate their bioequivalence to the reference listed drug (RLD) under fed conditions. Such food effect studies should be carried out for all orally administered drugs unless the drugs are immediate-release, or if their RLDs are labelled to be taken only on an empty stomach or has no labeling on food effect.

8.3.1.1 Study Design

BA studies should be designed as a randomized, balanced, single-dose, two-treatment (fed vs. fasting), two-period, two-sequence crossover in healthy subjects. In fed BE studies, a similar study design is used except that the two-treatment consists of the investigational vs. RLD, both administered to volunteers after a test meal (under fed conditions). If there are safety concerns with regards to the treatment investigated in healthy subjects, the volunteers may be drawn from the patient population. A minimum of 12 evaluable subjects should complete the study to achieve adequate power for statistical assessment [7].

A test meal should comprise high-calorie (approximately 800–1000 calories) and high-fat foods (approximately 50% of total caloric content of the meal), and be given to subjects following an overnight fast of at least 10 h. The caloric breakdown should be provided in the study report. The study drug is typically administered 30 min after the subject begins consuming the meal. For the fasted period, following an overnight fast of at least 10 h, the study drug may be administered with 240 ml of water and no food should be allowed for at least 4 h post-dose. There should be an adequate washout period between the two treatments, with the length of the washout period governed by the half-life of the drug (eg. at least 5 half-lives).

An equivalence approach is recommended by the FDA for food-effect studies during data analysis. The presence of food effect on the bioavailability of an investigational drug is demonstrated when the 90 percent confidence intervals for the ratio of population geometric means between fed and fasted treatments is beyond the equivalence limits of 80–125% for either AUC or C_{max}. Any changes to t_{max} and t_{lag} due to food effects must also be considered in terms of their clinical impact. Similarly, in BE studies, to conclude that the test drug is bioequivalent to the RLD under fed conditions, the 90 percent confidence intervals for the ratio of population geometric means between test and RLD should be within the BE limits of 80–125% for AUC and C_{max}.

8.3.2 Drug-Interaction Studies

PK evaluation of drug-drug interactions (DDI) via *in vitro* and clinical studies helps to determine if interactions exist between the concomitantly administered drugs, and if the interactions occur to an extent that necessitates dose adjustment of the drugs.

8.3.2.1 In Vitro Studies

In *in vitro* studies, understanding the principal routes of the drug's elimination, identifying the enzymes and transporters that are involved in the drug's metabolism and disposition, and determining how enzymes and transporters may be affected by the drug, will help to elucidate the potential DDI mechanisms.

The first step is to determine if the investigational drug is a substrate of metabolizing enzymes. Major metabolizing enzymes that should be routinely evaluated in *in vitro* phenotyping studies include CYP1A2, CYP2B6, CYP2C8, CYP2C9, CYP2C19, CYP2D6, and CYP3A4/5. Other additional enzymes include other CYP enzymes, including CYP2A6, CYP2J2, CYP4F2 and CYP2E1, phase I enzymes such as monoamine oxidase (MAO), Flavin monooxygenase (FMO), xanthine oxidase (XO) and alcohol/aldehyde dehydrogenase, and phase II enzymes including uridine diphosphate (UDP) glucuronosyl transferases (UGTs). If a specific metabolizing enzyme is responsible for >25% of the drug's elimination, then clinical DDI studies should be performed. The next step is to evaluate the potential of the investigational drug to inhibit (reversible inhibition or time-dependent inhibition) or induce the major metabolizing enzymes. If a significant interaction is found, mechanistic models may be applied to determine if one should proceed with clinical DDI studies. If the predicted ratio of AUC of a sensitive index substrate drug in the presence and absence of the investigation drug is ≤0.8 or ≥1.25 based on static mechanistic models, clinical DDI studies should be conducted using a sensitive index substrate.

8.3.2.2 Clinical Drug Interactions Studies

Clinical DDI studies compare substrate concentrations in the absence and presence of a perpetrator drug *in vivo*. They help to confirm the presence of the suspected DDI and guide the appropriate management of clinically significant DDI. To determine if an investigational drug is a 'victim' of DDI, it should be given with index perpetrators that predictably inhibit or induce drug metabolism or transport by a given pathway. Similarly, to test if an investigational drug is a perpetrator, one should use sensitive index substrates. Using a strong index perpetrator or sensitive substrate helps to create the "worst-case scenario" to evaluate the possible greatest magnitude of DDI of investigational drugs. As an example, to study the effects of potent CYP3A inhibitors on cancer drugs, ketoconazole is often used as the potent CYP3A inhibitor. If there is significant interaction with the strong inhibitors or inducers, or with the most sensitive substrates, additional studies may be conducted using less strong inhibitors or inducers, or with other substrates, selected based on likely co-administration [8]. A list of recommended index drugs for specific pathways is available on the FDA's website for Drug Development and Drug Interactions [9].

On the other hand, monoclonal antibodies are usually cleared in the reticuloendothelial system of the body or other protein degradation pathways. They are not subjected to usual drug metabolism for clearance, and are too large to be filtered in the glomerular membrane, and are therefore subjected to less potential for drug interactions.

8.3.2.3 Study Design

For most clinical DDI studies, healthy volunteers may be used unless there are safety concerns or the intention to evaluate PD endpoints that cannot be studied in healthy subjects. A randomized, two-way crossover study design helps to reduce inter-subject variability. The two treatments consist of substrate alone in the first period, and a second period with co-administration of the substrate and perpetrator. Parallel studies may be conducted instead if the drugs have a long half-life and a crossover design is not feasible. The choice of doses, dosing intervals, dosage forms, number of doses, routes and timing of co-administration should maximize the likelihood of finding a DDI, but with due safety consideration. For example, the dose of the perpetrator drug used should be the maximum dose, and with the shortest dosing interval. If the substrate demonstrates dose- or time-dependent non-linear PK, multiple-dose administration of the substrate and its perpetrator should be studied.

- The PK endpoints for DDI studies include changes in drug exposure parameters such as $AUC_{0\text{-}INF}$ and C_{max}. If the 90 percent confidence interval for these measured changes in systemic exposures in the DDI study falls completely within the no-effect boundaries, a conclusion of no clinically significant DDI is made. The no-effect boundaries are determined preferably based on exposure-response relationship derived from PK and PD analyses, and other available information on the substrate drug. Otherwise, by default, a no-effect boundary of 80–125% for AUC and C_{max} may be used. If the investigational drug is a CYP inhibitor or inducer, it can be classified based on the change in the substrate AUC. This classification helps to determine whether other drugs that have not been investigated in a DDI study with the investigational drug may have clinically significant DDIs with it. A strong, moderate and weak inhibitor increases the AUC of a sensitive index substrate by ≥5-fold, ≥2- to <5-fold, and ≥1.25- to <2-fold, respectively. An investigational drug is classified as a strong moderate or weak inducer if it decreases the AUC of a sensitive index CYP substrate by ≥80 percent, ≥50 to <80 percent, or by ≥20 to <50 percent, respectively [10].

8.4 Understanding Special Populations

8.4.1 Patients with Renal Impairment

Alterations in renal function can affect the clearance of anticancer drugs, especially if the drug is eliminated primarily through renal excretion. It can also affect hepatic and gut drug metabolism, and may change the drug's absorption, plasma protein binding and tissue distribution. Thus, the dose of anticancer drugs may need to be modified in patients with renal impairment as their PK may be affected.

For most drugs that are likely to be used on a chronic and systemic basic in patients with renal impairment, a PK study should be conducted to assess the need for dose adjustment in these patients. This includes drugs and cytokines that are not primarily excreted by the kidney. Drugs that are indicated for single-use, administered via inhalation route only and are primarily eliminated through the lungs, or are monoclonal antibodies, are unlikely to be altered in patients with renal impairment. Thus, PK study for these drugs is not necessary.

8.4.1.1 Full PK Study Design

A full PK study should be performed for drugs that are predominantly cleared by the kidney. For drugs that are not predominantly cleared by the kidney (i.e., predominantly cleared by hepatic metabolism or secreted in the bile), a "reduced PK study" design that compares the PK in patients at the extremes of renal function, may be initially performed. A full PK study is also warranted if the result of the "reduced PK study" is positive. (See Diagram 8.1).

There are several ways to define renal function. While the use of 24-h urine sample for measurement of creatinine clearance or the use exogenous markers such as cystatin C and EDTA, provide accurate estimation of glomerular filtration rate (GFR), in clinical practice, it is more practical to use serum-creatinine based equations to estimate GFR. The two commonly used serum-creatinine based equations used to estimate renal function are estimated creatinine clearance (CLcr) by the

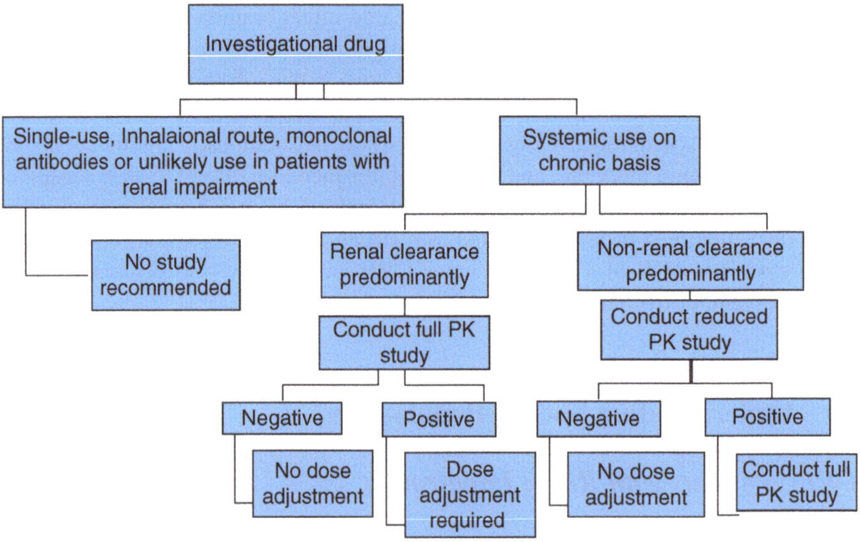

Diagram 8.1 Flowchart for PK study design in patients with renal impairment

Table 8.2 Classification of renal impairment as recommended by FDA [13]

Stage	Description	CLcr (ml/min) or eGFR (ml/min/1.73m^2)
1	Control (normal) GFR	≥90
2	Mild decrease in GFR	60–89
3	Moderate decrease in GFR	30–59
4	Severe decrease in GFR	15–29
5	End Stage renal disease (ESRD)	<15 not on dialysis
		Requiring dialysis

Cockcroft-Gault equation (C-G) [11] and estimated glomerular filtration rate (eGFR) from the Modification of Diet in Renal Disease (MDRD) Study [12]. Historically, C-G equation has been used to estimate renal function in PK studies. Either of the equations may be used to assign subjects to a renal impairment stage (see Table 8.2) based on their estimated renal function.

In order to have a sufficient representation of subjects with various degrees of renal impairment, an approximately equal number of subjects in stages 1–5 should be enrolled. For drugs with wide therapeutic range, subjects may be stratified based on GFR ≥ 60 ml/min (normal to mid decrease in GFR), 15–59 ml/min (moderate to severe renal damage), and ≤15 ml/min (End Stage Renal Disease (ESRD) not initiated on dialysis) [13].

The number of subjects enrolled in each group should be adequate to detect the level of renal impairment at which the PK may be changed significantly to warrant a dose adjustment. The PK variability within the subject group, as well as the PK/PD relationships for both therapeutic and adverse responses, will affect this decision. Of note, the controls with normal renal function used in such studies should be representative of the typical patient population.

A single-dose study may be conducted for drugs that have prior studies demonstrating that single-dose studies can satisfactorily determine their PK. In single-dose studies, the same dose can generally be administered to all patients in the study regardless of renal function because the peak concentration is not substantially affected by renal function. A multiple-dose study is recommended when the drug or its active metabolite exhibits nonlinear or time-dependent PK, and it is paramount to consider a lower or less frequent dosing in patients with impaired renal function to prevent accumulation of drug and its metabolites. The dosing should usually be continued long enough to achieve steady state, and sometimes, if the elimination half-life is markedly increased, a loading dose strategy may be considered to facilitate the process of reaching steady state. Plasma and urine samples should be analyzed for parent drug and its active metabolites. Plasma protein binding may be altered in patients with impaired renal function. Drug efficacy tends to be related to unbound drug concentrations at the site of action. Unbound concentrations should be measured in each plasma sample if the binding is concentration-dependent or if it is affected by metabolites or other time-varying factors. Otherwise, the unbound concentration may be evaluated with a single or limited number of samples in each patient. For drugs and metabolites with low extent of plasma protein binding (i.e., less than 80%), there will be little changes in their plasma protein binding when the renal function is impaired.

8.4.1.2 Reduced PK Study Design

A reduced PK study is essentially a "worst case" study where the PK parameters in patients with ESRD, but are not yet on dialysis are compared to the PK parameters of subjects with normal renal function. If reduced PK study shows a substantial effect (e.g., more than 50% increase in AUC, or a less effect in drugs with a narrow therapeutic index) in patients with renal impairment, a full PK study should be conducted. If no difference in PK are seen, no further study is required. When designing a reduced PK study, the same principles as in the full PK study apply.

8.4.1.3 Effect of Dialysis on PK Parameters

Dialysis may affect the PK of a drug to an extent such that dosage adjustment is required. As intermittent haemodialysis (HD) is the most common dialysis method in chronic ESRD patients, it is important to evaluate the effect of HD on PK. PK studies should also be considered in peritoneal dialysis if the drug is likely to be used in these patients and if peritoneal dialysis is likely to significantly affect the drug PK. PK study of the effect of dialysis on PK may be omitted if the drug is unlikely to be administered to ESRD patients treated with dialysis, or if the dialysis procedure is unlikely to result in significant elimination of drug or active metabolites. This includes drugs with large molecular weight, those that have a high plasma protein binding or large volume of distribution, or those that are primarily non-renally cleared.

For determining the effect of dialysis has on the drug elimination, PK parameters in patients under both dialysis and non-dialysis conditions are compared. During dialysis, concentration of the drug and its metabolites, total plasma proteins and drug free fraction in dialysate, and arterial and venous blood should be measured at several time points. Dialysis clearance (CL_D) can be calculated from the following equation:

$$CL_D = \text{Amount recovered} / AUC_{t0-t1} \tag{8.2}$$

where t_0 marks the start time and t_1 the termination of the haemodialysis session.

The fraction of the administered dose that is recovered in the dialysate is calculated in order to assess the need for administering supplemental drug doses to hemodialysis patients.

8.4.1.4 Data Analysis and Dosing Recommendation

After estimating the PK parameters of the drug and its active metabolites, the next step is to construct a mathematical model for the relationship between estimated renal function and the relevant PK parameters. The reported modeling results should include estimates of the parameters of the chosen model and measures of their precision (either standard errors or confidence intervals). Specific dosing recommendations can be made based on the study results using the model for the relationships between creatinine clearance or eGFR and relevant PK parameters.

8.4.2 Hepatic Impairment

The liver is responsible for drug clearance through various oxidative and conjugative metabolic pathways and through biliary excretion of unchanged drug or metabolites. In patients with liver dysfunction, their kidney functions may be affected as well. Hepatic impairment can lead to drug accumulation, and may less often, affect the formation of active metabolites.

A PK study should be conducted in patients with hepatic impairment if the drug or its active metabolites undergoes significant hepatic metabolism or excretion (i.e. >20% of the absorbed drug), if the drug or its active metabolite is eliminated to a lesser extent but has a narrow therapeutic range, or if the metabolism of the drug in unknown. PK study is not necessary if the drugs used are intended for single-dose administration, eliminated entirely via renal route, is primarily eliminated via the

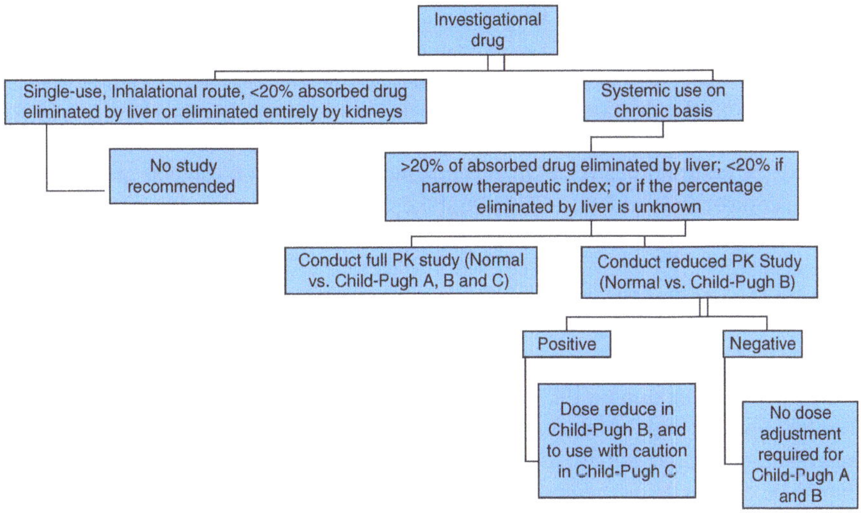

Diagram 8.2 Flowchart for PK study design in patients with hepatic impairment

lungs, or has wide therapeutic range and is metabolized in the liver to a small extent (<20%) (Diagram 8.2).

8.4.2.1 Full PK Study Design

Hepatic function may be measured using a variety of methods. An example is Child-Pugh classification that incorporate clinical signs (ascites and encephalopathy), measure of liver function (prothrombin time) and the levels of endogenous substances (albumin and bilirubin) in the estimation of hepatic function. FDA recommends that the Child-Pugh classification be used to categorize the degree of hepatic impairment in patients [14]. It is paramount that the alterations in the Child-Pugh components are due to the impaired hepatic function and not due to other causes. For example, in a patient with cancer metastasis to the peritoneum, ascites may not be secondary to hepatic impairment. To evaluate the effect on PK parameters across the entire spectrum of hepatic impairment, PK study should be carried out in controls and in patients with the following three Child-Pugh scores, namely mild, moderate and severe. There should be at least 6 subjects evaluated for each category [14].

The same principles for designing study for patients with renal impairment apply. The control group should be representative of the intended patient population. A single-dose or multiple-dose study may be carried out depending if the drug and its active metabolites exhibit linear and time-independent PK or non-linear and time-dependent PK, respectively. For drugs whose metabolism is mediated by enzymes known to exhibit genetic polymorphism, the metabolic status of the enrolled patients should be considered when analyzing the PK results.

8.4.2.2 Reduced PK Study Design

In a reduced PK study, the PK parameters in controls are compared to patients with moderate Child-Pugh score. The findings in the moderate category will apply to patients with a mild Child-Pugh category and dosing in the severe category would generally be contraindicated. FDA recommends that at least 8 subjects are recruited into the control and moderate Child-Pugh hepatic impairment arms.

8.4.2.3 Population PK Approach

Population PK screening in phases 2 and 3 can be useful in assessing the impact of altered hepatic function on PK if patients with hepatic impairment are not excluded from the phase 2 and 3 trials and if there is enough PK information collected about patients to characterize them reasonably well. The patients in phase 2 and 3 studies should be assessed for the components of the Child-Pugh score (serum albumin, serum bilirubin, prothrombin time, ascites and encephalopathy) or for a similar group of measures of hepatic function. Both parent drug and active metabolites, including their unbound concentrations, are typically measured.

8.4.2.4 Dosing Adjustment Recommendations

- The FDA recommends the use of a confidence interval approach, rather than a significance test in hepatic impairment PK studies. No effect of hepatic impairment on the drug's PK is supported when the PK parameters (AUC and Cmax) remains within the no-effect boundaries. These boundaries are defined based on PK information available for the investigational drug, or in absence of the information, a standard 90% confidence interval of 80–125%. If the effect of hepatic impairment on the PK of the drug is obvious (e.g., two-fold or greater increase in AUC), dosage adjustments should be recommended in the labeling.

8.5 Concluding Remarks

Well-designed PK studies during phase I drug development will allow an assessment of the impact of dosing and a preliminary evaluation of the patient variables that impact drug effect. The data would at most be considered preliminary as limited patient numbers restrict statistical robustness; and the data should still be iteratively analysed as more patients are included in later phases of drug development.

Key Expert Opinion Points

- Pharmacokinetic analysis is a valuable tool to understand and guide early development of investigational new drugs
- The design and conduct of PK studies requires careful thought and planning
- Drugs have considerable propensity for PK issues in real world use, and in such situations, understanding the influence of drugs, food, pharmacogenetics, renal or liver function on PK of a new drug is essential to prepare for its eventual use in the clinic.

References

1. Urien S, Barré J, Morin C, et al. Docetaxel serum protein binding with high affinity to alpha 1-acid glycoprotein. Investig New Drugs. 1996;14(2):147–51.
2. Bruno R, Olivares R, Berille J, et al. Alpha-1-acid glycoprotein as an independent predictor for treatment effects and a prognostic factor of survival in patients with non-small cell lung cancer treated with docetaxel. Clin Cancer Res. 2003;9(3):1077–82.
3. Goh BC, Lee SC, Wang LZ, et al. Explaining interindividual variability of docetaxel pharmacokinetics and pharmacodynamics in Asians through phenotyping and genotyping strategies. J Clin Oncol. 2002;20(17):3683–90.
4. Stage TB, Bergmann TK, Kroetz DL. Clinical pharmacokinetics of paclitaxel monotherapy: an updated literature review. Clin Pharmacokinet. 2018;57(1):7–19.
5. Fujita K, Sasaki Y. Optimization of cancer chemotherapy on the basis of pharmacokinetics and pharmacodynamics: from patients enrolled in clinical trials to those in the 'real world'. Drug Metab Pharmacokinet. 2014;29(1):20–8.
6. Yang H, Higgins B, Kolinsky K, et al. RG7204 (PLX4032), a selective BRAFV600E inhibitor, displays potent antitumor activity in preclinical melanoma models. Cancer Res. 2010;70(13):5518–27.
7. Food-Effect Bioavailability and Fed Bioequivalence Studies, Guidance for Industry. US Department of Health and Human Services Food and Drug Administration Center for Drug Evaluation and Research, 2002 at https://www.fda.gov/downloads/drugs/guidancecomplianceregulatoryinformation/guidances/ucm070241.pdf. Accessed 1 December 2018.
8. Rekić D, Reynolds KS, Zhao P, Zhang L, Yoshida K, Sachar M, Piquette Miller M, Huang SM, Zineh I. Clinical drug-drug interaction evaluations to inform drug use and enable drug access. J Pharm Sci. 2017;106(9):2214–8.
9. List of recommended index drugs for specific pathways is available on the FDA's website for Drug Development and Drug Interactions. https://www.fda.gov/Drugs/DevelopmentApprovalProcess/DevelopmentResources/DrugInteractionsLabeling/ucm093664.htm
10. Clinical Drug Interaction Studies – Study Design, Data Analysis, and Clinical Implications, Guidance for Industry. US Department of Health and Human Services Food and Drug Administration Center for Drug Evaluation and Research, Oct 2017. https://www.fda.gov/downloads/Drugs/GuidanceComplianceRegulatoryInformation/Guidances/UCM292362.pdf. Accessed 1 December 2018.
11. Cockcroft DW, Gault MH. Prediction of creatinine clearance from serum creatinine. Nephron. 1976;16(1):31–41.

12. Levey AS, Bosch JP, Lewis JB, Greene T, Rogers N, Roth D, et al. A more accurate method to estimate glomerular filtration rate from serum creatinine: a new prediction equation. Ann Intern Med. 130:461–70. https://doi.org/10.7326/0003-4819-130-6-199903160-00002.
13. Pharmacokinetics in Patients with Impaired Renal Function—Study Design, Data Analysis, and Impact on Dosing and Labeling, Guidance for Industry. US Department of Health and Human Services Food and Drug Administration Center for Drug Evaluation and Research, Mar 2010. https://www.fda.gov/downloads/Drugs/GuidanceComplianceRegulatoryInformation/Guidances/ucm072127.pdf. Accessed 1 December 2018.
14. Pharmacokinetics in patients with impaired hepatic function: study design, data analysis, and impact on dosing and labeling, guidance for industry. US Department of Health and Human Services Food and Drug Administration Center for Drug Evaluation and Research, May 2003.

Chapter 9
Development of Pharmacodynamic Biomarkers for Phase I Trials

María Vieito, Itziar Gardeazabal, Ignacio Matos, and Elena Garralda

Abstract According to the NCI experimental Therapeutics Program (NeXT) definition pharmacodynamic biomarkers (PD) are molecular indicators of the drug's effect on the target in an organism.

Using the pharmacological audit trail (PhAT) framework the role of PD in early drug development is to measure the effect of the drug against a certain target or pathway (proof-of-mechanism PD), or study the functional consequences of the drug-target interaction (proof-of-concept PD). Although regulatory and technical challenges to generalize the use of PD still remain we review some recent advances towards standardization and the fit-for model approach which can be used to determine the appropriate, use-specific, requirements of validation.

The validation of a PD biomarker should be started in the preclinical phase and continue during the early clinical development following a learn-predict-confirm approach to test the expected results against the clinical observations. PD biomarkers can be used to characterize the relationship between drug levels and biological effects or as part of adaptative clinical trial designs. Finally we review specific differences of on target-toxicity, tissue, blood based and imaging PD as well as review the role of PD biomarkers in the era of immunotherapy.

Keywords Pharmacodynamics · Pharmacological audit trail · biomarker qualification · Fit-for-purpose · Model-based drug-development

Key Points

1. According to the pharmacological audit trail, pharmacodynamic biomarkers should be used during the early phases of drug development to prove activity

M. Vieito (✉) · I. Gardeazabal · I. Matos · E. Garralda
Medical Oncology Department, Vall d'Hebron University Hospital, Autonomous University of Barcelona (UAB), Barcelona, Spain

Molecular Therapeutics Research Unit, Vall d'Hebron Institute of Oncology (VHIO), Barcelona, Spain
e-mail: mvieito@vhio.net; egarralda@vhio.net; imatos@vhio.net; igardeazabal@vhio.net

T. A. Yap et al. (eds.), *Phase I Oncology Drug Development*,
https://doi.org/10.1007/978-3-030-47682-3_9

against a particular target of a pathway, as well as downstream functional consequences of drug-target interaction.
2. Due to their complexity and lack clear of a coherent standardization pathway, the use of pharmacodynamic biomarkers has yet to be generalized.
3. Although the more widely used biomarkers are collected in blood or in other surrogate tissues, tissue based, image based and liquid biopsies are gaining importance.
4. The fit-for-purpose approach to biomarker qualification allows us to set different standards for biomarkers that are purely exploratory and companion diagnostics and also takes into account that not all modalities of biomarkers can be standardized to the same degree.
5. Model-based drug development expresses the expectations of a clinical trial as a mathematical equation in which the results, including pharmacodynamic biomarkers can either prove or disprove the model and lead to optimization through a iterative learn-predict-confirm approach.

9.1 Introduction: Integration of Pharmacodynamic Biomarkers in Early Drug Development

In recent years, early drug development in oncology has been transformed by new insights into the molecular biology of cancer and the role of the tumor environment. Fueled by a deeper understanding of the genomic and cell biology landscape, a new generation of drugs rationally designed to target genetic driver alterations is complementing conventional chemotherapy, dramatically altering the management of many cancers. Nonetheless, rational drug development remains a slow and costly process. Advocate groups and stakeholders have stressed the importance of biomarkers as a potentially valuable tools for selecting the optimal population for a given drug or as surrogate markers of efficacy endpoints in early clinical trials [1]. Despite many success stories, such as for *BRAF*-mutant melanoma or *HER2*-amplified breast cancer, barriers such as lack of standardization and validation pose major issues for biomarker-directed drug development [2].

A biomarker is typically defined as a characteristic that can be objectively measured and evaluated as an indicator of normal or pathogenic biological processes, or pharmacologic responses to a therapeutic intervention [3]. In this review we use the definition of pharmacodynamic (PD) biomarker following the NCI experimental Therapeutics Program (NeXT) which focuses on the link between the drug and its downstream biological effect. According to this definition, PD biomarkers are molecular indicators of the drug's effect on the target in an organism. A PD biomarker can be used to examine the link between a drug treatment, the target effects, and a biological tumor response [4].

Several factors contribute to the growing interest in PD biomarkers in phase I trials; the potential ability to correlate clinical data with target modulation, the development of tests that combine functional information with early assessment of tumor response, such as functional imaging studies (e.g. fluorodeoxyglucose–positron emission tomography [FDG-PET] or dynamic magnetic resonance imaging [MRI]) [5] and the possibility of combining them with conventional techniques such as pathological or biochemical analyses [6]. Finally, the failure of several late-stage investigational drugs has also motivated researchers to seek molecular and biochemical evidence of on-target engagement during early stages of drug development [7].

Some aspects of PD biomarkers remain controversial, such as the determination of "proof-of-mechanism", the optimal source of tissue for collecting PD biomarkers (especially in the phase I trial setting), the suitability of biomarkers as surrogate endpoints, the convenience of looking at one single analyte or measuring proteins in close functional proximity to the target, and even whether maximal target inhibition is indeed desirable for every drug [8]. Although PD biomarkers are nowadays integrated into most drug development programs, their potential usefulness during drug development is still underexploited [9]. Some key questions remain unanswered for many targeted drugs in development such as (1) defining the biologically optimal dose and schedule for phase II studies, (2) their use as surrogate endpoints of drug resistance, clinical toxicity or efficacy [1], and, as a consequence, (3) their clinical utility for defining the population likely to respond to the drug under investigation [10].

Developing and validating biomarkers is a complex process, and in some cases is proving to be almost as difficult as the development and approval of the new drug itself. This chapter focuses on PD biomarkers in the early phase of development during phase I trials, with the aim of illustrating the challenges and potential alternative approaches for their incorporation into the drug development process.

9.2 General Aspects of Pharmacodynamic Biomarker Validation: Technical and Regulatory Issues

(a) The Pharmacological Audit Trail (PhAT)

Originally proposed by Prof. Paul Workman in a series of articles in the early 2000s [8, 11, 12], the pharmacological audit trail (PhAT) is a framework of questions that should be answered during the process of developing a new drug to identify how much of the drug reaches a given location and the biological effect in the target tissue (Fig. 9.1). Although we will be briefly introducing the whole pharmacological audit trail, pharmacodynamic biomarkers will be used mostly to answer the later aspect.

The first set of questions uses predictive biomarkers discovered during preclinical testing to identify which is the target population of the study and what is the working hypothesis about the possible pharmacological effect. A second set of questions uses pharmacokinetic biomarkers to evaluate how the organism interacts with the drug, and ultimately to measure if biologically active concentrations are achieved in blood and, if possible, in the tumor.

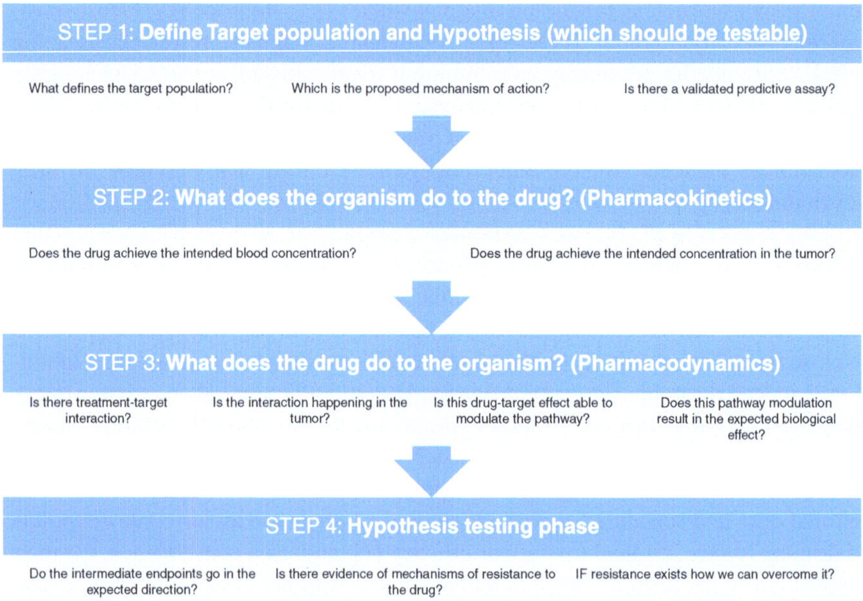

Fig. 9.1 The Pharmacologic Audit Trail (PhAT)

The third step, the evaluation of biological events happening in the organism as an effect of the drug, requires pPharmacodynamic biomarkers. eventsThe authors categorize them in (1) proof-of-mechanism PD biomarkers (when they measure the effect of the drug against a certain target or pathway), and (2) proof-of-concept biomarkers (when they show later effects on a hallmark cancer pathway, such a proliferation or angiogenesis). The later represent what the authors refer to as "functional consequences" of the drug-target interaction.

Workman et al. also introduce a third type of biomarkers that they call "intermediate endpoints of clinical response" that address the issue of whether the drug actually achieves the intended clinical effect. In this group they include biomarkers such as changes in tumor markers, circulating tumor cell (CTC) numbers and changes in circulating tumor DNA (ctDNA), as well as fludeoxyglucose (FDG)-PET [13].

Finally, the last set of questions tries to elucidate the mechanisms that cause therapeutic resistance, using resistance biomarkers phenomenon such as T790M mutation in EGFR mutant patients treated with TKIs, upregulation of compensatory oncogenic pathways (MET…) or other mechanisms [14].

The use of the PhAT is intended to guide the process of decision-making during drug development, allowing amongst other things, researchers to terminate (or modify) at an early stage the development of drugs if it is unlikely to be successful in later phases as well as to avoid the use of a drug at the wrong dose or in the wrong clinical context [8]. The PhAT establishes that phase I clinical trials are the optimal scenario for showing proof-of-mechanism with PD biomarkers. It could even be argued that allowing a drug that has not shown consistent target engagement to proceed to phase II trials could be considered a form of poor clinical science [15].

Although in the initial PhAT only proof-of-mechanism PD biomarkers were considered essential for early phases of drug-development, in revised versions and due to the paradigm shift experienced by phase I clinical trials, its authors incorporated also proof-of-concept PD biomarkers in "extended and stratified phase I trials" together with surrogate endpoints such as radiological response and progression-free survival [8].

(b) Regulatory Guidelines

The regulatory pathway for biomarkers has only recently begun to be standardized in a joint effort by the FDA, the EMA and the Critical Path Institute, a non-profit consortium of industry and academic stakeholders, although differences between the pathways recommended by the FDA and EMA are yet to be resolved. For the FDA, biomarkers used in the approval of a drug undergo a voluntary public qualification process that determines not only if the biomarker is approved but also the context of use (COU). The COU is defined by the FDA as a "a statement that fully and clearly describes the how the biomarker is to be used and its purpose of use".

FDA guidelines to validate a biomarker planned for use in a clinical trial setting are common to those used for other 'Drug Development Tools' such as Clinical Outcome Models and preclinical models [16]. The qualification process involves three stages. In the initiation stage, a letter of intent detailing the proposed biomarker is to be sent to the Biomarker Qualification Review Team (BQRT), then a group of experts will establish the appropriate scientific and regulatory background and issue a series of recommendations to the submitter [17]. During the consultation stage, a series of meetings between the BQRT and the submitter are held until a final agreement about the requirements for approval is reached. Finally, in the review phase, the full package of supporting evidence is sent to the BQRT which might request additional evidence in order to emit a recommendation for qualification which is then published by the FDA.

Since the launch of this initiative in 2014, as of June 2019 only 20 biomarkers, none of which was developed to guide anticancer treatments, have gone through the public qualification process and received FDA approval. An alternative, and more oftenly used approach is to include the potential biomarker in the investigational new drug (IND) application. In this path, a continuous discussion between the sponsor and the FDA goes on throughout the drug development process. If the evidence supporting the biomarker is judged to be appropriate, it can later become part of the new drug application (NDA) submission and the drug label [18].

In the COU statement, the application describes the following elements: (a) the identity of the biomarker, (b) the aspect of the biomarker that is measured and the form in which it is used for biological interpretation, (c) the characteristics of the subjects studied (d) the purpose of its use in drug development, (e) the drug development circumstances for applying the biomarker, and (f) the interpretation and decision/action based on the biomarker [16]. The FDA recommends a risk-based approach to evaluate the supporting evidence, where biomarkers that will be used to make decisions that will impact the approval of the drug (such as surrogate biomarkers) or that will limit the patient population, are subjected to increased regulatory scrutiny. In general, PD biomarkers fall into an intermediate part of the spectrum that goes from purely exploratory biomarkers to companion diagnostics [19].

In order to establish evidentiary standards, in 2008 the FDA's Center for Food Safety and Applied Nutrition (CFSAN), in conjunction with the Center for Drug Evaluation and Research (CDER), requested a report from the Institute of Medicine (IOM) containing recommendations for the process of biomarker development [18]. This report suggests a three-step process to ensure that a biomarker has (a) analytical validation, reflecting that biomarker tests need to present internal validity, including reliability, reproducibility and maintain adequate sensitivity and specificity; (b) qualification, which for the IOM biomarker qualification requires both [1] evidence of a link between the treatment and the biomarker and [2] between biomarker changes and changes on clinical endpoints of interest; (c) a defined utilization setting. The final decision about the intended use of a biomarker will depend on the context of use in addition to the strength of the available evidence, with stronger evidence and a higher compelling context needed for the use of a biomarker as a surrogate endpoint.

The FDA requires that biomarkers used in the enrichment of the target patient population and companion diagnostics follow such qualification process and has drafted specific guidelines to this effect. As such, if a biomarker will have a dual use, such as enrichment marker and eventually as companion diagnostic, it would have to follow additional requirements.

The EMA applies a similar approach but with a two-step process for biomarker qualification [20]. In the first step (which is not mandatory) the submitter can ask for Qualification Advice by sending a package detailing the context of use of the biomarker, the available supporting evidence and the proposed protocol and methods of qualification, and receives a non-binding opinion from the regulators. When the evidence submitted is promising, the EMA may publish a Letter of Support subject to the fulfillment of certain requirements. In the second step, if the submitter has fulfilled the requirements of the Qualification Advice or independently decides that the supporting evidence supports the requested context of use, a Qualification Opinion can be requested by submitting a dossier with the scientific evidence. If the EMA opinion is favorable, a draft approval will be published on the EMA website and after any comments and once suggestions from the scientific community have been addressed, the final opinion for the biomarker will be published. As it is in the case of the FDA and the US, only a few biomarkers (mostly the same ones that have gone through FDA regulatory approval) have received independent EMA approval [21].

It is to be hoped however, that in the future the trend will change as increasing number of drugs receive conditional approval using biomarkers that despite measuring the same biological process, have followed slightly different regulatory pathways. That is the case, for example, of the approval of different checkpoint inhibitors based on slightly different PD-L1 antibodies, that has led to confusing situation (there may be cases where, based on the label of the drug, the same patient could receive treatment with one inhibitor, but not with another [22]). If PD-L1- based evaluations had been subject to the proposed biomarker qualification process, the results of one test could be applicable to multiple settings and drugs.

(c) Quality Assurance and the Fit-for-Purpose Model
The fit-for-purpose approach to biomarker validation is based on the idea that the stringency of the evaluation process should depend on the intended use of the biomarker [23]. During the pre-validation process, the characteristics of the population and the parameter measured, the intended objective of studying the specific biomarker, and the COU determine the rigor applied to the assay validation. After the theoretical requirements have been defined and before proceeding with the validation, a protocol is used to minimize the pre-analytical sources of variability. This protocol should characterize each step of the process, including sample collection and storage conditions, standardizing the sourcing of the reagents and equipment, and a description of how changes in different parameters can influence the results [9].

The validation of a biomarker follows the general principles of bio-analytical method validation (Good Laboratory Practices [GLP] [24]), but major limitations apply to biomarkers due to their intrinsic variability introduced by the nature of the biological matrices in which they are measured and their own complexity. Because of this, it is mandatory to verify first the influence of the different biological matrices on the test's performance. The optimal biomarker would be is one that could be measured with accuracy in different tissue sources such as tumor tissues, CTCs and peripheral blood mononuclear cells (PBMCs).

The second step is the exploratory validation process which should occur early during the development of a biomarker. During the exploratory validation stage, the primary objective is to determine if the test achieves the desired sensitivity, specificity, precision and accuracy using suitable control samples. One of the objectives of this phase is to build a calibration curve and to determine the assay's dynamic range and limits of quantitation/detection.

Later, during the advanced validation process, the test is used in conditions that mimic potential interfering factors found in biological matrices (blood, tissue samples) such as the effects of hemolysis, storage, temperature, etc. The aim of the in-study validation step is to ensure that the properties of the test are consistent in real patient samples and that no difficulties, such as extreme baseline levels or high variability, arise when a biomarker is translated from animal models to human samples. Small scale assays with human samples before engaging in large scale testing of irreplaceable clinical samples is strongly advised in this phase of the program. It is important that biomarkers are not only internally validated but that biomarker analysis is initially centralized or a standardized process is implemented so that results obtained in different laboratories show concordant results [25]. An example of standardization of biomarkers between laboratories is seen with the NCI effort to establish measures to determine polymerization levels of PAR, Topo1 isomerase and apoptosis biomarkers [26] for assisting drug development programs.

9.3 Practical Integration of Pharmacodynamic Biomarkers into Early Drug Development

(a) Model-Based Drug Development

Traditional clinical trial design typically uses a pre-specified set of assumptions derived from observations from previous studies in a smaller populations, or in the case of early drug development, extrapolation from toxicology studies and preclinical models.

Model-based drug development, on the other hand, expresses the predicted outcomes as a mathematical systems and then uses an iterative process to test the model against the data using a learn-predict-confirm approach [27, 28] (Fig. 9.2). The first step is to use all available information from the preclinical testing that can be used for predicting clinical outcome and to choose the optimal biomarkers ("learn"). This information is used to create a mathematical model describing relationships between the different readouts (PK and PD biomarkers, toxicity assessments) and different conditions, and makes predictions about the intended outcomes ("predict"). When testing the model in the clinical setting one can then either validate the assumptions of the model or determine inconsistencies between predictions and reality ("confirm"). This would lead to revisit the process with a different set of assumptions. The advantage of having an explicit model is that it offers the opportunity to learn from any misconceptions and adapt the model. Model-based design can also provide insights on how differences in the baseline parameters of the study, such as biomarker prevalence, affect the sensitivity and power of the trial, which can, in turn, be used to redesign a more robust trial. Using model-based drug development, data from different sources (preclinical data, toxicology studies, phase 0 clinical trials) are incorporated into the mathematical model describing the drug effect.

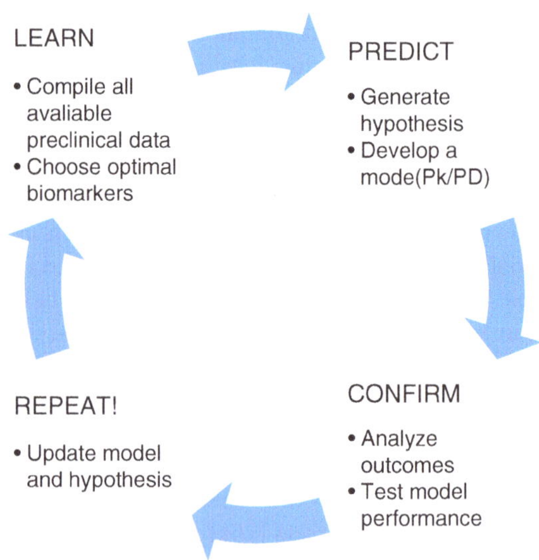

Fig. 9.2 Model-based clinical trial design

Predictions made in the model can then be tested in early clinical trials and adjusted according to the different aspects being studied (PK and PD biomarkers, clinical outcomes, toxicity assessments). Subsequent studies are then designed to test the model and confirm if it is able to describe the observed effects.

Model-based drug development makes use of pharmacometrics [29], the science of developing and applying mathematical and statistical methods to (a) characterize, understand, and predict a drug's PK and PD behavior, (b) quantify uncertainty of information about this behavior, and (c) rationalize data-driven decision-making in the drug development process and pharmacotherapy.

Using this learn-predict-confirm approach, some clinical trials could be substituted by *in silico trials* testing different hypothesis, reducing significantly the drug-development costs. For example, a model-based phase I clinical trial including the estimation of the dose-toxicity relationship being continuously fed by data from all enrolled patients could determine more effectively the maximum tolerated dose [30]. One recent example of the implementation of model-based clinical trial design and simulation of direct intrapatient dose escalation is KEYNOTE-001 trial, during the firsts clinical trials with Pembrolizumab [31].

(b) Pharmacokinetic/Pharmacodynamic Modeling

PK-PD models are mathematical models that describe the relationship between drug exposure (using PK parameters as surrogates) and drug activity (using PD markers as surrogates) [29]. PK-PD models allow determination of the minimum biological dose, dose needed to engage a biological pathway which is likely to be clinically relevant (minimal anticipated dose level [MABEL] [32]) thus optimizing the dose range in very early clinical trials. Other common models use toxicity as pharmacodynamics, like neutropenia in the case of chemotherapy agents. This was initially used with data from docetaxel, paclitaxel and etoposide trials, and more recently have for other drugs such as irinotecan and vinflunine. The application of toxicity as an indirect PD biomarker is being increasingly used in novel dose escalation phase I clinical trials to limit the probability of patients experiencing severe side effects [33].

The assumption that increasing drug exposure results in increasing drug engagement and clinical activity, though, is not always supported by the evidence. In many cases, instead of a linear relationship among these variables, there is a minimum threshold of exposure that must be achieved before a biological effect is detected and further increases in drug concentration above the plateau may not translate into increases in drug effect in what is described as a "sigmoidal curve".

(c) Adaptative Design

Adaptive design is based on the idea that clinical information collected during a trial could guide the further development of that trial. In a classic approach to early clinical trials, the main objective is to identify the maximum tolerated dose among a range of predefined dose levels having prespecified rules to guide dose escalation and recommended dose determination. These rules would be based almost exclusively on safety data occurring during the DLT period [34]. In an adaptive design, exemplified by different Bayesian dose escalation models, dose escalation is continuously guided by a model that takes into account the observed toxicity during the trial, including side effects beyond the DLT period.

Adaptive clinical trials offer a mechanism to adapt to different eventual scenarios during the trial with statistical support and scientific rationale. For example, the continuous reassessment method (CRM) and the escalation with overdose control (EWOC) method, the observed toxicity is incorporated into a mathematical model that is used to guide dosing decisions during the trial [35]. There are some other variations of adaptive designs that take into account more factors such as dose concentrations (especially useful for dose escalation in cases where preclinical PKs are expected to be less reliable) or pharmacodynamics readouts. These designs could facilitate, for example, changing the dosing schedule based on the PK profile and in response to observed PD biomarkers [34]. On the contrary, in traditional clinical trials, adapting the dose escalation in a protocol based on such findings would require a formal protocol amendment, involving considerable delays and increasing the study costs [36]. Recently, simplified versions of Bayesian adaptive designs based on toxicity that would not require a dedicated statistical team have been published [37].

The use of an adaptive design also allows to have the identification of the optimal biologic dose (OBD) or the optimal patient population as the main objective of the trial, facilitating optimal clinical development. Adaptive trials could be used, for example, to delimit the eligible population, adapting to the clinical responses seen in each biomarker-defined population, and ultimately exclude patients who are unlikely to respond based on the data [34]. The I-SPY 2 (NCT01042379) and BATTLE-2 protocols are phase II studies that have implemented a coordinated effort to test, analytically validate, and qualify companion biomarkers during the study, and further examples of ongoing clinical trials that follow an adaptive design have been summarized by Don Barry and colleagues [38].

(d) Window-of-Opportunity Studies and the Neoadjuvant Setting

One of the main advantages of performing clinical trials in the neoadjuvant setting early during drug development is the opportunity to correlate PD biomarkers with surrogates of clinical activity such as tumor response and pathological complete response (pCR) [2]. In neoadjuvant trials, baseline and post-treatment tumor samples can often be compared allowing identification of any changes in PD biomarkers without additional interventions. Neoadjuvant trials conducted in the biomarker-selected *HER2*-positive breast cancer subpopulation have become the basis for the approval of drugs in the early setting [39].

Window-of-opportunity (WOO) trials are also performed in the neoadjuvant setting but treatment duration is hort and they do not have a therapeutic intent. Patients with early-stage disease receive the drug for a brief period of time, before undergoing surgical treatment, being the objective of the treatment to explore PD biomarkers and early surrogates of potential antitumoral activity [2]. The rationale behind window-of periods in which tumors are treatment naïve, providing the opportunity to observe and characterize better the effects of the drug. Since the possibility of obtaining therapeutic is unknown in the case of early drugs used in the neoadjuvant setting, and minimal in WOO, some concerns have been raised on exposing patients with potentially curable diseases to unknown risks of toxicity, or delay or even compromise the patient's option to receive curative treatment [40]. In this regard, several requirements should be fulfilled before such trial in the neoadjuvant setting can be considered: the initial toxicity profile must be well established, the treatment should demonstrate some efficacy in the advanced-disease setting, there should be a strong rationale to include the specific population in the study, and the risk of delaying or compromising curative treatment should be minimal.

9.4 Pharmacodynamic Biomarker Approaches

(a) Tissue-Based Biomarkers

The established gold standard material for PD biomarker assessments is tumor specimens, which allow direct evaluation of the functional and molecular effects of new therapeutic agents within the tissue of interest. PD biomarkers that are optimally explored in tumor samples include protein markers of cell signaling such as expression and protein phosphorylation markers, measures of cellular proliferation/apoptosis, cell-cycle regulation biomarkers, and epigenetic changes [3]. Nonetheless, it is worth noting intrinsic limitations associated with the use of tumor tissues, such as the potential variability in drug exposure as well as inter- and intratumor heterogeneity. However, the principal limitations are the feasibility and costs associated with tumor sampling. To be ethically justified, these invasive procedures should be judged to represent an acceptable risk for patients in light of the potential benefits and the criticality of the biomarker information accrued. Although some studies have shown that clinical trial participants consider the potential biopsy-related complications to be acceptable, almost half of them do so based on the misconception that research-related biopsies have implications for their own treatment [41], a fact that highlights the importance of ensuring that patients are appropriately informed about the actual purpose of agreeing to provide biological samples. In this context, there is a strong need for non-invasive biomarkers as well as improved technological platforms that may serve to allow comprehensive molecular analyses on smaller (less invasive) specimens, such as fine-needle aspirates [2].

Pharmacodynamic markers collected in clinical trials through sequential tumor biopsies can elicit key aspects in the drug development program such as the degree of target engagement and its functional consequences. An illustrative example can be found in *BRAF*-mutant melanoma: in serial tumor biopsies (baseline and at day 15) obtained from selected patients in a phase I trial of vemurafenib, to assess changes in mitogen-activated protein kinase (MAPK) signaling, investigators observed reductions in tumor levels of phosphorylated extracellular signal-related kinase (p-ERK), cyclin D1 and Ki67 in all evaluated patients [42]. These results were key to establishing that the predominant PD effect of vemurafenib occurs via the on-target inhibition of MAPK signaling.

Nonetheless, obtaining serial tumor biopsies during treatment in the setting of early drug development trials is not always feasible or even ethical, which has enabled an interest in using easily accessible tissues such as skin, peripheral blood mononucleat cells (PBMCs) and plucked hair follicles as potential surrogate biomarkers. PD studies in surrogate tissues can provide insights into target inhibition (as a proof-of-mechanism) and the time course/duration of such effects, however it should not always be assumed that the effects of the drug on the tumor and the surrogate tissue will be identical. Potential limitations of using surrogate normal tissues for evaluating PD biomarkers in the place of tumor tissues include different drug penetration between the surrogate tissue and the tumor tissue, variations in key gene expression, absence of somatic mutations in the oncogenic target in normal tissues, differences in drug metabolism (such as abnormal drug efflux proteins) in tumor versus normal tissues and differences in terms of regulation of the signal transduction pathway in tumors (e.g., oncogene addiction) compared with normal cells [2]. Generally, only surrogate tissues which highly express the target of interest and where some correlation with effects in tumor have been observed should be used.

An illustrative example of the potential difficulties of using surrogate biomarkers is an early clinical study of an EGFR tyrosine kinase inhibitor which used skin biopsies as surrogate markers for PD assessments [43]. The skin biopsies revealed a decrease in EGFR phosphorylation with treatment, corresponding to target modulation. Despite target engagement (proof-of-mechanism), EGFR inhibitors were deemed insufficiently efficacious in unselected non-small cell lung cancer (NSCLC) populations [44]. It was later that it was subsequently recognized a different sensitivity between wild-type and mutant EGFR. In summary, pharmacodynamics markers, in tumor or surrogate tissues, can be used to confirm that an agent can cause target/pathway inhibition, as well as the time course of such inhibition, an important step towards effective antitumor use [2], and may need to be complemented with predictive markers to select the corrent patient population.

(b) Circulating Biomarkers: CTCs and ctDNA

Circulating biomarkers have the advantage of reducing the risks associated with invasive tumor biopsies and offer, due to their accessibility, the possibility of serial determination of parameters. Another advantage is that although biological fluids, especially blood are very complex, factors that influence biomarker testing are better understood and characterized, offering advantages over testing the same biomarker in the heterogeneous tumor microenvironment. Examples of circulating biomarkers that can be used in clinical trials range from markers of tumor cell death [45], unbound physiological ligands and soluble receptors [46], or changes in peripheral immune cell subpopulations following treatment with immunotherapy) [47].

Two reliable modalities of circulating biomarkers, circulating tumor cells (CTCs) and circulating tumor DNA (ctDNA), have emerged over the last decade, provoking strong interest on the basis of their potential as surrogate tumor biopsies. Advantages and drawbacks of CTCs as PD biomarkers have been extensively summarized elsewhere [48]. Currently the only FDA-validated method to quantify CTCs is the

CellSEARCH® system, which uses EpCAM-based immunomagnetic isolation and fluorescent staining for cytokeratins, CD45 and an additional marker to enumerate and characterize CTCs. The main limitation of this method resides in its reliance on the presence of these epithelial markers on the surface of the CTC to identify tumor cells, which limits its utility in tumor types for which such surface expression is absent or lost, and in tumor cells in which tumor resistance is driven by epithelial-mesenchymal transition. Circulating tumor cells could be used as PD (such as changes in the androgen receptor in CTCs of prostate cancer patients treated with androgen deprivation therapy) or as early surrogate of response (changes in CTC numbers during treatment) [49]. Alternative methods of determining CTCs that do not rely on the presence of epithelial markers and that allow comprehensive molecular characterization, including the establishment of tumor models [50] and the PD biomarkers are being evaluated, but their use in clinical trials is currently limited by their lack of validation [48].

ctDNA is found in the blood of cancer patients following necrosis or apoptosis of cancer cells and can potentially reflect more accurately the genomic and spatial heterogeneity of the tumor than current CTC methods, although there may be an implicit bias when assessing treatment-resistant clones that undergo less apoptosis [51]. While earlier methods such as Sanger sequencing and qPCR require the design of primers for each possible tumor mutation that may be detected which is costly, next generation sequencing (NGS) tests are not bound by such limitations, and furthermore the associated costs have been decreasing while sensitivity is increasing. The main limitation of using ctDNA as a PD biomarker is the inability of current techniques to detect functional changes that occur as a consequence of drug-target interactions. The prime indication for ctDNA is as a response biomarker thanks to its ability to detect changes in tumor dynamics, such as the apparition of a treatment-resistant clone [52].

(c) Image-Based Biomarkers

The increasing availability of imaging techniques that combine morphological and functional information, such as PET-CT and MRI with perfusion and diffusion techniques, has accelerated the use of imaging techniques as PD biomarkers and also as early surrogates of response [53]. Imaging biomarkers have some advantages (less invasive and safer than a tumor biopsy) and along with disadvantages (cost, technical complexity, use of ionizing radiation in some cases) but used as PD biomarkers they can complement, and in some cases replace, conventional PD biomarkers [54]. Depending on the imaging modality and the use of a labelling agent, imaging biomarkers can play different roles. For example, researchers have combined conventional FDG-PET with a radiolabeled-PARP inhibitor to show a correlation between drug distribution in the tumor tissue with a decrease in the metabolic activity of the tumor [55]. In contrast, the use of an MRI to measure drug perfusion in a clinical trial of an antiangiogenic agent is an example of pharmacodynamics marker, but may also be an early marker of response, such as in clear cell renal cancer patients treated with pazopanib in whom changes in perfusion parameters have been reported as predictive of treatment benefit [56].

Imaging can also be used to measure direct drug-target engagement, as reported by researchers who found that Z-endoxifen, a potent estrogen antagonist, significantly reduced the uptake of labelled 18F-fluoroestradiol, a physiological ligand, as early as 1 day post-drug administration [57].

(d) On-Target Toxicity
Some of the undesired clinical effects of the drug (side effects) are directly linked with the mechanism of action (on-target toxicity). In some instances, where a dynamic range can be established, these could be also used as PD biomarkers.

To standardize the collection of this information and for grading, the Common Toxicity Criteria-Adverse Events (CTCAE) was established by the National Cancer Institute. To better represent the changing toxicity profiles associated with new targeted treatments and immunotherapy agents, several updates have been developed (a new version of the CTCAE guidelines (v5.0) was published in December 2017 Toxicities receptor release [58]). A more comprehensive guideline was published in 2018 by the American Society of Clinical Oncology to standardize the grading and treatment of immune-related secondary effects [59].

To use toxicity-related data as pharmacodynamics markers, it is essential not only to use standardized grading criteria, but it is also important to ensure the quality of the data collected, that communication between the researcher and the drug development team is adequate, and that subjectivity in the classification of certain adverse events is reduced as much as possible (for example the same event could be reported as fatigue, asthenia or malaise).

In general, if on-target toxicity is seen earlier than expected or fails to appear when it is expected, this should raise questions for the drug development team as to whether the assumptions are correct. An example of unexpected toxicity that alerted researchers to an unpredicted interaction between pathways occurred during a phase I trial testing vemurafenib combined with ipilimumab in patients with *BRAF* V600 mutated melanoma. The trial was prematurely closed due to unexpected hepatotoxicity for reasons that are still unclear [60]. Surprisingly, further studies in which the immunotherapy was introduced after an induction period with vemurafenib did not find this hepatotoxicity [61].

9.5 The Changing Landscape: Immunotherapy and Beyond

The incorporation of immunotherapy into the therapeutic paradigm is widely recognized as the main advance in oncology in recent decades. However, it seems that our ability to understand the mechanisms involved in the response to immune therapy has lagged behind its use. Only very recently, researchers have started to understand that achieving a response with immunotherapy requires both an immunogenic tumor (in some instances associated with a high tumoral mutational burden), as well as a competent immune system (that could be exemplified by a T cell inflamed gene expression profile) [62]. Single markers, such as PD-L1 expression correlate somehow with aspects of the immune response, but offer limited information and will probably be replaced by robust, multiplex biomarkers such as TMB and GEP.

Although researchers are beginning to understand why some patients are more likely to have a response to conventional immunotherapy, little is understood about the consequences of the treatment (i.e., pharmacodynamics) for the patient [63]. Recently the Methodology for the Development of Innovative Cancer Therapies task force marked the development of robust validated PD biomarkers as a priority for early clinical trials with immunotherapy agents and combinations [64].

Other challenges that need to be better addressed when developing PD biomarkers for immunotherapy include the relationship between dose, response and toxicity. It is becoming more apparent that in many instances there is not a lineal or sinusoidal dose/effect relationship, but a threshold over which dose increases only lead to marginal gains [65].

Paired tumor biopsies have becomingly increasingly standard in early clinical trials with immunotherapy, and to date the changes in the composition of tumor-infiltrating immune cells [66] and transcriptional changes [67] seem to offer high potential for a role as immunotherapy PD biomarkers. Dynamic changes in soluble biomarkers such as CD25 and IL-2 and circulating immune subpopulations including CD8 and NK are also being used to design rational immunotherapy combinations [68]. Interestingly PD-L1 can be characterized in CTCs where it seems to be highly upregulated as a mechanism to overcome immune-vigilance. Persistence of high levels of PD-L1 expression in CTCs after treatment with a checkpoint inhibitor was associated with worse long-term outcomes in patients with NSCLC [69]. Thus, changes in surface biomarkers associated with the immune response in liquid biopsies have the potential to become biomarkers for immunotherapy, combining the advantages of tumor biopsies and peripheral samples.

In conclusion, the number of compounds in clinical oncology development is today growing almost exponentially, posing a challenge for drug development and prioritization of resources. Pharmacodynamics have an essential role to play in early clinical trials, adding an important set of data for go/no go decisions.

In particular, developing pharmacodynamic biomarkers for immunotherapy is critical to move from single-agent trial to combinatorial strategies and to understand why some clinical trials have failed. Although the use of PD biomarkers has been limited in the past, regulatory pressure, combined with the growing availability of PD biomarkers that offer "more bang for their buck", such as liquid biopsy and NGS testing, combined with the necessity of making informed go-no go decisions guarantee major developments in this area over the coming years.

In the future, the gold standard practice for drug development will include not only PD biomarkers used to show proof-of-mechanism during early clinical trials, but also a complete strategy of pharmacodynamic biomarkers to characterize downstream drug activity and understand phenomenons such as intrinsic treatment resistance and on-target toxicity.

Key Expert Opinion Points

- The number of compounds in clinical oncology development is today growing almost exponentially, posing a challenge for drug development and prioritization of resources.
- Pharmacodynamic biomarkers have an essential role to play in early clinical trials, adding an important set of data for go/no go decisions.
- In particular, developing pharmacodynamic biomarkers for immunotherapy is critical to move from single-agent trial to combinatorial strategies and to understand why some clinical trials have failed.
- Although the use of PD biomarkers has been limited in the past, regulatory pressure, combined with the growing availability of PD biomarkers that offer "more bang for their buck", such as liquid biopsy and NGS testing, guarantee major developments in this area over the coming years.
- In the future, the gold standard practice for drug development will include not only PD biomarkers used to show proof-of-mechanism but also a complete strategy of pharmacodynamic biomarkers to characterize downstream drug activity and understand phenomenons such as intrinsic treatment resistance and on-target toxicity.

References

1. Kelloff GJ, Bast RC, Coffey DS, D'Amico AV, Kerbel RS, Park JW, et al. Biomarkers, surrogate end points, and the acceleration of drug development for cancer prevention and treatment: an update prologue. Clin Cancer Res. 2004 Jun;10(11):3881–4.
2. Gainor JF, Longo DL, Chabner BA. Pharmacodynamic biomarkers: Falling short of the mark? Clin Cancer Res [Internet]. 2014 [cited 2018 Aug 29];20(10):2587–94. Available from: http://www.ncbi.nlm.nih.gov/pubmed/24831281
3. Biomarkers Definitions Working Group. Biomarkers and surrogate endpoints: preferred definitions and conceptual framework. Clin Pharmacol Ther. 2001;69(3):89–95.
4. National Cancer Institute. Pharmacodynamic Biomarkers | Development | NExT Resources | NExT [Internet]. [cited 2019 Jun 3]. Available from: https://next.cancer.gov/developmentResources/pd_biomarker.htm
5. Cerfolio RJ, Bryant AS, Winokur TS, Ohja B, Bartolucci AA. Repeat FDG-PET after neoadjuvant therapy is a predictor of pathologic response in patients with non-small cell lung cancer. Ann Thorac Surg. 2004;78(6):1903–9. discussion 1909
6. Duffy MJ, Harbeck N, Nap M, Molina R, Nicolini A, Senkus E, et al. Clinical use of biomarkers in breast cancer: updated guidelines from the European Group on Tumor Markers (EGTM). Eur J Cancer. 2017;75:284–98.
7. Seruga B, Ocana A, Amir E, Tannock IF. Failures in phase III: causes and consequences. Clin Cancer Res. 2015 Oct;21(20):4552–60.
8. Banerji U, Workman P. Critical parameters in targeted drug development: the pharmacological audit trail. Semin Oncol [Internet]. 2016 Aug 1 [cited 2018 Aug 29];43(4):436–45. Available from: https://www.sciencedirect.com/science/article/pii/S0093775416300306?via%3Dihub
9. De Gramont A, Watson S, Ellis LM, Rodón J, Tabernero J, De Gramont A, et al. Pragmatic issues in biomarker evaluation for targeted therapies in cancer. Nat Rev Clin Oncol. 2015;12:197–212.

10. Goulart BHL, Clark JW, Pien HH, Roberts TG, Finkelstein SN, Chabner BA. Trends in the use and role of biomarkers in phase I oncology trials. Clin Cancer Res. 2007;13(22):6719–26.
11. Workman P. How much gets there and what does it do?: The need for better pharmacokinetic and pharmacodynamic endpoints in contemporary drug discovery and development. Curr Pharm Des [Internet]. 2003 [cited 2018 Sep 9];9(11):891–902. Available from: http://www.ncbi.nlm.nih.gov/pubmed/12678873.
12. Workman P. Challenges of PK/PD measurements in modern drug development [Internet]. Eur J Cancer. 2002 [cited 2018 Sep 9];38: 2189–93. Available from: http://linkinghub.elsevier.com/retrieve/pii/S0959804902003957
13. Bradley E. Incorporating biomarkers into clinical trial designs: points to consider. Nat Biotechnol [Internet]. 2012 Jul 1 [cited 2018 Aug 24];30(7):596–9. Available from: http://www.nature.com/articles/nbt.2296
14. Holohan C, Van Schaeybroeck S, Longley DB, Johnston PG. Cancer drug resistance: an evolving paradigm. Nat Rev Cancer [Internet]. 2013 Oct 24 [cited 2019 Jun 24];13(10):714–26. Available from: http://www.ncbi.nlm.nih.gov/pubmed/24060863
15. Rossanese O, Eccles S, Springer C, Swain A, Raynaud FI, Workman P, et al. The pharmacological audit trail (PhAT): use of tumor models to address critical issues in the preclinical development of targeted anticancer drugs. Drug Discov Today Dis Model [Internet]. 2016 Sep 1 [cited 2018 Aug 29];21(2016):23–32. Available from: https://www.sciencedirect.com/science/article/pii/S1740675717300270
16. FDA. Guidance: Qualification Process for Drug Development Tools. FDA [Internet]. 2014 [cited 2018 Dec 20]. Available from: http://www.fda.gov/cder/guidance/index.htm
17. Mattes WB, Goodsaid F. Regulatory landscapes for biomarkers and diagnostic tests: qualification, approval, and role in clinical practice. Exp Biol Med [Internet]. 2018 Feb 7 [cited 2018 Dec 20];243(3):256–61. Available from: http://www.ncbi.nlm.nih.gov/pubmed/29110507
18. Amur S, Lavange L, Zineh I, Buckman-Garner S, Woodcock J. Biomarker qualification: toward a multiple stakeholder framework for biomarker development, regulatory acceptance, and utilization. Clin Pharmacol Ther [Internet]. 2015 [cited 2018 Dec 20];98(1):34–46. Available from: https://www.fda.gov/downloads/Drugs/NewsEvents/UCM470575.pdf
19. Leptak C, Menetski JP, Wagner JA, Aubrecht J, Brady L, Brumfield M, et al. What evidence do we need for biomarker qualification? [Internet]. Vol. 9, Science translational medicine. 2017 [cited 2018 Dec 20]. pii. eaal4599. Available from: http://www.ncbi.nlm.nih.gov/pubmed/29167393
20. Advice S, Party W, Adoption S, Agreed F, Ema K, Novel C. Qualification of novel methodologies for drug development: guidance to applicants. 2012;44(January):1–16.
21. Manolis E, Koch A, Deforce D, Vamvakas S. The European Medicines Agency experience with biomarker qualification. In: Methods in molecular biology (Clifton, NJ) [Internet]. 2015 [cited 2018 Dec 20]. 255–72. Available from: http://www.ncbi.nlm.nih.gov/pubmed/25384751.
22. Udall M, Rizzo M, Kenny J, Doherty J, Dahm S, Robbins P, et al. PD-L1 diagnostic tests: a systematic literature review of scoring algorithms and test-validation metrics. Diagn Pathol [Internet]. 2018 Feb 9 [cited 2018 Dec 20];13(1):12. Available from: http://www.ncbi.nlm.nih.gov/pubmed/29426340.
23. Lee JW, Devanarayan V, Barrett YC, Weiner R, Allinson J, Fountain S, et al. Fit-for-purpose method development and validation for successful biomarker measurement. Pharm Res. 2006;23:312–28.
24. FDA. CFR - Code of Federal Regulations Title 21, 21CFR172.110 [Internet]. 2014. 2014. 5–6. Available from: http://www.accessdata.fda.gov/scripts/cdrh/cfdocs/cfCFR/CFRSearch.cfm?fr=172.110
25. Yee LM, Lively TG, McShane LM. Biomarkers in early-phase trials: fundamental issues. Bioanalysis [Internet]. 2018 Jun [cited 2018 Aug 24];10(12):933–44. Available from: https://www.future-science.com/doi/10.4155/bio-2018-0006
26. Kinders R, Ferry-Galow K, Wang L, Srivastava AK, Ji JJ, Parchment RE. Implementation of validated pharmacodynamic assays in multiple laboratories: challenges, successes, and limita-

tions. Clin Cancer Res [Internet]. 2014 May 15 [cited 2018 Nov 9];20(10):2578–86. Available from.: http://www.ncbi.nlm.nih.gov/pubmed/24831280.
27. Shen L, Kantarjian H, Guo Y, Lin E, Shan J, Huang X, et al. DNA methylation predicts survival and response to therapy in patients with myelodysplastic syndromes. J Clin Oncol [Internet]. 2010 Feb 1 [cited 2016 Sep 19];28(4):605–13. Available from: http://www.ncbi.nlm.nih.gov/pubmed/20038729.
28. Lalonde RL, Kowalski KG, Hutmacher MM, Ewy W, Nichols DJ, Milligan PA, et al. Model-based drug development. Clin Pharmacol Ther [Internet]. 2007 Jul 23 [cited 2018 Dec 20];82(1):21–32. Available from.: http://www.ncbi.nlm.nih.gov/pubmed/17522597.
29. Williams PJ, Ette EI. Pharmacometrics: impacting drug development and pharmacotherapy. In: Pharmacometrics: the science of quantitative pharmacology [Internet]. Hoboken, NJ: Wiley; 2006 [cited 2018 Dec 20]. 1–21. Available from: http://doi.wiley.com/10.1002/9780470087978.ch1
30. Kimko H, Pinheiro J. Model-based clinical drug development in the past, present and future: a commentary. Br J Clin Pharmacol [Internet]. 2015 Jan [cited 2018 Dec 20];79(1):108–16. Available from: http://www.ncbi.nlm.nih.gov/pubmed/24527997
31. Elassaiss-Schaap J, Rossenu S, Lindauer A, Kang S, de Greef R, Sachs J, et al. Using model-based "learn and confirm" to reveal the pharmacokinetics-pharmacodynamics relationship of pembrolizumab in the KEYNOTE-001 trial. CPT Pharmacometrics Syst Pharmacol [Internet]. 2017 Jan 1 [cited 2018 Dec 20];6(1):21–8. Available from: http://doi.wiley.com/10.1002/psp4.12132
32. Agoram BM. Use of pharmacokinetic/ pharmacodynamic modelling for starting dose selection in first-in-human trials of high-risk biologics. Br J Clin Pharmacol [Internet]. 2009 Feb [cited 2018 Dec 20];67(2):153–60. Available from: http://www.ncbi.nlm.nih.gov/pubmed/19076987
33. Bender BC, Schindler E, Friberg LE. Population pharmacokinetic-pharmacodynamic modelling in oncology: a tool for predicting clinical response. Br J Clin Pharmacol [Internet]. 2015 Jan [cited 2018 Dec 20];79(1):56–71. Available from.: http://www.ncbi.nlm.nih.gov/pubmed/24134068
34. Lorch U, O'Kane M, Taubel J. Three steps to writing adaptive study protocols in the early phase clinical development of new medicines. BMC Med Res Methodol [Internet]. 2014 Dec 30 [cited 2018 Dec 20];14(1):84. Available from: http://bmcmedresmethodol.biomedcentral.com/articles/10.1186/1471-2288-14-84
35. Petroni GR, Wages NA, Paux G, Dubois F. Implementation of adaptive methods in early-phase clinical trials. Stat Med [Internet]. 2017 Jan 30 [cited 2018 Dec 20];36(2):215–24. Available from: http://doi.wiley.com/10.1002/sim.6910
36. Mandrekar SJ, Sargent DJ. Design of clinical trials for biomarker research in oncology. Clin Investig (Lond) [Internet]. 2011 Dec [cited 2018 Aug 24];1(12):1629–36. Available from: http://www.ncbi.nlm.nih.gov/pubmed/22389760
37. Yan F, Mandrekar SJ, Yuan Y. Keyboard: a novel Bayesian toxicity probability interval design for phase I clinical trials. Clin Cancer Res [Internet]. 2017 Aug 1 [cited 2017 Aug 1];23(15):3994–4003. Available from: http://clincancerres.aacrjournals.org/content/23/15/3994?rss=1
38. Berry DA. The Brave New World of clinical cancer research: Adaptive biomarker-driven trials integrating clinical practice with clinical research. Mol Oncol [Internet]. 2015 May 1 [cited 2018 Nov 12];9(5):951–9. Available from: https://www.sciencedirect.com/science/article/pii/S1574789115000472
39. Swain SM, Kim SB, Cortés J, Ro J, Semiglazov V, Campone M, et al. Pertuzumab, trastuzumab, and docetaxel for HER2-positive metastatic breast cancer (CLEOPATRA study): overall survival results from a randomised, double-blind, placebo-controlled, phase 3 study. Lancet Oncol. 2013;
40. Generali D, Ardine M, Strina C, Milani M, Cappelletti MR, Zanotti L, et al. Neoadjuvant treatment approach: The rosetta stone for breast cancer? J Natl Cancer Inst - Monogr [Internet]. 2015 May 1 [cited 2018 Dec 20];2015(51):32–5. Available from: https://academic.oup.com/jncimono/article-lookup/doi/10.1093/jncimonographs/lgv019

41. Agulnik M, Oza AM, Pond GR, Siu LL. Impact and perceptions of mandatory tumor biopsies for correlative studies in clinical trials of novel anticancer agents. J Clin Oncol. 2006 Oct;24(30):4801–7.
42. Flaherty KT, Puzanov I, Kim KB, Ribas A, McArthur GA, Sosman JA, et al. Inhibition of mutated, activated BRAF in metastatic melanoma. N Engl J Med. 2010 Aug;363(9):809–19.
43. Malik SN, Siu LL, Rowinsky EK, deGraffenried L, Hammond LA, Rizzo J, et al. Pharmacodynamic evaluation of the epidermal growth factor receptor inhibitor OSI-774 in human epidermis of cancer patients. Clin Cancer Res. 2003 Jul;9(7):2478–86.
44. Shepherd FA, Rodrigues Pereira J, Ciuleanu T, Tan EH, Hirsh V, Thongprasert S, et al. Erlotinib in previously treated non–small-cell lung cancer. N Engl J Med. 2005 Jul;353(2):123–32.
45. Greystoke A, O'Connor JPB, Linton K, Taylor MB, Cummings J, Ward T, et al. Assessment of circulating biomarkers for potential pharmacodynamic utility in patients with lymphoma. Br J Cancer [Internet]. 2011 Feb 18 [cited 2018 Dec 20];104(4):719–25. Available from: http://www.ncbi.nlm.nih.gov/pubmed/21245866
46. DePrimo SE, Bello CL, Smeraglia J, Baum CM, Spinella D, Rini BI, et al. Circulating protein biomarkers of pharmacodynamic activity of sunitinib in patients with metastatic renal cell carcinoma: modulation of VEGF and VEGF-related proteins. J Transl Med [Internet]. 2007 Jul 2 [cited 2018 Dec 20];5(1):32. Available from: http://translational-medicine.biomedcentral.com/articles/10.1186/1479-5876-5-32
47. Gros A, Parkhurst MR, Tran E, Pasetto A, Robbins PF, Ilyas S, et al. Prospective identification of neoantigen-specific lymphocytes in the peripheral blood of melanoma patients. Nat Med [Internet]. 2016 Apr 22 [cited 2018 Dec 21];22(4):433–8. Available from.: http://www.ncbi.nlm.nih.gov/pubmed/26901407
48. Yap TA, Lorente D, Omlin A, Olmos D, de Bono JS. Circulating tumor cells: a multifunctional biomarker. Clin Cancer Res [Internet]. 2014 May 15 [cited 2018 Dec 20];20(10):2553–68. Available from.: http://www.ncbi.nlm.nih.gov/pubmed/24831278
49. Miyamoto DT, Lee RJ, Stott SL, Ting DT, Wittner BS, Ulman M, et al. Androgen receptor signaling in circulating tumor cells as a marker of hormonally responsive prostate cancer. Cancer Discov [Internet]. 2012 Nov 1 [cited 2018 Dec 20];2(11):995–1003. Available from.: http://www.ncbi.nlm.nih.gov/pubmed/23093251
50. Hodgkinson CL, Morrow CJ, Li Y, Metcalf RL, Rothwell DG, Trapani F, et al. Tumorigenicity and genetic profiling of circulating tumor cells in small-cell lung cancer. Nat Med [Internet]. 2014 Aug 1 [cited 2018 Dec 20];20(8):897–903. Available from.: http://www.ncbi.nlm.nih.gov/pubmed/24880617
51. Siravegna G, Marsoni S, Siena S, Bardelli A. Integrating liquid biopsies into the management of cancer. Nat Rev Clin Oncol [Internet]. 2017 Mar 2 [cited 2018 Dec 20];14(9):531–48. Available from: http://www.nature.com/doifinder/10.1038/nrclinonc.2017.14
52. Wan JCM, Massie C, Garcia-Corbacho J, Mouliere F, Brenton JD, Caldas C, et al. Liquid biopsies come of age: towards implementation of circulating tumour DNA. Nat Rev Cancer [Internet]. 2017 Feb 24 [cited 2017 Feb 24];17(4):223–38. Available from: http://www.nature.com/articles/nrc.2017.7
53. Jackson RC. Pharmacodynamic modelling of biomarker data in oncology. ISRN Pharmacol [Internet]. 2012 Feb 16 [cited 2018 Aug 29];2012:1–12. Available from: https://www.hindawi.com/archive/2012/590626/
54. Merchant S, Witney TH, Aboagye EO. Imaging as a pharmacodynamic and response biomarker in cancer. Clin Transl Imaging [Internet]. 2014 Feb 11 [cited 2018 Aug 29];2(1):13–31. Available from: http://link.springer.com/10.1007/s40336-014-0049-z
55. Carney B, Kossatz S, Lok B, Poirier J, Weber W, Rudin C, Reiner T. In vivo characterization of two PARP inhibitors using a recently developed PET imaging agent in small cell lung cancer. J Nucl Med. 2016;57:334.
56. Sweis RF, Medved M, Towey S, Karczmar GS, Oto A, Szmulewitz RZ, et al. Dynamic contrast-enhanced magnetic resonance imaging as a pharmacodynamic biomarker for pazopanib in metastatic renal carcinoma. Clin Genitourin Cancer [Internet]. 2017 Apr 1 [cited

2018 Dec 20];15(2):207–12. Available from: https://www.sciencedirect.com/science/article/pii/S1558767316302452
57. Lin FI, Gonzalez EM, Kummar S, Do K, Shih J, Adler S, et al. Utility of 18F-fluoroestradiol (18F-FES) PET/CT imaging as a pharmacodynamic marker in patients with refractory estrogen receptor-positive solid tumors receiving Z-endoxifen therapy. Eur J Nucl Med Mol Imaging [Internet]. 2017 Mar 21 [cited 2018 Dec 20];44(3):500–8. Available from: http://link.springer.com/10.1007/s00259-016-3561-8
58. Cancer Institute N. Common Terminology Criteria for Adverse Events v3.0 (CTCAE). In: Principles and Practice of Clinical Trial Medicine [Internet]. 2008. 461–533. Available from: https://linkinghub.elsevier.com/retrieve/pii/B9780123736956000223
59. Brahmer JR, Lacchetti C, Schneider BJ, Atkins MB, Brassil KJ, Caterino JM, et al. Management of immune-related adverse events in patients treated with immune checkpoint inhibitor therapy: American Society of Clinical Oncology Clinical Practice Guideline. J Clin Oncol [Internet]. 2018 Jun 10 [cited 2018 Dec 20];36(17):1714–68. Available from: http://ascopubs.org/doi/10.1200/JCO.2017.77.6385
60. Ribas A, Hodi FS, Callahan M, Konto C, Wolchok J. Hepatotoxicity with Combination of Vemurafenib and Ipilimumab. N Engl J Med [Internet]. 2013 Apr 4 [cited 2018 Dec 20];368(14):1365–6. Available from.: http://www.ncbi.nlm.nih.gov/pubmed/23550685
61. Amin A, Lawson DH, Salama AK, Koon HB, Guthrie T, Thomas SS, et al. Phase II study of vemurafenib followed by ipilimumab in patients with previously untreated BRAF-mutated metastatic melanoma. J Immunother Cancer. 2016; https://doi.org/10.1186/s40425-016-0148-7.
62. Cristescu R, Mogg R, Ayers M, Albright A, Murphy E, Yearley J, et al. Pan-tumor genomic biomarkers for PD-1 checkpoint blockade-based immunotherapy. Science [Internet]. 2018 Oct 12 [cited 2018 Oct 18];362(6411):eaar3593. Available from.: http://www.ncbi.nlm.nih.gov/pubmed/30309915
63. Ochoa de Olza M, Oliva M, Hierro C, Matos I, Martin-Liberal J, Garralda E. Early-drug development in the era of immuno-oncology: are we ready to face the challenges? Ann Oncol [Internet]. 2018 Aug 1 [cited 2018 Aug 17];29(8):1727–40. Available from: https://academic.oup.com/annonc/article/29/8/1727/5045458
64. Smoragiewicz M, Bogaerts J, Calvo E, Marabelle A, Perrone A, Seymour L, et al. Design and conduct of early clinical studies of immunotherapy agent combinations: recommendations from the task force on methodology for the development of innovative cancer therapies. Ann Oncol [Internet]. 2018 Nov 1 [cited 2018 Dec 20];29(11):2175–82. Available from: https://academic.oup.com/annonc/article/29/11/2175/5094492
65. Parchment RE, Voth AR, Doroshow JH, Berzofsky JA. Immuno-pharmacodynamics for evaluating mechanism of action and developing immunotherapy combinations. Semin Oncol. 2016;43(4):501–13.
66. Tumeh PC, Harview CL, Yearley JH, Shintaku IP, Taylor EJM, Robert L, et al. PD-1 blockade induces responses by inhibiting adaptive immune resistance. Nature. 2014 Nov;515(7528):568–71.
67. Chen PL, Roh W, Reuben A, Cooper ZA, Spencer CN, Prieto PA, et al. Analysis of immune signatures in longitudinal tumor samples yields insight into biomarkers of response and mechanisms of resistance to immune checkpoint blockade. Cancer Discov. 2016;6(8):827–37.
68. van Brummelen E, Lassen U, Melero I, Tabernero J, Homicsko K, Angevin E, et al. 1181PPharmacokinetics (PK) and Pharmacodynamics (PD) of cergutuzumab amunaleukin (CA), a carcinoembryonic antigen (CEA)-targeted interleukin 2 variant (IL2v) with abolished binding to CD25. Ann Oncol [Internet]. 2017 Sep 1 [cited 2018 Dec 20];28(suppl_5). Available from: http://academic.oup.com/annonc/article/doi/10.1093/annonc/mdx376.046/4109260/1181PPharmacokinetics-PK-and-Pharmacodynamics-PD
69. Nicolazzo C, Raimondi C, Mancini M, Caponnetto S, Gradilone A, Gandini O, et al. Monitoring PD-L1 positive circulating tumor cells in non-small cell lung cancer patients treated with the PD-1 inhibitor Nivolumab. Sci Rep [Internet]. 2016 Oct 24 [cited 2018 Dec 20];6(1):31726. Available from.: http://www.ncbi.nlm.nih.gov/pubmed/27553175

Chapter 10
Efficacy Considerations in Phase I Trials

Kanan Alshammari, Kirsty Taylor, and Lillian L. Siu

Abstract The traditional goals of phase I trials are to determine safety and tolerability, maximum tolerated dose (MTD) and recommend phase II dose (RP2D) for a new drug or drug combination, and assessments for antitumor activity have been considered ancillary. Changes in the drug development landscape have been rapid, especially with the emergence of precision oncology that enables genotype-drug matching, and immuno-oncology that harnesses host immunity. The need to make go-no-go decisions at an earlier time point in a drug's developmental path, and the urgency to bring effective compounds to patients, have fueled the growing role of efficacy considerations in phase I trials. In this chapter, key distinctive features of standard imaging based response criteria are reviewed. In addition, alternative ways to determine antitumor activity, such as new imaging based approaches, time based efficacy evaluations and biomarker driven strategies are highlighted. Innovative clinical trial methodology including enrichment for target patient populations, phase 0 trials, use of expansion cohorts and seamless designs, as well as appropriate patient selection through the application of validated prognostic indices, may optimize the efficacy read-out in patients who participate in phase I trials.

Keywords Phase I · Clinical trial methodology · Efficacy · Objective response Time-based analysis · RECIST · iRECIST · Biomarker · Radiomics · Expansion cohort · Seamless design · Prognostic index

---

K. Alshammari · K. Taylor
Division of Medical Oncology and Hematology, Princess Margaret Cancer Centre, University Health Network, Toronto, ON, Canada

Department of Medicine, University of Toronto, Toronto, ON, Canada
e-mail: alshammarika@ngha.med.sa; ktaylor13@qub.ac.uk

L. L. Siu (✉)
Division of Medical Oncology and Hematology, Princess Margaret Cancer Centre, University Health Network, Toronto, ON, Canada

Department of Medicine, University of Toronto, Toronto, ON, Canada

Princess Margaret Cancer Centre, Toronto, ON, Canada
e-mail: lillian.siu@uhn.ca

T. A. Yap et al. (eds.), *Phase I Oncology Drug Development*,
https://doi.org/10.1007/978-3-030-47682-3_10

Key Points

1. Efficacy considerations including objective tumor response (ORR), time-based endpoints such as progression-free survival (PFS), and biomarker-based evaluation of antitumor effects are increasingly observed in phase I trials.
2. Key distinguishing features of various response criteria including RECIST 1.1, iRECIST, specific considerations for solid tumors (e.g. ovarian cancer, prostate cancer) and hematological malignancies (e.g. lymphoma, multiple myeloma) are reviewed.
3. Predictive biomarker-based strategies to enable patient selection and pharmacodynamic biomarker-based assessments of target engagement using tumor and blood samples in phase I trials are discussed.
4. Phase I clinical trial design elements such as enrichment for specific target populations, use of expansion cohorts and seamless trials, are often used to maximize the opportunity for efficacy assessments in the early drug development process.
5. Prognostic indices exist that may be applied to ensure appropriate patients are enrolled into phase I trials who are suitable for safety evaluation beyond DLT period and for efficacy assessment.

10.1 Introduction

Traditionally, the goals of a phase I clinical trial have been to determine the safety, tolerability, and maximally tolerated dose (MTD) of the studied drug or drug combinations, the basis upon which a phase II dose is recommended (RP2D). More recently, these goals have been evolving, and many phase I trials now encompass a more comprehensive study of the "body's effect on the drug" i.e. pharmacokinetic evaluations; and the "drugs' effect on the body" i.e. pharmacodynamic biomarkers for proof of mechanism, and early reporting of objective tumor responses or efficacy for proof of concept. With the implementation of more realistic *in vivo* models (such as genomically characterized patient-derived xenografts), novel clinical trial designs [such as seamless phase I/II studies, adaptive designs, etc. (reviewed in Chap. 10)] and clearly defined go-no-go decisions, less than promising drugs are terminated early in their development and potentially active agents are being selected to proceed to phase I trials [1]. Also, advances in knowledge have been unprecedented, including the understanding of molecular oncology pathways, the host immune system and its interaction with the tumor microenvironment, coupled with progress in technology such as molecular characterization of tumors for precision oncology and immunophenotyping. From a methodological perspective, strategic applications of enrichment designs with specific histologic characteristics and biomarkers have been associated with higher probability of clinical benefit [2]. Furthermore, careful selection of patients using validated prognostic indices such as the Royal Marsden Hospital index can help identify patients who are expected to survive during their participation in phase I trials. In this chapter, the endpoint of efficacy considerations within the context of phase I clinical trials is discussed. Besides conventional response evaluation using different validated criteria, efficacy assessments using alternative imaging based methods and biomarker based studies are considered.

10.2 Conventional Validated Response Evaluation

10.2.1 RECIST 1.1 v iRECIST

Response evaluation to assess the efficacy of cytotoxic chemotherapy in clinical practice and all phases of clinical trials has been well established, validated and consistent since the Response Evaluation Criteria in Solid Tumors (RECIST) working group simplified the 1981 World Health Organization (WHO) response criteria in 2000. These were then revised and refined to RECIST 1.1 in 2009 and remain the criteria used by US Food and Drug Administration (FDA) and other regulatory agencies to grant license and approval for new therapies [3]. The application of RECIST 1.1 in phase I trials for efficacy assessment is generally to report on tumor size changes during the experimental period when the investigational agent is administered. The evaluation of tumor growth rate, which compares tumor growth kinetics by RECIST 1.1 between the washout period before the introduction of the investigational drug (reference period) and the experimental period, has been advocated by some groups, though it remains underused in phase I trials [4].

The introduction of molecularly targeted agents, often resulting in stabilization of disease, questioned the applicability of RECIST 1.1 to measure the antitumor activity of these drugs. A RECIST working group analysis of pooled individual patient data from phase II and III clinical trials evaluated molecularly targeted agents in solid tumors, demonstrated comparable results for these compounds and cytotoxic chemotherapy without modification [5]. However, with the changing landscape of anti-cancer agents to include immunotherapy, unique patterns of response are observed that are not adequately captured by these traditional response criteria. Pseudoprogression, the increase in tumor measurements as a result of immune cell infiltration, can lead to premature withdrawal of therapy, from which patients may actually benefit [6]. The past decade has seen a number of novel response criteria developed to evaluate patients who receive immune-modulating drugs. In 2009 Wolchok et al. proposed the immune-related response criteria (irRC) based on the original WHO criteria [7], and in 2013 revised guidance was published using unidimensional measurements in line with the original RECIST criteria, termed immune-related RECIST (irRECIST) [8]. These criteria are typically used in conjunction with RECIST 1.1 in the clinical trial setting, each with their own differences and limitations. Their application has not always been consistent and raised concerns among researchers and clinicians alike regarding the comparability of data and results between clinical trials.

In an effort to standardize and validate immune response criteria, the RECIST working group evaluated data collected from prospective clinical trials using immunotherapy and RECIST 1.1, to develop guidelines for modified RECIST, termed immune RECIST (iRECIST) [9]. The continued use of RECIST 1.1 is recommended to define lesions that are measurable and non-measurable, the standard clinical imaging methods for measurement and the broad principles used to establish objective tumor response. The major difference is the concept of reassessing disease burden following initial progression in clinically stable patients, to annotate whether there is subsequent tumor shrinkage versus confirmed progression. Tables 10.1 and 10.2 outline the key differences between these 2 criteria and immune time point responses, respectively [9].

Table 10.1 Comparison of RECIST 1.1 and iRECIST

	RECIST 1.1	iRECIST
Definition of measurable disease; numbers and site of target disease	Measurable lesions are ≥10 mm in diameter (≥15 mm for nodal lesions); maximum of 5 lesions (2 per organ); all other disease is considered non-target (must be ≥10 mm in short axis for nodal disease)	As per RECIST 1.1; however, new lesions are assessed as per RECIST 1.1 but recorded separately (not included in the sum of lesions for target lesions identified at baseline)
Complete response (CR), partial response (PR), or stable disease (SD)	Cannot have met criteria for progression before CR, PR or SD	Can have previous iUPD (one or more instances), but not iCPD, prior to confirmed iCR, iPR, or iSD
Confirmation of CR or PR	Required for non-randomized trials only	As per RECIST 1.1
Confirmation of SD	Not required	As per RECIST 1.1
New lesions	Result in progression; recorded but not measured	iUPD at first appearance, iCPD only assigned if at next assessment additional new lesions confirmed or an increase of new lesions (≥5 mm sum of new lesions target or any increase in new lesion non-target); new lesions when none previously recorded can also confirm iCPD.
Independent blinded review and central collection of scans	Recommended in some circumstances (e.g. trials with progression-based endpoints planned for marketing approval)	Collection of scans but not independent review for all trials
Confirmation of progression	Not required (unless equivocal)	Required
Consideration of clinical status	Not included in assessment	Aids determination of continuation after iUPD

"i" indicates immune responses using iRECIST. *RECIST* response evaluation criteria in solid tumors; *iUPD* unconfirmed progression; *iCPD* confirmed progression; *iCR* complete response; *iPR* partial response; *iSD* stable disease

Table 10.2 Assignment of time point response using iRECIST

	Time point response with no previous iUPD	Time point response with previous iUPD[a]
Target lesions: iCR; Non-target lesions: iCR; New lesions: no	iCR	iCR
Target lesions: iCR; Non-target lesions: non-iCR/ non-iUPD; New lesions: no	iPR	iPR
Target lesions: iPR; Non-target lesions: non-iCR/ non-iUPD; New lesions: no	iPR	iPR
Target lesions: iSD; Non-target lesions: non-iCR/ non-iUPD; New lesions: no	iSD	iSD
Target lesions: iUPD, or decrease from last time point; Non-target lesions: iUPD, or decrease from last time point; New lesions: yes	N/A	New lesions confirm iCPD if new lesions were previously identified and have increased in size (≥5 mm in sum of measures for new lesion target or any increase for new lesion non-target) or number; If no change in new lesions (size or number) from last time point, remains iUPD
Target lesions: iSD, iPR, iCR; Non-target lesions: iUPD; New lesions: no	iUPD	Remains iUPD unless iCPD confirmed based on further increase in the size of non-target disease (does not need to meet RECIST 1.1 criteria for unequivocal progression)
Target lesions: iUPD; Non-target lesions: non-iCR/non-iUPD, or iCR; New lesions: no	iUPD	Remains iUPD unless iCPD confirmed based on further increase in sum of measures ≥5 mm, otherwise remains iUPD
Target lesions: iUPD; Non-target lesions: iUPD; New lesions: no	iUPD	Remains iUPD unless iCPD confirmed based on a further increase in previously identified target lesion iUPD in sum of measures ≥5 mm or non-target lesion iUPD (previous assessment does not need to show unequivocal progression)

Table 10.2 (continued)

	Time point response with no previous iUPD	Time point response with previous iUPD[a]
Target lesions: iUPD; Non-target lesions: iUPD; New lesions: yes	iUPD	Remains iUPD unless iCPD confirmed based on further increase in previously identified target lesion iUPD sum of measures ≥5 mm, previously identified non-target lesion iUPD (does not need to be unequivocal), or an increase in the size or number of new lesions previously identified
Target lesions: non-iUPD or progression; Non-target lesions: non-iUPD or progression; New lesions: yes	iUPD	Remains iUPD unless iCPD is confirmed on the basis of an increase in the size or number of new lesions previously identified

[a]Target lesions, non-target lesions, and new lesions defined according to RECIST 1.1; if no pseudoprogression occurs, RECIST 1.1 and iRECIST categories for complete response, partial response, and stable disease are the same

Another unique response seen with immune checkpoint inhibitors is that of hyperprogressive disease (HPD), accelerated tumor growth rate (TGR) compared with pretreatment kinetics. This is not yet well characterized, with variability in both the definition of HPD and in the calculation of TGR across investigators, limiting direct comparison [10]. Unlike pseudoprogression, immune response criteria are not well adapted to identify this phenomenon and no consistent predictor has been identified in early phase immunotherapy trials [11–13] with further prospective clarification required.

The iRECIST guidelines aid in the assessment of unique pseudo-responses with immunotherapy, offer guidance on assessment of patient stability and provide a framework for consistency of evaluation and data management among clinical trials [9]. At present the recommendation remains that randomized studies planned for licensing application continue to use RECIST 1.1 as the primary criteria for response-based end points, with iRECIST continuing to be an exploratory endpoint. However, in early phase trials it is reasonable to consider using primarily iRECIST as appropriate to guide the therapeutic development of immuno-oncology agents [14].

10.2.2 Specific Solid Tumor Populations

In addition to RECIST 1.1 there are a number of validated response assessment scores specific to individual solid cancer types, commonly included in efficacy evaluation of early phase trials.

10.2.2.1 Ovarian Cancer

CA125 is an accurate, readily available and validated response marker for patients with ovarian cancer [15, 16]. The Gynecological Cancer Intergroup (GCIG) [17, 18] recommend that for trials of relapsed ovarian cancer, response according to CA125 be used in addition to RECIST 1.1. CA125 response is defined as at least a 50% reduction in pre-treatment CA125 levels, which must be ≥2 times ULN (upper limit of normal) within 2 weeks of commencing treatment. Reduction must be confirmed and maintained for 28 days. A CA125 level reduced to within the normal range is considered a CA125 complete response. Of note, patients are considered non-evaluable if there has been peritoneal intervention within the previous 28 days. Patients may be measurable by one or both RECIST 1.1 and CA125 criteria, and may have different time point responses. The date of the overall efficacy outcome assessment is determined by the earlier of the two events, and specific guidance is provided by GCIG depending on nadir CA125.

10.2.2.2 Prostate Cancer

Updated response criteria have been defined by the Prostate Cancer Clinical Trials Working Group (PCWG3) [19, 20] and are used in assessing eligibility for early phase clinical trials and in conjunction with RECIST 1.1 for efficacy assessment. They aim to move drug development closer to the unmet needs in clinical practice, focusing on the concept of clinical benefit, to highlight the difference between first evidence of progression and clinical need to discontinue treatment. PCWG3 criteria classify patients by number and sequence of previous lines of therapy, stratify by histological subtype and define best imaging practices. Computed Tomography (CT) or Magnetic Resonance Imaging (MRI) of the abdomen and pelvis, along with nuclear medicine bone scan remain the standard imaging modalities for prostate cancer patients, but with increased frequency of initial monitoring and specific guidance on distinguishing true disease progression from initial disease flare in cases with bone only metastases.

PSA response is also incorporated with best PSA response monitored throughout treatment and categorized as response, non-response or progression. "Response" requires a 50% decrease from baseline, maintained for ≥4 weeks; "non-response" is defined as a failure to achieve PSA response; and "progression" is defined as a ≥ 25% increase of PSA value from the nadir and an absolute increase of ≥2 μg/L, confirmed by a second value ≥3 weeks later. With the delivery of systemic treatment, early PSA rises ≤12 weeks after commencing treatment are not uncommon and should not be considered for the classification of best response. Provided there is no clinical evidence of progression, patients should remain on treatment until definitive progression is confirmed.

10.2.3 Hematological Malignancies

The hematological malignancies comprise a heterogeneous collection of conditions with varying clinical behaviors and response profiles. Objective means of evaluating treatment efficacy through response criteria have evolved as the combination of medical imaging and molecular techniques can provide more functional information. The respective international working groups have revised, standardized and validated new response criteria in some of these hematological malignancies, while others face challenges in the implementation of such guidelines to recognize emerging treatments, technologies and evolving endpoints [21].

10.2.3.1 Lymphoma

The Lugano Classification has been the standard response criteria for evaluating response in lymphoma since 2014, based on CT and Positron Emission Tomography-CT (PET-CT) imaging, the latter preferred for ^{18}F-Fluorodeoxyglucose (FDG)-avid lymphomas [22, 23]. This classification modifies the Deauville five-point scoring system (D5PS), which grades the intensity of ^{18}F-FDG uptake, and assists in both overall and interim response assessments, enabling improved determinations of prognosis and earlier treatment modifications [24, 25].

The increase in approved and investigational agents being administered to lymphoma patients as standard of care or within the context of early and late phase clinical trials, led to an effort by the International Working Group in 2017 to harmonize the Lugano Criteria with RECIST; Response Evaluation Criteria in Lymphoma (RECIL) optimizes the use of FDG-PET uptake in combination with single dimension tumor measurement of target lesions to assess tumor burden. The authors defined frequency of response assessment and in line with solid tumor clinical trial efficacy assessment, RECIL accommodates for potential pseudoprogression in those receiving immune-modulating agents by requiring confirmation on consecutive scans [26].

10.2.3.2 Multiple Myeloma

In 2014, the International Myeloma Working Group (IMWG) diagnostic criteria changed the definition of multiple myeloma from a disease defined by symptoms to a disease defined by biomarkers including serum and urine paraproteins, free light chains and bone marrow clonal plasma cells. In response to this in 2016 the IMWG updated their response criteria, outlining treatment response assessment and also included minimal residual disease (MRD) as the deepest level of treatment response in multiple myeloma, correlating with longer progression-free and overall survival [27]. The magnitude of change in paraprotein and the normalization of the free light chain ratio (rFLC) form the basis of these response criteria. A retrospective review of 87 patients with relapsed or refractory multiple myeloma, with sufficient data for analysis, enrolled in 19 early-phase clinical trials demonstrated a statistically significant improvement in both PFS and OS at sequential time points; validating the use of IMWG response criteria in the phase I trial setting and suggesting the use of these criteria as viable biomarkers for surrogate endpoints in early phase clinical trials and drug development [28].

10.3 Alternative Evaluations of Efficacy

10.3.1 Alternative Imaging Based Evaluation of Response

It remains a significant challenge to improve the efficacy output of early phase clinical trials by effectively identifying patients who are likely to derive benefit from specific treatments. Objective tumor responses to different therapeutic agents are variable based on patient and tumor characteristics, thus innovative predictors of response to enable subject selection are needed to improve treatment outcomes.

Evaluation of the characteristics of human tissue non-invasively by medical imaging, most commonly with CT or MRI which assess tissue density in one or two dimensional qualitative descriptors, remains the standard of care. Advances in image acquisition and analysis allowing objective and quantitative imaging descriptors to be extracted, have led to the development of novel techniques to predict and monitor tumor response to systemic anti-cancer therapies. These new techniques avail of routine imaging scheduled as standard longitudinal response assessments and are being incorporated as exploratory endpoints in clinical trial protocols in all phases.

Radiomics, defined as high-throughput extraction of quantitative features resulting in the conversion of images into mineable data to generate imaging biomarkers, is the most developed technique in the field of medical image analysis [29]. Tissue-specific spatial information can be extracted, to include tumor texture, density, shape and other parameters, which can then be analyzed to build predictive models. Radiomics employs advanced image processing methods through machine learning algorithms to compute, quantify and classify such spatial information [30]. This technique has demonstrated success in developing algorithms that significantly correlate with a number of clinical, histological and molecular parameters [31–33]. For example, a robust association has been shown between radio-phenotypes and gene expression in glioblastomas, including a link with epidermal growth factor receptor (EGFR) overexpression [34] and allowing for survival prediction and stratification of treatment outcomes of disease with better accuracy than existing radiological risk models [35]. In patients with non-small cell lung cancer (NSCLC), EGFR mutation status in pre-surgical patients [36] and response to the EGFR inhibitor gefitinib [37] were reflected in radiomic features. These pilot radiomics studies have to date largely been carried out in patients with localized disease. The application of radiomics in the metastatic setting, to include early phase trial participants, brings new challenges. The presence of inter and intra-tumor heterogeneity due to disease evolution and treatment selection pressures can confound the development of robust radiomic signatures in patients with advanced cancers.

In addition, in the immunotherapy era, radiomic signatures to differentiate between true and pseudoprogression and to clarify radiographic toxicity from treatment such as pneumonitis, are being actively sought [38–40]. A study from Gustave Roussy recently investigated a radiomic estimator of tumor infiltrating CD8 T-cells, to assess association with tumor immune phenotype and evaluate outcomes in mixed solid tumor patients enrolled in phase I monotherapy trials of inhibitors of programmed death protein or its ligand (PD1/PD-L1). They found the final radiomic score to be associated with gene expression signature of CD8 T-cells; and that a higher radiomic score at baseline correlated with both objective response rate (ORR) and overall survival (OS) in patients treated with immunotherapy. The eight variable radiomic signature was validated in three independent cohorts. This promising study was able to predict clinical outcomes of patients treated with immune checkpoint inhibitors in a non-invasive manner by successfully integrating radiomic and genomic features [41–43].

The field of radiomics is evolving, however, the current level of evidence is insufficient, and lacks standardized evaluation. Further work is required for validation in prospective studies and to develop evaluation criteria before routine incorporation in clinical trials for efficacy assessment can be considered.

10.3.2 Time Based Efficacy Endpoints

Time based efficacy endpoints such as time to progression (TTP), progression-free survival (PFS), and OS are frequently used in phases II and III, but rarely phase I, clinical trials. The lack of a comparator control arm in most phase I clinical trials renders time-based endpoints challenging as a reliable readout for efficacy. Furthermore, these efficacy endpoints are difficult to interpret especially during the dose escalation process, due to the enrollment of patients with different histologies and other disease characteristics, heterogeneity in patients' prior therapies, and variations in dose and/or schedule being tested. However, the reporting of time-based endpoints does occur in some phase I trials (Table 10.3), typically as a secondary or exploratory objective to provide a preliminary efficacy read-out. Interestingly, PFS was used as a primary endpoint in the WINTHER trial (NCT01856296), a precision medicine trial which matched patients to suggested therapies based on genomic and transcriptomic results. In this study, patients' PFS on immediate prior standard therapy (PFS1) was compared to their PFS on WINTHER-oriented therapy (PFS2), with a ratio of PFS2/PFS1 of >1.5 defining a positive outcome [48]. Similarly, the MOSCATO-01 trial which used high-throughput genomic analyses to match patients to suggested therapies also used PFS as its primary endpoint. However, unlike in WINTHER, a PFS2/PFS1 ratio of more than 1.3 was considered positive [49]. Other scenarios in which endpoints such

Table 10.3 Examples of reporting of time-based efficacy endpoints in phase I trials

Agent	Mechanism of action	Patient population	Sample size	Time-based endpoints	Design and Reference
Crizotinib	Inhibition of ROS1 signaling	NSCLC with ROS1 rearrangement	50	ORR, PFS	Single-arm expansion cohort of phase I trial [44]
Larotrectinib	Inhibition of TRK signaling	Advanced solid tumors with TRK rearrangement	55	ORR, PFS	Compilation of results from 3 single-arm phase I, I/II, II trials [45]
Pembrolizumab	Inhibition of PD-1	Locally advanced or metastatic NSCLC	495	ORR, PFS, OS	Seamless trial design with multiple expansion cohorts including use of randomization in some cohorts [46]
Atezolizumab	Inhibition of PD-L1	Metastatic RCC	70	ORR, PFS, OS	Seamless trial design with multiple expansion cohorts [47]

NSCLC non-small cell lung cancer; *RCC* renal cell carcinoma; *ORR* objective response rate; *PFS* progression free survival; *OS* overall survival

as PFS or OS are reported in phase I trials include histology based or biomarker specific expansion cohorts after initial dose escalation, often through the application of seamless trial design with multiple expansion cohorts that may or may not involve randomization. PFS or OS data in single-arm expansion cohorts in phase I trials must be interpreted with caution, as they are similar in their limitations as single-arm phase II trials without randomization and control, where selection and other biases can affect efficacy outcome. Attention should be paid to the pre-specified statistical analysis plans for these expansion cohorts, and any amendments in trial assumptions and sample size during protocol conduct must be justified appropriately.

10.3.3 Biomarker Based Approaches to Evaluate Antitumor Activity

10.3.3.1 Biomarker Based Strategies

There have been major advances in the studies of molecular biology, as well as improvements in the understanding of signaling and survival pathways associated with certain cancers. This knowledge has been expanded by initiatives such as the International Cancer Genome Consortium (ICGC), and The Cancer Genome Atlas (TCGA) which provided access to cancer genomic data for drug development research [50, 51]. Modern medicinal chemistry has contributed to the ability to target specific "druggable" and "actionable" aberrations in cancers, made possible due to next generation sequencing and other molecular characterization techniques. "Targetable/druggable genomic alteration" has been defined as one that encodes an altered protein against which a drug exists or can be synthesized, whereas "actionable genomic alterations" include both targetable alterations and genomic alterations that cannot be directly targeted but that lead to dysregulation of a pathway in which there are possible targets (for example alteration of the *PTEN* tumor suppression gene can be targeted with PI3K/AKT inhibitors) [52]. This precision medicine approach using a biomarker based strategy has been associated with higher response rates when compared to non-biomarker based treatments [2]. More recently the American Association of Cancer Research (AACR) launched an initiative known as Genomics Evidence Neoplasia Information Exchange (GENIE) project, which is a publicly accessible annotated cancer genome database with the objective of accelerating precision cancer medicine. In contrast to ICGC and TCGA, which predominantly consisted of surgical specimens from patients with primary diagnosis of their cancers, GENIE has a higher proportion of recurrent or metastatic tumors. Such initiative can help advance research in identifying new drug targets, designing biomarker driven trials and providing specific genomic determinants of response to therapy [53].

A meta-analysis to determine the utility of biomarker based drug development examined 58 cancer drugs from first entry into human testing until approval. Based on trials published between September 1998 and June 2013, this meta-analysis assessed and specifically examined whether the development of these drugs was biomarker based or not, and compared them to non-biomarker based drugs. The authors defined "biomarker based strategy" as when a cognate biomarker was used to select patients for treatment, or when at least 50% of selected patients are known to harbor the cognate biomarker—with an example of hairy cell leukemia being known to harbor a *BRAF* mutation in almost 100% of cases. The studied drugs were all molecularly targeted agents in the biomarker based group, whereas they comprised 65% of the non-biomarker based group, with cytotoxic agents accounting for the remaining 35%. ORR, PFS, and OS were reported to be higher in the drugs that have been developed using biomarker based approaches [54]. Another meta-analysis that examined phase I oncology clinical trials published between January 2011 and December 2013 also found that studies using biomarker based anti-cancer agents were associated with significantly higher ORR and PFS [55]. Again, most of the precision oncology studies used targeted agents, whereas the non-precision oncology studies used targeted and cytotoxic drugs. Furthermore, another study that examined all published phase I trials between January 2014 and June 2015 found that ORR was higher in trials that investigated drugs targeting tumors with specific histological characteristics, or were biomarker based [2]. Altogether, these results indicate that oncology phase I clinical trials with enrichment designs using biomarkers that are predicated on strong scientific rationale and robust preclinical data have been associated with a greater probability of clinical benefit than those that have not.

10.3.3.2 Tumor Biopsies and Circulating Biomarkers

Tumor biopsies providing proof of pharmacodynamic effects of target inhibition can be informative in early phase studies. Serial tumor biopsies may include those procured pre-treatment, on-treatment, and even at the time of disease progression, to enable investigators to study molecular and immune effects of the investigational drug directly on the tissue of interest and in the surrounding tumor microenvironment [56]. Selected examples of phase I trials with tumor biopsies for pharmacodynamic studies (for proof of mechanism) are shown in Table 10.4 [56].

For example, serial tumor biopsies were done in the early trials of vemurafenib in *BRAF* mutated malignant melanoma to assess for changes in the mitogen activated protein kinase signaling (MAPK) pathway. After exposure to vemurafenib, observed reductions in tumor levels of phosphorylated extracellular signal-related-kinase (p-ERK), as well as reductions in cell proliferation markers such as cyclin

Table 10.4 Selected PD markers in tumors (and surrogate tissues) in phase I trials

Pharmacodynamic marker	Drug target	PD measurement	Phase I trial
Protein phosphorylation marker	mTOR	p-eIF-4G, p-4E-BP1	Phase I pharmacodynamic study of everolimus. Results helped determine schedule/dosing of everolimus—daily vs weekly [57]
	EGFR	p-EGFR, p-ERK	Phase I study of OSI-774 (erlotinib) [58, 59]
	MET	p-MET, p-FAK	Phase I study of ARQ 197 (tivantinib) [60]
	MEK	p-ERK	Phase I study of BAY86-9766 (refametinib) [61]
	BRAF	p-ERK	Phase I study of PLX4032 (vemurafenib) [62]
	BCR-ABL	p-CRKL	Phase I study of AMN107 (nilotinib) [63]
Epigenetic markers	HDAC	Acetylated histone 3	Phase I study of JNJ-26481585 (quisinostat) [64]
	DNA methyltransferase	MAGE1A CpG island methylation, 5-methyl-2′-deoxycytidine levels, HbF expression	Phase I study of 5-aza-2′-deoxycytidine (decitabine) and carboplatin [65]
Tumor infiltrating immune cells	PD-L1	Tumor infiltrating immune cells, PD-L1 expression	Phase 1 study of MPDL3280A (atezolizumab) [66]

p-eIF-4G phosphorylated eukaryotic initiation factor 4G; *p-4E-BP1* phosphorylated 4E binding protein 1; *p-ERK* phosphorylated extracellular signal-related-kinase; *FAK* focal adhesion kinase; *MEK* mitogen activated protein/extracellular signal-regulated kinase; *HDAC* histone deacetylase

Table 10.5 Selected NSCLC trials with tumor biopsies identifying resistance mechanisms

Molecularly targeted agent(s)	Brief description of trial	Resistance mechanisms discovered
EGFR inhibitors—gefitinib and erlotinib	Prospective trial of 155 patients who progressed on EGFR inhibitors	T790M mutation, MET amplification, HER2 amplification, small cell transformation [70]
ALK inhibitor—crizotinib	Case series of 18 patients with progression on crizotinib	Multiple mutations including point mutations in L1196M, C1156Y, L1152R and others [69]
EGFR inhibitors—erlotinib and gefitinib	Case series of 37 patients with progression on erlotinib and gefitinib	T790M, MET amplification, EGFR amplification, PIK3CA mutation, transformation to SCLC [71]

D1 and Ki67, led to confirmation of the mechanistic effects of vemurafenib and its inhibition of MAPK signaling [67]. Serial biopsies have also been used to identify resistance to other targeted therapies. For example, in *EGFR* mutated NSCLC treated with EGFR inhibitor tyrosine kinase inhibitors, repeat biopsies revealed that 50% of patients harbored *EGFR T790M* as a secondary mutation [68]. This discovery led to the development of a third generation EGFR inhibitor osimertinib which has been effective in treating patients with this acquired *T790M* mutation. Similarly, in NSCLC with echinoderm microtubule-associated protein-like 4-Anaplastic Lymphoma Kinase (*EML4-ALK*) translocation, serial tumor biopsies have helped identify resistance to crizotinib, a small molecule selective oral inhibitor of c-MET and ALK [69]. Table 10.5 shows selected studies in NSCLC that used tumor biopsies to identify resistance mechanisms to targeted agents.

In contrast, some experts have argued against the use of tumor biopsies for pharmacodynamic studies and their role in accelerating drug development. An analysis that examined 72 phase I trials from 2003 to 2010 reported that there were a high number of non-diagnostic biopsies, and only 5 studies resulted in a statistically significant biomarker result that was cited in subsequent publications. Tumor heterogeneity, risks attributable to the biopsy procedure, and associated costs are all concerns and should be considered in phase I trials with tumor biopsies [72].

The development of non-invasive liquid biopsies such as circulating tumor DNA (ctDNA) and circulating tumor cells (CTC), may ultimately replace invasive procedures such as tumor biopsies by providing a more globalized picture of the evolving genomic landscape in advanced tumors under the selective pressures of anti-cancer therapeutics (reviewed in Chap. 17). Many ctDNA based gene panels are now commercially available that can be used pre-treatment as predictive biomarkers to detect mutations, copy number variations and gene fusions for treatment assignment. Circulating biomarkers may be used to monitor molecular changes on-treatment such as expansion of an existent subclone or the emergence of a new clone that may occur as a result of acquired resistance [73]. In addition, ctDNA has been studied and used as a prognostic tool in various cancers [73–75], as a readout for treatment efficacy (reflected by a decline in CTC or ctDNA quantity), or as a pharmacodynamic measure to evaluate mechanistic effects.

10.4 Optimizing Efficacy Read-Out in Early Phase Trials

10.4.1 Identifying Target Populations

Despite extensive preclinical research, the majority of phase I trials test drugs for which target tumor types have not yet been identified. Therefore, patients with various different cancers are enrolled, especially during dose escalation. When new drugs are being combined with known active regimes in phase Ib trials then patients with cancers that are deemed appropriate for these combinations are chosen, to increase the chance of deriving benefit and to follow a logical strategy for subsequent combinatorial development. The enrichment with patient populations whose tumors harbor specific molecular characteristics such as druggable or actionable mutations may be of benefit as early as in phase I trials. However, this may not always be possible in many cancers since complex molecular pathways and interactions are often the drivers of oncogenesis, and not single mutations or "targets". Molecularly targeted agents when given to patients with tumors that are oncogenically addicted to a specific druggable or actionable target have the potential of demonstrating objective antitumor responses [76]. As an example, larotrectinib, an oral and selective inhibitor of tropomyosin receptor kinases (TRK), has been studied in adult and pediatric cancer patients in a phase I/II trial in 17 different tumors harboring *NTRK* gene fusions, and demonstrated ORR as high as 75–80% which were durable. These results led to the New Drug Application (NDA) being filed with the US FDA in December of 2017, and the FDA granting priority review of the application in May 2018, with resultant approval on November 26th, 2018 [45]. In the phase I study of crizotinib, NSCLC patients whose tumors harbor the *EML4-ALK* gene rearrangement were found to derive significant benefit. This target population was enriched successfully, and ultimately led to FDA approval based on this strategy [77]. Well executed enrichment designs using appropriately selected target populations based on robust preclinical data and biomarker studies may provide a higher probability of clinical benefit and an expeditious drug development path.

10.4.2 Phase 0 Studies

Phase 0 studies are exploratory investigational new drug studies that may help determine whether a drug is promising by preliminary assessment of its pharmacokinetics and target inhibition. By doing so, drugs that are not promising can be aborted early before formal toxicity and dose finding studies via phase I clinical trials [78]. The concept of phase 0 studies has been endorsed by the US FDA to address the problems of high expense and failure rate associated with drug development, which led to a decline in new drug applications. These studies involve giving a micro dose of the investigational drug to a small group of patients, generally 10 to 15, and performing studies that evaluate the mechanisms of action including target modulation, assessing pharmacokinetic and pharmacodynamic relationships, and optimizing a target assay. Risk of toxicity is low since only micro dosing is used. However, due to this, it is expected that no or minimal therapeutic benefit can be achieved which poses an ethical challenge to applying such studies in oncology patients. Once biomarker assays and imaging studies are incorporated and target inhibition is proven, the study can then proceed to a phase I trial with further dose escalations, and perhaps also an early examination of the drug's efficacy. This process of conducting phase 0 studies may also shorten the time of drug development [79]. Phase 0 studies may be of interest with immuno-oncology agents whereby intratumoral injection of new drugs at low doses can be given to determine if host immune response can be triggered locally. Despite these potential opportunities, phase 0 studies remain underused, largely due to concerns for patients being exposed to subtherapeutic doses of drugs with a minimal chance to derive clinical benefit.

10.4.3 Judicious Use of Expansion Cohorts and Seamless Phase I/II Trials

Using expansion cohorts is an important tool that has been associated with increased approval of investigational drugs in phase I clinical trials. A systematic review in 2017 examined 533 phase I trials assessing 381 drugs found that trials with expansion cohorts involving 2 to 20 patients were associated with higher rates of success in phase II trials, and a higher rate of FDA approval compared to phase I trials with no expansion cohorts [80]. However, this study had some limitations, including the possibility of overestimating the benefit of expansion cohorts due to publication bias and also the caveat of attributing expansion cohort as a cause rather than an effect of promising antitumor activity. Expansion cohorts, when used effectively and safely, may indeed expedite the drug approval process [81]. An example of this is the phase I study of the anti-PD1 antibody pembrolizumab with expansion cohorts in melanoma patients who progressed on single agent Ipilimumab or BRAF inhibitors (if *BRAF V600* mutated) in the KEYNOTE-001 study [82]. Investigational New Drug (IND) application was submitted in December of 2010 with the initial plan of testing the drug on 18 patients with melanoma in a "3+3" dose escalation protocol, followed by an additional 14 patients with melanoma and renal cell cancer in 2 disease specific expansion cohorts. However, in reality, 8 amendments resulted in 9 expansion cohorts ensued over the course of 2.5 years and resultant 1235 patients being enrolled. One of the amendments to the protocol added objectives of antitumor activity measurement resulted in an open label, randomized 1:1, dose comparative expansion cohort embedded within KEYNOTE-001 of 173 advanced melanoma patients, with results showing an objective response rate of 26% that were durable. Data were taken from three large cohorts and submitted to FDA for accelerated approval which was granted in September of 2014. Multiple trials were then designed and undertaken to further test and verify the clinical benefit of pembrolizumab in the studied patient population, which is required by the FDA to grant regular approval. These confirmatory trials add strength to the accelerated approval pathway [83].

Historically, phase I clinical trials focused solely on drug safety, and determining the MTD, so it can be used to decide on a RP2D for subsequent efficacy evaluations. Phase I and phase II trials are traditionally planned and performed separately and independently. However, in recent years, newer trial models have been proposed that combine phase I and II trials in an effort to expedite the drug development process [84]. When this is done, efficacy of the investigational drug is also specifically examined. This "seamless" transition from phase I to phase II trials is known as seamless phase I/II trials [85]. These trials have many advantages which include operational efficiency, cost reduction, rapidity of accrual due to multiple expansions, and earlier detection of efficacy which may allow for accelerated approvals of the investigational drugs if antitumor activity signals are compelling. In these trial designs protocol amendments frequently happen—as opposed to writing new protocols—to add expansion cohorts for new histologies or biomarker based groups when deemed appropriate based on promising scientific findings, observations in dose escalation, or results from other ongoing clinical trials of similar compounds [86]. These protocols may also use expansion cohorts to further assess and confirm efficacy of the tested drug. KEYNOTE-001, described above, represented one of the first examples of seamless phase I/II trials, where an earlier assessment of efficacy was observed and led to amendments to the protocol that added multiple phase II trial-like expansion cohorts and resulted in the rapid accrual of many patients [83]. Another example is the CHECKMATE-040 trial where the safety of the anti-PD1 antibody nivolumab was studied in patients with unresectable hepatocellular carcinoma [87]. Modifications to the study protocol added cohorts that evaluated activity in patients pre-treated with sorafenib. Further amendments to the protocol added expansion cohorts where nivolumab efficacy and safety were assessed in Child-Pugh B patients.

Despite the benefits of seamless phase I/II trial design, some concerns have emerged. These include the lack of a formal statistical analytical plan for expansion cohorts and over-emphasis of non randomized efficacy estimates. Another concern is that such designs may expand rapidly and open in multiple different investigator sites without a formal process of review of safety data, and an excessive number of patients may be exposed to ineffective or potentially toxic treatments. Advantages and disadvantages of seamless designs versus traditional phase I trials are described in Table 10.6.

10.4.4 Use of Prognostic Indices

Selection of patients for phase I clinical trials can be challenging. Patients who are candidates for phase I trials are generally those who have progressed on multiple lines of therapy and have no further standard therapeutic options. These patients can be unwell due to their advanced cancer state, and are at an increased risk of toxicity.

Table 10.6 Advantages versus disadvantages in seamless phase I/II trial designs and traditional phase I designs

	Seamless phase I/II trial	Traditional phase I trial
Advantages	• Reduced time duration between phases • Compelling activity can lead to accelerated approval • Rapid accrual of patients • Randomization across expansion cohorts can help determine clinical benefit early	• Feasible as trial is typically activated in a limited number of investigator sites • Pre-specified statistical analyses, with clear endpoints • Established framework for safety reporting and monitoring
Disadvantages	• Complex when activates in multiple investigator sites • Can lack formal design for expansion cohorts • Difficult safety monitoring with multiple expansion cohorts in many sites • Challenges in disseminating new safety information to patients, investigators, institutional review boards, regulators, etc. in a timely manner • Diluted clinical experience due to large number of participating sites	• Pauses between phases, and hence longer duration of study • Requires additional protocols and institutional review board approvals • Often lacks randomization, and therefore hard to detect clinical benefit

Typically, patients needed for phase I trials are ones who have an adequate performance status, organ functions, and are expected to live for more than 3 months such that it is possible to evaluate them for dose limiting toxicity and other treatment-emergent adverse events. Despite applying these criteria, almost 15% of all phase I cancer patients die within the first 3 months of enrollment [88]. There have been prognostic indicators that examined this population to enable the selection of appropriate patients for phase I clinical trials by assessing multiple patient-based and disease-based risk factors that impact on their life expectancy. The Royal Marsden Hospital drug development group has created a prognostic score (RMH index) that incorporates measurements of lactate dehydrogenase (LDH), albumin, and number of metastases to categorize patients into high risk or low risk groups based on their expected survival [89]. It has been prospectively validated at the same center and externally, and is one of the most utilized indices [90, 91]. The Princess Margaret Cancer Center drug development group has also developed their prognostic index (PMHI) in predicting the 90-day mortality of patients enrolled in phase I studies [92]. The PMHI included serum albumin levels, number of metastatic sites, and ECOG performance status. However, it has not been prospectively validated. The Gustave Roussy group has likewise created their prognostic score (GR Im-score), which included albumin, LDH, as well as neutrophil to lymphocyte ratio, and this index has recently been validated internally [93]. GR Im-score differs from existent indices in that it is aimed at estimating survival for patients enrolled to receive immune checkpoint inhibitors in phase I trials. It has been found to be superior than the RMH index in this group with regards to predicting OS. Other prognostic scores have been created by different groups, however these remain underused [94–96]. General application of prognostic indices can be a simple way of choosing appropriate patients with expected survival of more than 3 months in phase I clinical trials, such that longer-term safety as well as efficacy evaluations can be feasible in such patients.

10.5 Conclusions

There has been an increasing frequency in the consideration of efficacy endpoints in phase I trials of investigational new drugs or drug combinations, to accompany the traditional endpoints of safety, tolerability and RP2D determination. This changing landscape is driven by the interest to make go-no-go decisions at an earlier time point in the drug development process and also by the urgency to bring effective therapies to patients. While imaging based methods remain the primary basis of efficacy assessment, there are continued efforts in biomarker based explorations to ascertain antitumor activity and pharmacodynamic effects using tumor biopsies and blood samples. Innovations in clinical trial designs and patient selection strategies are needed to optimize efficacy read-out in phase I trials in the modern era.

Key Expert Opinion Points

1. The key deliverables of modern phase I trials are no longer limited to safety and RP2D determinations, but also include efficacy considerations to make go-no-go decisions to expedite the drug development process. As the lines between trial phases become blurred, phase I trialists are increasingly confronted with making such decisions based on limited data.
2. New response criteria or supplements to existent criteria have emerged to meet the needs of novel anti-cancer agents such as immuno-oncology drugs that may exhibit different effects on tumor growth kinetics compared to cytotoxic or targeted therapies. Observations of unique characteristics of new agents need to be reported to inform the continuous refinement and validation of response assessment tools.
3. Efficacy determinations in the phase I trial setting are often complicated by heterogeneous patient populations and single arm designs without comparators. These concerns have led to the emergence of expansion cohorts to enroll more homogeneous patient subsets based on histology or biomarker selection. Randomization is being used in some cases to provide a contemporaneous control. The statistical analytic plan specifying objectives, endpoints and sample size must be clearly articulated a priori in phase I trials with these elements, this stipulation applies also to study protocols undergoing amendments during their conduct.
4. Patient selection strategies based on robust preclinical data and strong scientific rationale are crucial as efficacy considerations play an increasing role in the phase I trial setting. However, there are mixed views related to the contribution

of information from tumor biopsies in guiding dose selection and target patient identification. There needs to be a better way to integrate preclinical, clinical and correlative sciences data from phase I studies to reduce redundancies and maximize their utility.

5. Innovative technologies such as radiomics, circulating biomarkers, etc. are being intensely evaluated in clinical trials, including in the phase I trial setting and may ultimately become an important component of efficacy considerations.

References

1. Yu J, Qin B, Moyer AM, Sinnwell JP, Thompson KJ, Copland JA 3rd, et al. Establishing and characterizing patient-derived xenografts using pre-chemotherapy percutaneous biopsy and post-chemotherapy surgical samples from a prospective neoadjuvant breast cancer study. Breast Cancer Res. 2017;19(1):130.
2. Chakiba C, Grellety T, Bellera C, Italiano A. Encouraging trends in modern phase 1 oncology trials. N Engl J Med. 2018;378(23):2242–3.
3. Eisenhauer EA, Therasse P, Bogaerts J, Schwartz LH, Sargent D, Ford R, et al. New response evaluation criteria in solid tumours: revised RECIST guideline (version 1.1). Eur J Cancer. 2009;45(2):228–47.
4. Ferte C, Fernandez M, Hollebecque A, Koscielny S, Levy A, Massard C, et al. Tumor growth rate is an early indicator of antitumor drug activity in phase I clinical trials. Clin Cancer Res. 2014;20(1):246–52.
5. Litiere SIG, De Vries E, Bogaerts J, Chen AP, Dancey J, Ford R, Gwyther SJ, Hoekstra OS, Huang E, Lin NU, Mandrekar SJ, Schwartz LH, Shankar L, Therasse P, Seymour L. Validation of RECIST 1.1 for use with cytotoxic agents and targeted cancer agents (TCA): results of a RECIST Working Group analysis of a 50 clinical trials pooled individual patient database. J Clin Oncol. 2017;35:2534.
6. Chiou VL, Burotto M. Pseudoprogression and immune-related response in solid tumors. J Clin Oncol. 2015;33(31):3541–3.
7. Wolchok JD, Hoos A, O'Day S, Weber JS, Hamid O, Lebbe C, et al. Guidelines for the evaluation of immune therapy activity in solid tumors: immune-related response criteria. Clin Cancer Res. 2009;15(23):7412–20.
8. Nishino M, Giobbie-Hurder A, Gargano M, Suda M, Ramaiya NH, Hodi FS. Developing a common language for tumor response to immunotherapy: immune-related response criteria using unidimensional measurements. Clin Cancer Res. 2013;19(14):3936–43.
9. Seymour L, Bogaerts J, Perrone A, Ford R, Schwartz LH, Mandrekar S, et al. iRECIST: guidelines for response criteria for use in trials testing immunotherapeutics. Lancet Oncol. 2017;18(3):e143–e52.
10. Champiat S, Ferrara R, Massard C, Besse B, Marabelle A, Soria JC, et al. Hyperprogressive disease: recognizing a novel pattern to improve patient management. Nat Rev Clin Oncol. 2018;15(12):748–62.
11. Champiat S, Dercle L, Ammari S, Massard C, Hollebecque A, Postel-Vinay S, et al. Hyperprogressive disease is a new pattern of progression in Cancer patients treated by anti-PD-1/PD-L1. Clin Cancer Res. 2017;23(8):1920–8.
12. Kato S, Goodman A, Walavalkar V, Barkauskas DA, Sharabi A, Kurzrock R. Hyperprogressors after immunotherapy: analysis of genomic alterations associated with accelerated growth rate. Clin Cancer Res. 2017;23(15):4242–50.
13. Kanjanapan Y, Day D, Wang L, Al-Sawaihey H, Abbas E, Namini A, Siu LL, Hansen A, Razak AA, Spreafico A, Leighl N, Joshua AM, Butler MO, Hogg D, Chappell MA, Soultani L, Chow

K, Boujos S, Bedard PL. Hyperprogressive disease in early-phase immunotherapy trials: clinical predictors and association with immune-related toxicities. Cancer. 2018;125:1341–9.
14. Carter BW, Bhosale PR, Yang WT. Immunotherapy and the role of imaging. Cancer. 2018;124(14):2906–22.
15. Rustin GJ, Nelstrop AE, McClean P, Brady MF, McGuire WP, Hoskins WJ, et al. Defining response of ovarian carcinoma to initial chemotherapy according to serum CA 125. J Clin Oncol. 1996;14(5):1545–51.
16. Guppy AE, Rustin GJ. CA125 response: can it replace the traditional response criteria in ovarian cancer? Oncologist. 2002;7(5):437–43.
17. Rustin GJ, Bast RC Jr, Kelloff GJ, Barrett JC, Carter SK, Nisen PD, et al. Use of CA-125 in clinical trial evaluation of new therapeutic drugs for ovarian cancer. Clin Cancer Res. 2004;10(11):3919–26.
18. Rustin GJ, Vergote I, Eisenhauer E, Pujade-Lauraine E, Quinn M, Thigpen T, et al. Definitions for response and progression in ovarian cancer clinical trials incorporating RECIST 1.1 and CA 125 agreed by the gynecological Cancer Intergroup (GCIG). Int J Gynecol Cancer. 2011;21(2):419–23.
19. Scher HI, Halabi S, Tannock I, Morris M, Sternberg CN, Carducci MA, et al. Design and end points of clinical trials for patients with progressive prostate cancer and castrate levels of testosterone: recommendations of the prostate Cancer Clinical Trials Working Group. J Clin Oncol. 2008;26(7):1148–59.
20. Scher HI, Morris MJ, Stadler WM, Higano C, Basch E, Fizazi K, et al. Trial design and objectives for castration-resistant prostate Cancer: updated recommendations from the prostate Cancer Clinical Trials Working Group 3. J Clin Oncol. 2016;34(12):1402–18.
21. Bloomfield CD, Estey E, Pleyer L, Schuh AC, Stein EM, Tallman MS, et al. Time to repeal and replace response criteria for acute myeloid leukemia? Blood Rev. 2018;32(5):416–25.
22. Cheson BD, Fisher RI, Barrington SF, Cavalli F, Schwartz LH, Zucca E, et al. Recommendations for initial evaluation, staging, and response assessment of Hodgkin and non-Hodgkin lymphoma: the Lugano classification. J Clin Oncol. 2014;32(27):3059–68.
23. Cheson BD. Staging and response assessment in lymphomas: the new Lugano classification. Chin Clin Oncol. 2015;4(1):5.
24. Moghbel MC, Kostakoglu L, Zukotynski K, Chen DL, Nadel H, Niederkohr R, et al. Response assessment criteria and their applications in lymphoma: part 1. J Nucl Med. 2016;57(6):928–35.
25. Moghbel MC, Mittra E, Gallamini A, Niederkohr R, Chen DL, Zukotynski K, et al. Response assessment criteria and their applications in lymphoma: part 2. J Nucl Med. 2017;58(1):13–22.
26. Younes A, Hilden P, Coiffier B, Hagenbeek A, Salles G, Wilson W, et al. International Working Group consensus response evaluation criteria in lymphoma (RECIL 2017). Ann Oncol. 2017;28(7):1436–47.
27. Landgren O, Rajkumar SV. New developments in diagnosis, prognosis, and assessment of response in multiple myeloma. Clin Cancer Res. 2016;22(22):5428–33.
28. Barbee MS, Nooka A, Kaufman JL, Kim S, Chen Z, Heffner LT Jr, et al. Predictors of survival outcomes in phase 1 relapsed or refractory multiple myeloma patients. Cancer. 2015;121(6):853–62.
29. Yankeelov TE, Mankoff DA, Schwartz LH, Lieberman FS, Buatti JM, Mountz JM, et al. Quantitative imaging in cancer clinical trials. Clin Cancer Res. 2016;22(2):284–90.
30. Gillies RJ, Kinahan PE, Hricak H. Radiomics: images are more than pictures, they are data. Radiology. 2016;278(2):563–77.
31. Aerts HJ, Velazquez ER, Leijenaar RT, Parmar C, Grossmann P, Carvalho S, et al. Decoding tumour phenotype by noninvasive imaging using a quantitative radiomics approach. Nat Commun. 2014;5:4006.
32. Zhang Y, Oikonomou A, Wong A, Haider MA, Khalvati F. Radiomics-based prognosis analysis for non-small cell lung cancer. Sci Rep. 2017;7:46349.
33. Vallieres M, Kay-Rivest E, Perrin LJ, Liem X, Furstoss C, Aerts H, et al. Radiomics strategies for risk assessment of tumour failure in head-and-neck cancer. Sci Rep. 2017;7(1):10117.

34. Lee J, Narang S, Martinez J, Rao G, Rao A. Spatial habitat features derived from multiparametric magnetic resonance imaging data are associated with molecular subtype and 12-month survival status in glioblastoma multiforme. PLoS One. 2015;10(9):e0136557.
35. Kickingereder P, Burth S, Wick A, Gotz M, Eidel O, Schlemmer HP, et al. Radiomic profiling of glioblastoma: identifying an imaging predictor of patient survival with improved performance over established clinical and radiologic risk models. Radiology. 2016;280(3):880–9.
36. Liu Y, Kim J, Qu F, Liu S, Wang H, Balagurunathan Y, et al. CT features associated with epidermal growth factor receptor mutation status in patients with lung adenocarcinoma. Radiology. 2016;280(1):271–80.
37. Aerts HJ, Grossmann P, Tan Y, Oxnard GR, Rizvi N, Schwartz LH, et al. Defining a radiomic response phenotype: a pilot study using targeted therapy in NSCLC. Sci Rep. 2016;6:33860.
38. Colen RR, Fujii T, Bilen MA, Kotrotsou A, Abrol S, Hess KR, et al. Radiomics to predict immunotherapy-induced pneumonitis: proof of concept. Investig New Drugs. 2018;36(4):601–7.
39. Limkin EJ, Sun R, Dercle L, Zacharaki EI, Robert C, Reuze S, et al. Promises and challenges for the implementation of computational medical imaging (radiomics) in oncology. Ann Oncol. 2017;28(6):1191–206.
40. Trebeschi S, Kurilova I, Călin AM, Lambregts DMJ, Smit EF, Aerts H, et al. Radiomic biomarkers for the prediction of immunotherapy outcome in patients with metastatic non-small cell lung cancer. J Clin Oncol. 2017;35(15 suppl):e14520.
41. Sun R, Limkin EJ, Vakalopoulou M, Dercle L, Champiat S, Han SR, et al. A radiomics approach to assess tumour-infiltrating CD8 cells and response to anti-PD-1 or anti-PD-L1 immunotherapy: an imaging biomarker, retrospective multicohort study. Lancet Oncol. 2018;19(9):1180–91.
42. El Naqa I, Ten Haken RK. Can radiomics personalise immunotherapy? Lancet Oncol. 2018;19(9):1138–9.
43. Nalley C. Radiomics-based imaging tool may predict response to immunotherapy. Oncol Times. 2018;40(6):13.
44. Shaw AT, Ou SH, Bang YJ, Camidge DR, Solomon BJ, Salgia R, et al. Crizotinib in ROS1-rearranged non-small-cell lung cancer. N Engl J Med. 2014;371(21):1963–71.
45. Drilon A, Laetsch TW, Kummar S, DuBois SG, Lassen UN, Demetri GD, et al. Efficacy of Larotrectinib in TRK fusion-positive cancers in adults and children. N Engl J Med. 2018;378(8):731–9.
46. Garon EB, Rizvi NA, Hui R, Leighl N, Balmanoukian AS, Eder JP, et al. Pembrolizumab for the treatment of non-small-cell lung cancer. N Engl J Med. 2015;372(21):2018–28.
47. McDermott DF, Sosman JA, Sznol M, Massard C, Gordon MS, Hamid O, et al. Atezolizumab, an anti-programmed death-ligand 1 antibody, in metastatic renal cell carcinoma: long-term safety, clinical activity, and immune correlates from a phase Ia study. J Clin Oncol. 2016;34(8):833–42.
48. Rodon J, Soria J-C, Berger R, Miller WH, Lazar V, Rubin E, et al. WINTHER: an international WIN Consortium precision medicine trial using genomic and transcriptomic analysis in patients with advanced malignancies. J Clin Oncol. 2018;36(15 Suppl):12011.
49. Massard C, Michiels S, Ferte C, Le Deley MC, Lacroix L, Hollebecque A, et al. High-throughput genomics and clinical outcome in hard-to-treat advanced cancers: results of the MOSCATO 01 trial. Cancer Discov. 2017;7(6):586–95.
50. Joly Y, Dove ES, Knoppers BM, Bobrow M, Chalmers D. Data sharing in the post-genomic world: the experience of the international Cancer genome consortium (ICGC) data access compliance office (DACO). PLoS Comput Biol. 2012;8(7):e1002549.
51. Tomczak K, Czerwinska P, Wiznerowicz M. The Cancer genome atlas (TCGA): an immeasurable source of knowledge. Contemp Oncol (Pozn). 2015;19(1A):A68–77.
52. Yates LR, Seoane J, Le Tourneau C, Siu LL, Marais R, Michiels S, et al. The European Society for Medical Oncology (ESMO) precision medicine glossary. Ann Oncol. 2018;29(1):30–5.
53. The AACR Project GENIE Consortium. AACR project GENIE: powering precision medicine through an international consortium. Cancer Discov. 2017;7(8):818–31.

54. Jardim DL, Schwaederle M, Wei C, Lee JJ, Hong DS, Eggermont AM, et al. Impact of a biomarker-based strategy on oncology drug development: a meta-analysis of clinical trials leading to FDA approval. J Natl Cancer Inst. 2015;107(11) https://doi.org/10.1093/jnci/djv253.
55. Schwaederle M, Zhao M, Lee JJ, Lazar V, Leyland-Jones B, Schilsky RL, et al. Association of biomarker-based treatment strategies with response rates and progression-free survival in refractory malignant neoplasms: a meta-analysis. JAMA Oncol. 2016;2(11):1452–9.
56. Gainor JF, Longo DL, Chabner BA. Pharmacodynamic biomarkers: falling short of the mark? Clin Cancer Res. 2014;20(10):2587–94.
57. Tabernero J, Rojo F, Calvo E, Burris H, Judson I, Hazell K, et al. Dose- and schedule-dependent inhibition of the mammalian target of rapamycin pathway with everolimus: a phase I tumor pharmacodynamic study in patients with advanced solid tumors. J Clin Oncol. 2008;26(10):1603–10.
58. Hidalgo M, Siu LL, Nemunaitis J, Rizzo J, Hammond LA, Takimoto C, et al. Phase I and pharmacologic study of OSI-774, an epidermal growth factor receptor tyrosine kinase inhibitor, in patients with advanced solid malignancies. J Clin Oncol. 2001;19(13):3267–79.
59. Malik SN, Siu LL, Rowinsky EK, de Graffenried L, Hammond LA, Rizzo J, et al. Pharmacodynamic evaluation of the epidermal growth factor receptor inhibitor OSI-774 in human epidermis of cancer patients. Clin Cancer Res. 2003;9(7):2478–86.
60. Yap TA, Olmos D, Brunetto AT, Tunariu N, Barriuso J, Riisnaes R, et al. Phase I trial of a selective c-MET inhibitor ARQ 197 incorporating proof of mechanism pharmacodynamic studies. J Clin Oncol. 2011;29(10):1271–9.
61. Weekes CD, Von Hoff DD, Adjei AA, Leffingwell DP, Eckhardt SG, Gore L, et al. Multicenter phase I trial of the mitogen-activated protein kinase 1/2 inhibitor BAY 86-9766 in patients with advanced cancer. Clin Cancer Res. 2013;19(5):1232–43.
62. Flaherty KT, Puzanov I, Kim KB, Ribas A, McArthur GA, Sosman JA, et al. Inhibition of mutated, activated BRAF in metastatic melanoma. N Engl J Med. 2010;363(9):809–19.
63. La Rosee P, Holm-Eriksen S, Konig H, Hartel N, Ernst T, Debatin J, et al. Phospho-CRKL monitoring for the assessment of BCR-ABL activity in imatinib-resistant chronic myeloid leukemia or Ph+ acute lymphoblastic leukemia patients treated with nilotinib. Haematologica. 2008;93(5):765–9.
64. Venugopal B, Baird R, Kristeleit RS, Plummer R, Cowan R, Stewart A, et al. A phase I study of quisinostat (JNJ-26481585), an oral hydroxamate histone deacetylase inhibitor with evidence of target modulation and antitumor activity, in patients with advanced solid tumors. Clin Cancer Res. 2013;19(15):4262–72.
65. Appleton K, Mackay HJ, Judson I, Plumb JA, McCormick C, Strathdee G, et al. Phase I and pharmacodynamic trial of the DNA methyltransferase inhibitor decitabine and carboplatin in solid tumors. J Clin Oncol. 2007;25(29):4603–9.
66. Herbst RS, Soria JC, Kowanetz M, Fine GD, Hamid O, Gordon MS, et al. Predictive correlates of response to the anti-PD-L1 antibody MPDL3280A in cancer patients. Nature. 2014;515(7528):563–7.
67. Trunzer K, Pavlick AC, Schuchter L, Gonzalez R, McArthur GA, Hutson TE, et al. Pharmacodynamic effects and mechanisms of resistance to vemurafenib in patients with metastatic melanoma. J Clin Oncol. 2013;31(14):1767–74.
68. Kobayashi S, Boggon TJ, Dayaram T, Janne PA, Kocher O, Meyerson M, et al. EGFR mutation and resistance of non-small-cell lung cancer to gefitinib. N Engl J Med. 2005;352(8):786–92.
69. Katayama R, Shaw AT, Khan TM, Mino-Kenudson M, Solomon BJ, Halmos B, et al. Mechanisms of acquired crizotinib resistance in ALK-rearranged lung cancers. Sci Transl Med. 2012;4(120):120ra17.
70. Yu HA, Arcila ME, Rekhtman N, Sima CS, Zakowski MF, Pao W, et al. Analysis of tumor specimens at the time of acquired resistance to EGFR-TKI therapy in 155 patients with EGFR-mutant lung cancers. Clin Cancer Res. 2013;19(8):2240–7.
71. Sequist LV, Waltman BA, Dias-Santagata D, Digumarthy S, Turke AB, Fidias P, et al. Genotypic and histological evolution of lung cancers acquiring resistance to EGFR inhibitors. Sci Transl Med. 2011;3(75):75ra26.

72. Sweis RF, Drazer MW, Ratain MJ. Analysis of impact of post-treatment biopsies in phase I clinical trials. J Clin Oncol. 2016;34(4):369–74.
73. Rossi G, Mu Z, Rademaker AW, Austin LK, Strickland KS, Costa RLB, et al. Cell-free DNA and circulating tumor cells: comprehensive liquid biopsy analysis in advanced breast cancer. Clin Cancer Res. 2018;24(3):560–8.
74. Xu-Welliver M, Carbone DP. Blood-based biomarkers in lung cancer: prognosis and treatment decisions. Transl Lung Cancer Res. 2017;6(6):708–12.
75. Creemers A, Krausz S, Strijker M, van der Wel MJ, Soer EC, Reinten RJ, et al. Clinical value of ctDNA in upper-GI cancers: a systematic review and meta-analysis. Biochim Biophys Acta Rev Cancer. 2017;1868(2):394–403.
76. Ivy SP, Siu LL, Garrett-Mayer E, Rubinstein L. Approaches to phase 1 clinical trial design focused on safety, efficiency, and selected patient populations: a report from the clinical trial design task force of the national cancer institute investigational drug steering committee. Clin Cancer Res. 2010;16(6):1726–36.
77. Kwak EL, Camidge DR, Clark J, Shapiro GI, Maki RG, Ratain MJ, et al. Clinical activity observed in a phase I dose escalation trial of an oral c-met and ALK inhibitor, PF-02341066. J Clin Oncol. 2009;27(15S):3509.
78. Coloma PM. Phase 0 clinical trials: theoretical and practical implications in oncologic drug development. Open Access J Clin Trials. 2013;2013:119–26.
79. Kummar S, Kinders R, Rubinstein L, Parchment RE, Murgo AJ, Collins J, et al. Compressing drug development timelines in oncology using phase '0' trials. Nat Rev Cancer. 2007;7(2):131–9.
80. Bugano DDG, Hess K, Jardim DLF, Zer A, Meric-Bernstam F, Siu LL, et al. Use of expansion cohorts in phase I trials and probability of success in phase II for 381 anticancer drugs. Clin Cancer Res. 2017;23(15):4020–6.
81. Theoret MR, Pai-Scherf LH, Chuk MK, Prowell TM, Balasubramaniam S, Kim T, et al. Expansion cohorts in first-in-human solid tumor oncology trials. Clin Cancer Res. 2015;21(20):4545–51.
82. Robert C, Ribas A, Wolchok JD, Hodi FS, Hamid O, Kefford R, et al. Anti-programmed-death-receptor-1 treatment with pembrolizumab in ipilimumab-refractory advanced melanoma: a randomised dose-comparison cohort of a phase 1 trial. Lancet. 2014;384(9948):1109–17.
83. Kang SP, Gergich K, Lubiniecki GM, de Alwis DP, Chen C, Tice MAB, et al. Pembrolizumab KEYNOTE-001: an adaptive study leading to accelerated approval for two indications and a companion diagnostic. Ann Oncol. 2017;28(6):1388–98.
84. Wages NA, Tait C. Seamless phase I/II adaptive design for oncology trials of molecularly targeted agents. J Biopharm Stat. 2015;25(5):903–20.
85. Hobbs BP, Barata PC, Kanjanapan Y, Paller CJ, Perlmutter J, Pond GR, Prowell TM, Rubin EH, Seymour L, Wages NA, Yap TA, Feltquate D, Garrett-Mayer E, Grossman W, Hong DS, Ivy SP, Siu LL, Reeves S, Rosner GL. Seamless designs: current practice and considerations for early-phase drug development in oncology. JNCI. 2019;111:118–28.
86. Siu LL, Ivy SP, Dixon EL, Gravell AE, Reeves SA, Rosner GL. Challenges and opportunities in adapting clinical trial design for immunotherapies. Clin Cancer Res. 2017;23(17):4950–8.
87. El-Khoueiry AB, Sangro B, Yau T, Crocenzi TS, Kudo M, Hsu C, et al. Nivolumab in patients with advanced hepatocellular carcinoma (CheckMate 040): an open-label, non-comparative, phase 1/2 dose escalation and expansion trial. Lancet. 2017;389(10088):2492–502.
88. Penel N, Delord JP, Bonneterre ME, Bachelot T, Ray-Coquard I, Blay JY, et al. Development and validation of a model that predicts early death among cancer patients participating in phase I clinical trials investigating cytotoxics. Investig New Drugs. 2010;28(1):76–82.
89. Arkenau HT, Olmos D, Ang JE, de Bono J, Judson I, Kaye S. Clinical outcome and prognostic factors for patients treated within the context of a phase I study: the Royal Marsden Hospital experience. Br J Cancer. 2008;98(6):1029–33.

90. Arkenau HT, Barriuso J, Olmos D, Ang JE, de Bono J, Judson I, et al. Prospective validation of a prognostic score to improve patient selection for oncology phase I trials. J Clin Oncol. 2009;27(16):2692–6.
91. Garrido-Laguna I, Janku F, Vaklavas C, Falchook GS, Fu S, Hong DS, et al. Validation of the Royal Marsden Hospital prognostic score in patients treated in the phase I clinical trials program at the MD Anderson Cancer Center. Cancer. 2012;118(5):1422–8.
92. Chau NG, Florescu A, Chan KK, Wang L, Chen EX, Bedard P, et al. Early mortality and overall survival in oncology phase I trial participants: can we improve patient selection? BMC Cancer. 2011;11:426.
93. Bigot F, Castanon E, Baldini C, Hollebecque A, Carmona A, Postel-Vinay S, et al. Prospective validation of a prognostic score for patients in immunotherapy phase I trials: the Gustave Roussy immune score (GRIm-score). Eur J Cancer. 2017;84:212–8.
94. Penel N, Vanseymortier M, Bonneterre ME, Clisant S, Dansin E, Vendel Y, et al. Prognostic factors among cancer patients with good performance status screened for phase I trials. Investig New Drugs. 2008;26(1):53–8.
95. Wheler J, Tsimberidou AM, Hong D, Naing A, Jackson T, Liu S, et al. Survival of patients in a phase 1 clinic: the M. D Anderson Cancer Center experience. Cancer. 2009;115(5):1091–9.
96. Han C, Braybrooke JP, Deplanque G, Taylor M, Mackintosh D, Kaur K, et al. Comparison of prognostic factors in patients in phase I trials of cytotoxic drugs vs new noncytotoxic agents. Br J Cancer. 2003;89(7):1166–71.

Chapter 11
Considerations for the Development of Novel Chemotherapies and Antibody Drug Conjugates in Phase I Trials

Vivek Subbiah and Roman Groisberg

Abstract The notion of using chemicals to treat diseases has been around since the turn of the twentieth century, with early discoveries coming serendipitously. By the 1950s, a Cancer Chemotherapy National Service Center (CCNSC) had begun to screen compounds for antitumor activity. It was from this effort that we derive our modern clinical trials methods in oncology as well. Modern chemotherapy is predominantly based on our understanding of the cell cycle, and most active agents interfere with pre-mitotic phases or mitosis. Models such as the "log-kill" hypothesis explained tumor kinetics and were based on leukemia cell growth. Based on this early understanding, chemotherapy was pushed to a maximal tolerated dose (MTD) and this became the benchmark endpoint for early phase clinical trials. The "log-kill" hypothesis proved inadequate for describing behavior of solid tumors. Norton and Simon showed that a Gompertzian curve was more representative of solid tumor kinetics. Based on this observation, chemotherapy "dose-density" was developed with investigators giving less recovery time between cycles of chemotherapy to maximize tumor volume reduction.

Many of today's most recognized chemotherapeutic agents were developed in the mid-twentieth century under the CCNSC. New agents have continued to be developed in the twenty-first century, as alternative formulations of old chemotherapies or entirely new compounds derived from unusual places such as the ocean. Alternative formulations have been especially successful, improving patient convenience or reducing toxicity with oral, long-lasting (PEGylation), or liposomal formulations.

V. Subbiah (✉)
Division of Cancer Medicine, Department of Investigational Cancer Therapeutics (Phase I Clinical Trials Program), Unit #455, University of Texas MD Anderson Cancer Center, Houston, TX, USA
e-mail: vsubbiah@mdanderson.org

R. Groisberg
Department of Melanoma/Sarcoma Medical Oncology, Rutgers Cancer Institute of New Jersey, New Brunswick, NJ, USA
e-mail: roman.groisberg@rutgers.edu

T. A. Yap et al. (eds.), *Phase I Oncology Drug Development*,
https://doi.org/10.1007/978-3-030-47682-3_11

Antibody-drug conjugates (ADCs) are novel chemotherapies and delivery mechanisms. They allow for the targeted delivery of extremely potent chemotherapeutic agents directly to the tumor, sparing the patient from significant toxicity. The development of ADCs combines targeting of specific tumor cell surface markers by antibodies with super-potent chemotherapeutic agents, such as auristatins. Joining the antibody with the chemotherapeutic payload is a stable linker mechanism that releases the agent upon entry into the cancer cell.

Future development of chemotherapies will take many forms and continues to be a vibrant and exciting area of cancer research.

Keywords Chemotherapy · Cell cycle · Maximal tolerated dose · Dose density Antibody-drug conjugate · Auristatin · Liposomal formulation · Pegylation

Key Points

- Chemotherapy targets dividing cells in the pre-mitotic phases or mitosis
- logarithmic kinetics describe leukemic cancer cell growth as well as chemotherapy induced cell death, an essential concept for understanding multiple cycle chemotherapy and maximum tolerated dose
- Kinetics of solid tumors are better described using a "Gompertzian" curve, the basis for "dose-dense" chemotherapy
- Modern chemotherapy development involves seeking compounds in new places and devising more convenient and less toxic formulations of existing agents
- Antibody-drug conjugates are a burgeoning field of drug discovery blending traditional chemotherapy with targeted therapy

11.1 Historical Development of Chemotherapy

The term "chemotherapy" dates back over a century, when the esteemed chemist Paul Ehrlich began using chemicals to treat diseases. Dr. Ehrlich's great contribution to cancer drug development was the use of animal models to screen chemicals for effectiveness against a disease [1]. Early research on cancer revolved predominantly around the development of such model systems to study tumors.

Still, the earliest advances in cancer chemotherapy did not come from the study of animal models and were instead serendipitous. For example, the observation that mustard gas caused marrow depletion led to the first use of chemotherapy to treat lymphoma with nitrogen mustard and the synthesis of related alkylating compounds such as chlorambucil and cyclophosphamide [2, 3]. Other drugs, most notably methotrexate, were developed from nutritional literature on the depletion of folic acid and the negative effect on bone marrow production [4]. Still other chemotherapies were accidental byproducts of burgeoning antimicrobial and anti-malarial development in the post-World War II era.

By the 1950s, sufficient animal models for cancer had been developed and the Cancer Chemotherapy National Service Center (CCNSC) was founded as a branch of the National Cancer Institute. This entity would be a centralized organization that could screen new chemical compounds for antitumor activity in these newly developed model organisms. Beyond the discovery of novel agents, CCNSC set the guidelines for design and conduct of clinical trials, statistical methods, and trial protocols [1].

11.1.1 Chemotherapy Principles and Cell Biology

Modern chemotherapy is based fundamentally on the principles of cell biology, specifically the cell cycle. Briefly, eukaryotic cells exist in either a resting phase, interphase, or cell division phase. The resting phase, referred to as Gap 0 (G0), is the inactive stage. Most human cells exist in this state at a given time and only the most non-specific agents are able to kill a cell in this state. When cells divide, they proceed through interphase (Gap 1, Synthesis, Gap 2) and into cell division (Mitosis). The majority of chemotherapeutic agents target cells in these stages of division. Agents such as cytarabine, methotrexate, fluorouracil, mercaptopurine, and hydroxyurea target cells in Synthesis (S-phase), while bleomycin targets cells in Gap 2 (G2) and Mitosis (M-phase) [5] (modern pharmacology, Chap. 55).

The earliest cancer models were based on leukemia cells with predictable exponential growth dynamics and consistent fraction of cells killed by chemotherapy. These cell lines would double in size no matter what the tumor volume was. Skipper, Schabel, and Wilcox proposed the "log-kill" hypothesis which stated that a certain dose of chemotherapy kills the same fraction of cancer cells regardless of tumor size [6] (Fig. 11.1). Since only a fraction of cells is killed instead of an absolute number, successive cycles of chemotherapy are necessary. The larger the fraction of killed cells, the fewer number of cycles are needed to eradicate all of the cancer cells.

11.1.2 Maximum Tolerated Dose

The kill fraction of a cytotoxic chemotherapy is directly related to the dose of a cytotoxic agent. Unfortunately, the lack of selectivity by antineoplastic agents means that the effect on normal human tissue is equivalent to the effect on tumor cells. The concept of maximal tolerated dose (MTD) was introduced to achieve maximum kill fraction and have low enough toxicity to be acceptable for use in

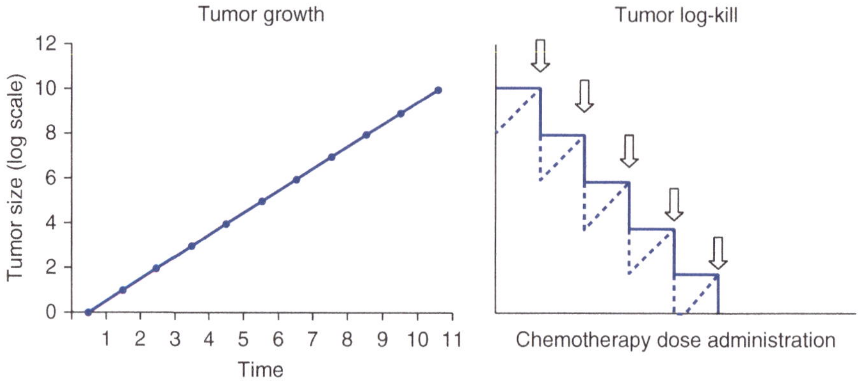

Fig. 11.1 Adapted from Traina and Norton [6]

humans. Sontag et al. originally defined the MTD as "highest dose of the test agent during the chronic study that can be predicted not to alter the animals' longevity from effects other than carcinogenicity." [7]. MTD was proposed for animal studies, but has since been revised and adapted by clinical investigators for use in humans. In early phase dose finding clinical trials (phase 1), the MTD is the highest dose of a drug that does not cause unacceptable side effects (NCI Dictionary of Cancer Terms). Increasing doses of a drug are administered to subsequent subjects until unacceptable adverse effects occur. The goal is to achieve a maximum amount of drug delivered to the patient, while still maintaining an acceptable level of tolerability. By the classic "3+3" trial design described elsewhere in this book, an acceptable threshold for severe toxicity is 33% [8].

11.1.3 Norton-Simon, the Gompertzian Growth Curve, and Dose Schedules

The log-kill hypothesis represents leukemic cells well, but falls short in describing solid tumors, whose growth plateaus due to nutrient depletion and hypoxia. The true growth rate of a tumor is better described by a Gompertzian curve. Benjamin Gompertz was a British actuary, who in 1825 described the population growth that occurs in nature [9]. Initially, populations including tumor cells grow exponentially, but as their numbers increase and nutrients become scarce, the growth plateaus giving the entire growth curve a sigmoid appearance (Fig. 11.2). Furthermore, when tumors are treated with a cytotoxic agent, their growth kinetics also change. Recognizing these growth patterns, Norton and Simon proposed a new model that was generally applicable, independent of restrictive assumptions, and could describe

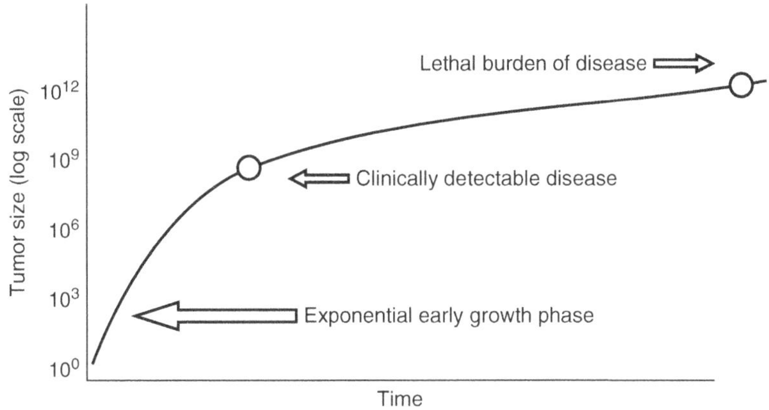

Fig. 11.2 Adapted from Traina and Norton [10]

the entire growth history of the tumor including the response to therapy [11]. Following the Gompertzian curve, one can extrapolate that larger tumors have smaller fractions of dividing cells and are less sensitive to drugs targeting the cell cycle. Similarly, smaller tumors grow at a faster rate. The important observation of Norton and Simon was that treating a larger and slower growing tumor with chemotherapy results in a smaller and faster re-growing tumor. It becomes entirely conceivable, and indeed observed, that tumors may completely regrow to their original size between cycles of chemotherapy.

The major clinical implication of the Norton-Simon hypothesis was the introduction of dose density into chemotherapy administration schedules. The superiority of a dose dense regimen was demonstrated by Citron and colleagues. Surgically resected breast cancer patients were given adjuvant doxorubicin and cyclophosphamide in either a dose-dense every 2-week schedule or a conventional every 3-week schedule. The every 2-week schedule showed significantly fewer disease relapses [12]. Reflecting on this trial and the Norton-Simon hypothesis, the maximum dose of chemotherapy must be delivered as quickly as possible, allowing less time for tumor regrowth.

11.2 Chemotherapy Development in the Twenty-First Century

In the modern era, traditional cell-cycle targeting chemotherapy development has continued (Fig. 11.3).

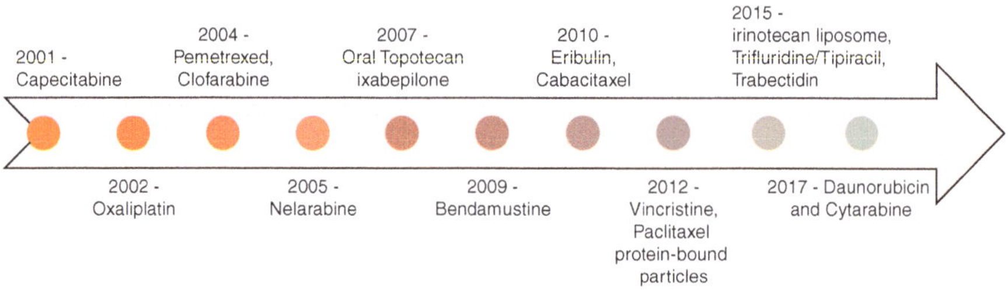

Fig. 11.3 Chemotherapy development after 2000

11.2.1 Going to New Places to Discover

During the middle decades of the last century, the Cancer Chemotherapy National Service Center, a branch of the national cancer institute, screened thousands of compounds from plants, animals, and bacteria to find compounds with anticancer activity. In the twenty-first century, drug developers have had to look in new places, such as the ocean, for sources of novel agents.

Trabectedin was derived from the sea squirt *Ecteinascidia turbinate* and further determined to be from the symbiotic bacterium *Candidatus Endoecteinascidia frumentensis* [13, 14]. This agent acts predominantly as a DNA minor groove binder, interfering with transcription and forming DNA double-strand breaks [13]. Trabectedin was approved in 2015 for the treatment of soft-tissue sarcomas. The sea has contributed other important chemotherapeutic agents such as cytarabine, eribulin, and Monomethyl auristatin E (MMAE, Vedotin). [15] Eribulin is derived from the sea sponge *Halichondria,* which produces the microtubule disrupting mitotic inhibitor halichondrin B [16, 17]. Eribulin was approved in 2010 for the treatment of metastatic breast cancer, and later for liposarcomas in 2016. MMAE is derived from the marine mollusk *Dolabella auricularia,* belonging to a class of drugs called dolastatins [18]. The dolastatins act as tubulin destabilizers, by binding to the *Vinca* domain [19]. MMAE's toxicity made it impossible to use as a stand-alone drug, but it has become tremendously important in the development of antibody-drug conjugates discussed below.

11.2.2 Alternative Formulations

The success of the National Cancer Institute screening programs led many contemporary drug developers to conclude that new agents are too difficult, if not impossible to find. Development has instead turned to reformulation of existing chemotherapies, focusing on convenience of administration, increased activity, or reduced toxicity. Drugs such as capecitabine, topotecan, and trifluridine/tipiracil have focused on oral administration of established drugs: 5-FU, camptothecin, and 5-FU respectively. The development of nanoparticle encapsulation technology has aimed to achieve all three goals of reformulation.

Nanoparticle technology reached the market in the form of liposomal encapsulation. First described in 1961, liposomes are lipid bilayers that form spheres with an aqueous center. The lipid bilayer can be modified by the addition of sterols to influence membrane permeability and therefore drug delivery characteristics [20]. Liposomes have become easy to manufacture and load. Hydrophilic drugs can be encapsulated in the aqueous inner layer and hydrophobic drugs can be incorporated into the membrane, making the number of possible payload candidates almost limitless. Membrane modification for charge, size, and permeability allows the liposome to be targeted to certain tissues as well as control the clearance time. One of the major drawbacks of liposomes is their propensity to accumulate in the reticuloendothelial system, especially the liver, reducing their circulation time [21]. The addition of polyethylene glycol (PEGylation) increases time in circulation, reducing dosing frequency as well as toxicity [22].

The first such clinically successful chemotherapeutic agent to be developed was Doxil®, a PEGylated liposomal formulation of doxorubicin, which was approved in 1995 for the treatment of breast and ovarian cancer, as well as AIDS-related Kaposi's sarcoma. Doxorubicin is one of the most potent and versatile chemotherapeutic agents with application in diverse cancers: leukemias, lymphomas, breast, uterine, ovarian, gastric, bladder, and sarcomas [23]. Toxicities include myelosuppression, nausea, stomatitis, and cardiotoxicity, which causes an irreversible congestive heart failure when cumulative doses greater than 550 mg/m^2 are used. Doxorubicin causes oxidative stress by the formation of free radicals and in the body is preferentially attracted to cardiolipin contained within mitochondrial membranes. The high cardiolipin content in cardiac muscle is thought to be the reason for doxorubicin's cardiotoxicity [24]. After a major clinical failure with OLV-DOX, a first generation liposomal doxorubicin, Doxil® emerged from the lessons learned. The new drug achieved several clinical milestones: it was stable for long periods of time in human plasma arriving to the tumor intact, small enough (less than 100 nm) to extravasate into the tumor from the vasculature, and effectively released doxorubicin upon arrival at the tissue [25]. Doxil® was better tolerated than traditional doxorubicin with a reduced risk of cardiotoxicity and improved response rates as well as progression-free survival in breast cancer [26]. The successful development of Doxil® showed the feasibility and advantages of a liposomal drug delivery system. Since then, many drugs have been reformulated including daunorubicin (DaunoXome®), cytarabine (Depocyt®), vincristine (Marquibo®), irinotecan (Onyvide®), and daunorubicin with cytarabine (Vyxeos®) (Fig. 11.4).

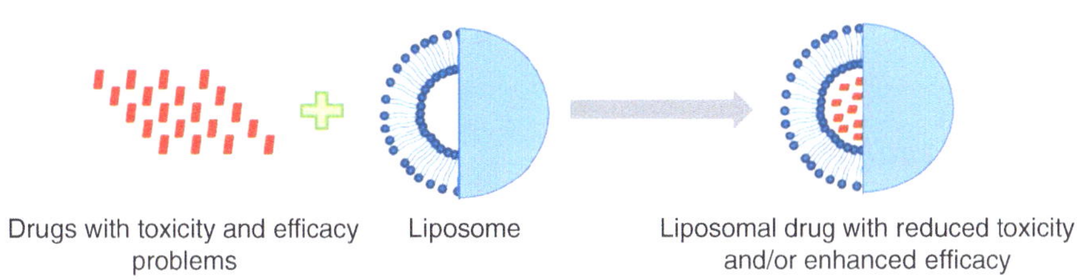

Fig. 11.4 Adapted from Bulbake et al. [20]

11.3 Development of Antibody-Drug Conjugates

The significant toxicity of systemic chemotherapy is often the limiting factor in how much drug can be delivered, how many cycles can be administered to a patient, and ultimately what fraction of cancer cells are eradicated. A chemotherapy that could be delivered only to the tumor and spare healthy tissues is ideal. One way to achieve this is by linking the chemotherapy to a tumor directed antibody, making an antibody-drug conjugate (ADC).

The first trial of an ADC in man was with vindesine-anti-CEA. The drug was able to localize to the desired tumor and avoided undue toxicity, but ultimately was not developed further [27]. A series of ADCs were developed using various established chemotherapeutic agents, each showed acceptable tolerability in early trials, but without significant clinical efficacy. The first agent to show antitumor activity in human tumor xenograft models was BR96-doxorubicin, a Lewis antigen directed antibody conjugated to doxorubicin, which cured 70 percent of mice with lung adenocarcinoma [28]. Unfortunately, doxorubicin has a relatively low potency and therefore required high number of drug to antibody ratios with as many as eight molecules of doxorubicin attached to one BR96 antibody. This, along with non-specificity of the antibody and lability of the linker led to severe toxicity and off-target effects, ultimately stopping further drug development [29].

Lessons learned from countless failed ADCs led to the successful development of gemtuzumab ozogamicin (Mylotarg®), an ADC directed at CD33 which is expressed on acute myeloid leukemia cells. Patients who received gemtuzumab ozogamicin achieved significant rates of remission after their disease had relapsed [30]. Unfortunately, the drug was withdrawn from the market in 2010 because of concern for high number of fatal events [30]. It was re-introduced to the market again in 2017 when subsequent studies showed the drug had acceptable toxicity [31]. A decade after the approval of Mylotarg® in 2001, brentuximab-vedotin (Adcetris®) was approved for the treatment of relapsed Hodgkin's lymphoma and anaplastic large cell lymphoma [31]. Brentuximab-vedotin incorporated a spacer between the linker and the toxin monomethyl auristatin E (MMAE), allowing up to five molecules of MMAE to be stably attached to one antibody. Another ADC to be approved was ado-trastuzumab emtansine (Kadcyla®) which used an established therapy for HER2 expressing breast cancer, trastuzumab, linked to the cytotoxic agent emtansine. The conjugate was approved in 2013 for HER2 positive breast cancer that had progressed on trastuzumab alone.

The development of a successful ADC is complex and requires three essential parts to work together perfects: the antibody, payload, and linker between them.

11.3.1 Antibody-Antigen

Before the 1980s, ADC development was not possible, hindered by the inability to produce sufficient quality and quantity of antibodies. The production of a monoclonal antibody was first described by Milstein in 1975, followed by a recombinant chimeric antibody by Morrison in 1984 and a humanized antibody by Jones [32].

The antibody and its target antigen must have certain properties to be successful as an ADC. An antigen must be highly expressed on the tumor to attract the antibody to its target. Similarly, the antigen must have low expression in normal tissues to minimize on-target effects, leading to toxicity. This can be achieved by finding an antigen that is expressed solely on the tumor. Unfortunately, because tumors are derived from human cells, they share antigens with their cell of origin as well as other tissues in the body. The expression of a given antigen may be higher on a tumor cell, but the aggregate of cells in an organ system may still have higher expression of the antigen resulting in on-target toxicity to this organ [33]. BR96-doxurubicin and bivatuzumab-mertansine, both had significant and unexpected on-target effects leading to hemorrhagic gastritis and fatal skin toxicity respectively, halting their development [34, 35].

Ideally, an antigen will be uniformly expressed across a tumor allowing for even distribution of an ADC. However, due to tumor heterogeneity this is unlikely to occur. In practice this is not a major problem as free toxin is released after a tumor cell is killed, entering neighboring cells and resulting in bystander kill [36]. A threshold number of antigen binding sites must exist per cell, but beyond that, level of expression does not correlate with tumor eradication [37].

Upon binding to an antigen, the antibody complex should be efficiently internalized. An optimal level of internalization exists for tumor kill. Slowly internalized targets are preferred for penetration of drug into distal regions of the tumor [38]. The antibody can be "tuned" by changing the binding site of an IgG to its antigen, FcγRs, complement component, or FcRn. Often, the conjugation of a cytotoxic payload to the antibody increases internalization versus the antibody alone [39]. The selection of an IgG subtype is important when designing an antibody alone as a drug. IgG1 is able to cause complement-dependent cellular cytotoxicity, while IgG2 and IgG4 don't. However, this may not be important when designing ADCs as the killing is accomplished by the payload rather than the antibody or complement [29].

11.3.2 Payload

Early ADCs carried an established chemotherapy such as doxorubicin. These drugs served as a poor payload choice as they had limited potency and required high drug to antibody ratios. A solution was found in the high potency microtubule destabilizing agents maytansines, auristatins, and dolastatins. Until recently, the limitation on drug to antibody ratios resulted in almost all ADCs using one of these compounds. Unfortunately, microtubule destabilizing agents have a limited spectrum of activity, reducing their utility to a few diseases [33]. An alternative payload option is the DNA minor groove binding agent calicheamicin, as employed by gemtuzumab-ozogamycin [40]. Another novel payload is duocarmycin and its analogues, which exert cell kill in a cell cycle independent way by alkylating adenine bases and disrupting the DNA architecture [41]. These agents may ultimately be more successful as ADC payload since they exhibit activity across many different tumor types in-vitro, while maintaining high potency and activity at nanomolar concentrations.

11.3.3 Linker

Seemingly the least interesting part of an ADC may be the most important. The linker must be able to hold a sufficient amount of drug (drug-antibody ratio, DAR) to deliver a sufficiently cytotoxic dose to a tumor cell. Overloading the linker with too much payload results in off-target toxicity such as neutropenia, diarrhea, and hepatotoxicity [42]. The linker must remain stable in blood or similar off-target effects will be experienced by free-floating cytotoxin. Concurrently, the linker must release its payload upon entering the target cell. When an antibody binds to an antigen on the cell surface the entire conjugate is internalized by endocytosis. The conjugate is degraded inside the endosome, releasing free toxin into the cell cytoplasm and resulting in cell kill [29]. Newer linker technologies are in development that will allow stable DAR of 20 or more, perhaps expanding the possibility of payload options. However, as discussed above, more payload may not be necessary as additional high potency toxins are employed.

The current generation of ADCs have used a random conjugation process that results in variable amounts of drug attached to each antibody as well as random sites of attachment. The net effect of this volatility is unpredictable stability and pharmacokinetics [43]. Future generations of ADCs will have predictable sites of drug binding to antibody. This will result in predictable pharmacokinetics, stable release of drug at the tumor site, and reduced toxicity (Figs. 11.5 and 11.6).

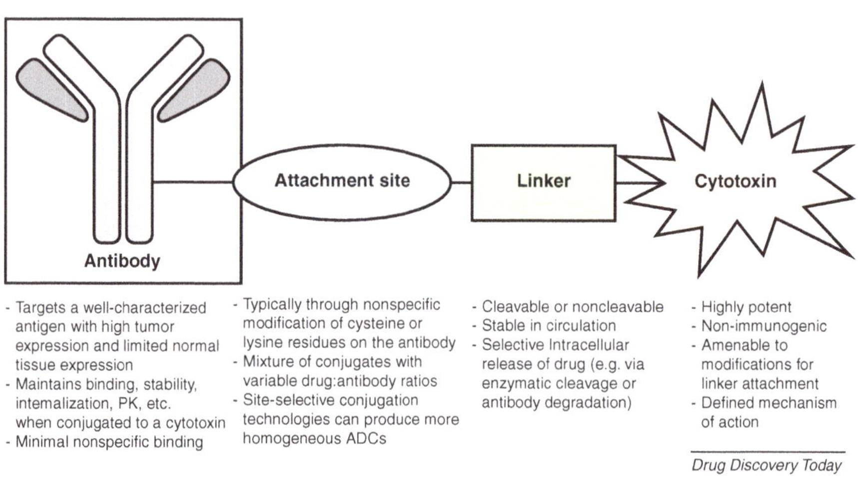

Fig. 11.5 Adapted from Perez et al. [29]

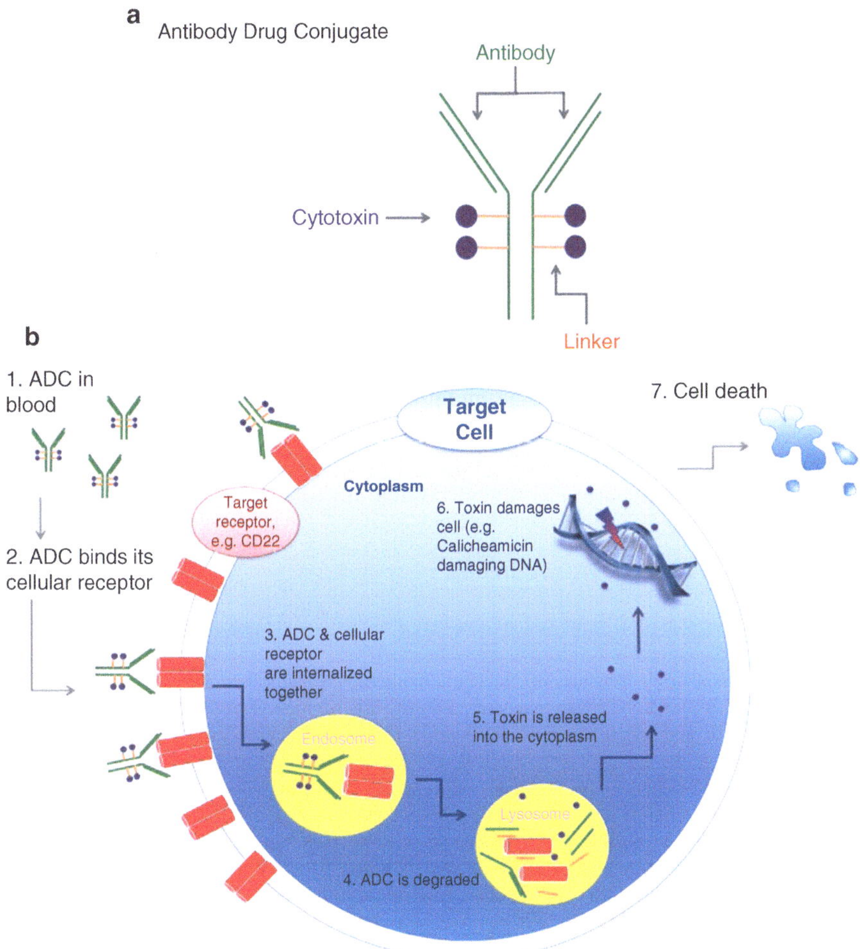

Fig. 11.6 Adapted from Feld, oncotarget 2013 [42]

11.4 Conclusions

Despite the advent of small molecules and immunotherapies, traditional cytotoxic chemotherapy is still relevant and continues to be developed today. Novel agents take many forms. Some are new drugs derived from organisms living in exotic places. Others are reformulations of existing drugs, making them easier to administer, less frequent in dosing, or with reduced toxicity. Reformulations are aided by development of companion delivery systems such as liposomes, PEGylation, or antibody drug conjugates. Although the drugs may be new, the lessons we keep from past successes and failures still apply.

Key Expert Opinion Points

- Despite the advent of small molecules and immunotherapies, novel ways to administer cytotoxics with reduced toxicity to the "right patient at the right time" in the form of antibody drug conjugates (ADC) will be a part of precision oncology.
- The development of a successful ADC will continue to evolve, with improvements in the technologies and delivery systems that include all the components of ADCs: the antibody, payload, and linker between them.
- Because the development of a patient selection strategy linked to target expression on the tumor is crucial, efforts are underway using RNASeq from TCGA for estimating the prevalence of ADC target expression that can guide the future development of companion diagnostics.
- Since ADC payloads cause immunogenic cell death in their targets, combining ADCs with immune checkpoint inhibitors opens up the possibility of reversing the elusive strategies that cancers exploit to bypass immunosurveillance.
- Optimization of ADC use in oncology includes establishing combination therapies with agents that arm the immune system for treating diverse cancers.

References

1. DeVita VT Jr, Chu E. A history of cancer chemotherapy. Cancer Res. 2008;68(21):8643–53.
2. Goodman LS, et al. Nitrogen mustard therapy: use of methyl-bis(beta-chloroethyl)amine hydrochloride and tris(beta-chloroethyl)amine hydrochloride for hodgkin's disease, lymphosarcoma, leukemia and certain allied and miscellaneous disorders. J Am Med Assoc. 1946;132(3):126–32.
3. Marshall EK Jr. Historical perspectives in chemotherapy. Adv Chemother. 1964;13:1–8.
4. Farber S, Diamond LK. Temporary remissions in acute leukemia in children produced by folic acid antagonist, 4-aminopteroyl-glutamic acid. N Engl J Med. 1948;238(23):787–93.
5. Craig CR, Stitzel RE. Modern pharmacology: clinical applications. Philadelphia, PA; London: Lippincott Williams & Wilkins; 2003.
6. Traina TA, Norton L. Log-Kill Hypothesis. In: Schwab M, editor. Encyclopedia of cancer. Berlin, Heidelberg: Springer; 2017. p. 2537–9.
7. Sontag J. Guidelines for carcinogen bioassay in small rodents. Natl Cancer Inst Carcinog Tech Rep Ser. 1976;1:1–65.
8. Le Tourneau C, Lee JJ, Siu LL. Dose escalation methods in phase I cancer clinical trials. JNCI. 2009;101(10):708–20.
9. Gompertzian growth curve. In: Schwab V, editor. Encyclopedia of cancer. Berlin, Heidelberg: Springer; 2011. p. 1576.
10. Traina TA, Norton L. Norton-Simon hypothesis. In: Schwab M, editor. Encyclopedia of cancer. Berlin Heidelberg: Springer; 2017. p. 3142–4.
11. Norton L, Simon R. Growth curve of an experimental solid tumor following radiotherapy. JNCI. 1977;58(6):1735–41.
12. Citron ML, et al. Randomized trial of dose-dense versus conventionally scheduled and sequential versus concurrent combination chemotherapy as postoperative adjuvant treatment of node-positive primary breast cancer: first report of Intergroup Trial C9741/Cancer and Leukemia Group B Trial 9741. J Clin Oncol. 2003;21(8):1431–9.

13. Le VH, et al. Ecteinascidins. A review of the chemistry, biology and clinical utility of potent tetrahydroisoquinoline antitumor antibiotics. Nat Prod Rep. 2015;32(2):328–47.
14. Schofield MM, et al. Identification and analysis of the bacterial endosymbiont specialized for production of the chemotherapeutic natural product ET-743. Environ Microbiol. 2015;17(10):3964–75.
15. Malve H. Exploring the ocean for new drug developments: marine pharmacology. J Pharm Bioallied Sci. 2016;8(2):83–91.
16. Towle MJ, et al. In vitro and in vivo anticancer activities of synthetic macrocyclic ketone analogues of halichondrin B. Cancer Res. 2001;61(3):1013–21.
17. Bai RL, et al. Halichondrin B and homohalichondrin B, marine natural products binding in the vinca domain of tubulin. Discovery of tubulin-based mechanism of action by analysis of differential cytotoxicity data. J Biol Chem. 1991;266(24):15882–9.
18. Dosio F, Brusa P, Cattel L. Immunotoxins and anticancer drug conjugate assemblies: the role of the linkage between components. Toxins. 2011;3(7):848.
19. Avendaño C, Menéndez JC. Chapter 8 - Anticancer drugs targeting tubulin and microtubules. In: Avendaño C, Menéndez JC, editors. Medicinal chemistry of anticancer drugs. Amsterdam: Elsevier; 2008. p. 229–49.
20. Bulbake U, et al. Liposomal formulations in clinical use: an updated review. Pharmaceutics. 2017;9(2):1.
21. Torchilin VP. Recent advances with liposomes as pharmaceutical carriers. Nat Rev Drug Discov. 2005;4:145.
22. Veronese FM, Pasut G. PEGylation, successful approach to drug delivery. Drug Discov Today. 2005;10(21):1451–8.
23. Weiss RB. The anthracyclines: will we ever find a better doxorubicin? Semin Oncol. 1992;19(6):670–86.
24. Rahman AR, et al. Comparative pharmacokinetics of free doxorubicin and doxorubicin entrapped in cardiolipin liposomes. Cancer Res. 1986;46(5):2295–9.
25. Barenholz Y. Doxil(R)—the first FDA-approved nano-drug: lessons learned. J Control Release. 2012;160(2):117–34.
26. Xing M, et al. Efficacy and cardiotoxicity of liposomal doxorubicin-based chemotherapy in advanced breast cancer: a meta-analysis of ten randomized controlled trials. PLoS One. 2015;10(7):e0133569.
27. Ford CH, et al. Localisation and toxicity study of a vindesine-anti-CEA conjugate in patients with advanced cancer. Br J Cancer. 1983;47:35.
28. Trail PA, et al. Cure of xenografted human carcinomas by BR96-doxorubicin immunoconjugates. Science. 1993;261(5118):212–5.
29. Perez HL, et al. Antibody–drug conjugates: current status and future directions. Drug Discov Today. 2014;19(7):869–81.
30. Sievers EL, et al. Efficacy and safety of gemtuzumab ozogamicin in patients with CD33-positive acute myeloid leukemia in first relaps*e*. J Clin Oncol. 2001;19(13):3244–54.
31. Rowe JM, Löwenberg B. Gemtuzumab ozogamicin in acute myeloid leukemia: a remarkable saga about an active drug. Blood. 2013;121(24):4838.
32. Shen W-C. Antibody-drug conjugates: a historical review. In: Wang J, Shen W-C, Zaro JL, editors. Antibody-drug conjugates: the 21st century magic bullets for cancer. Cham: Springer; 2015. p. 3–7.
33. Tolcher AW. Antibody drug conjugates: lessons from 20 years of clinical experience. Ann Oncol. 2016;27(12):2168–72.
34. Saleh MN, et al. Phase I trial of the anti-Lewis Y drug immunoconjugate BR96-doxorubicin in patients with lewis Y-expressing epithelial tumors. J Clin Oncol. 2000;18(11):2282–92.
35. Tijink BM, et al. A phase I dose escalation study with anti-CD44v6 bivatuzumab mertansine in patients with incurable squamous cell carcinoma of the head and neck or esophagus. Clin Cancer Res. 2006;12(20 Pt 1):6064–72.

36. Kovtun YV, et al. Antibody-drug conjugates designed to eradicate tumors with homogeneous and heterogeneous expression of the target antigen. Cancer Res. 2006;66(6):3214.
37. Polson AG, Ho WY, Ramakrishnan V. Investigational antibody-drug conjugates for hematological malignancies. Expert Opin Investig Drugs. 2011;20(1):75–85.
38. Ackerman ME, Pawlowski D, Wittrup KD. Effect of antigen turnover rate and expression level on antibody penetration into tumor spheroids. Mol Cancer Therap. 2008;7(7):2233.
39. Carter PJ. Potent antibody therapeutics by design. Nat Rev Immunol. 2006;6:343.
40. Hinman LM, et al. Preparation and characterization of monoclonal antibody conjugates of the calicheamicins: a novel and potent family of antitumor antibiotics. Cancer Res. 1993;53(14):3336.
41. Boger DL, Johnson DS. CC-1065 and the duocarmycins: unraveling the keys to a new class of naturally derived DNA alkylating agents. Proc Natl Acad Sci USA. 1995;92(9):3642–9.
42. Feld J, et al. Linked-in: design and efficacy of antibody drug conjugates in oncology. Oncotarget. 2013;4(3):397–412.
43. Boylan NJ, et al. Conjugation site heterogeneity causes variable electrostatic properties in Fc conjugates. Bioconjugate Chem. 2013;24(6):1008–16.

Chapter 12
Development of Molecularly Targeted Agents in Early Phase Clinical Trials

Pedro C. Barata and Timothy A. Yap

Abstract There are a significant number of signaling networks that play a key role in living organisms, but which are commonly hijacked during oncogenesis. The identification of these drivers of cancer has led to the clinical development and subsequent regulatory approval of multiple molecularly targeted agents. Nonetheless, drug resistance is almost inevitable due to the development of signaling crosstalk, disruption of negative feedback loops and other mechanisms. In order to overcome these challenges, there has been an expansion of clinical trials investigating novel therapies and rational combinations of different targeted agents. Here, we describe the features of successful early phase clinical trials: strong scientific rationale leading to their initiation; robust preclinical data from model systems; inclusion of pharmacokinetic (PK) and pharmacodynamic (PD) proof-of-mechanism studies; use of optimal trial designs; and incorporation of predictive biomarkers of response to optimize patient selection to these trials. Such approaches may optimize and accelerate the drug development process and lead to monotherapy and combination strategies that benefit patients with different cancers.

Keywords Early-phase trials · Signaling pathways · Molecularly targeted agents Combination regimens · Drug resistance

---

P. C. Barata
Tulane Medical School, Deming Department of Medicine, Section of Hematology and Medical Oncology, New Orleans, LA, USA

T. A. Yap (✉)
Department of Investigational Cancer Therapeutics (Phase I Program), The University of Texas MD Anderson Cancer Center, Houston, TX, USA

Khalifa Institute for Personalized Cancer Therapy, The University of Texas MD Anderson Cancer Center, Houston, TX, USA

The Institute for Applied Cancer Science, The University of Texas MD Anderson Cancer Center, Houston, TX, USA

Department of Thoracic/Head and Neck Medical Oncology, The University of Texas MD Anderson Cancer Center, Houston, TX, USA
e-mail: tyap@mdanderson.org

T. A. Yap et al. (eds.), *Phase I Oncology Drug Development*,
https://doi.org/10.1007/978-3-030-47682-3_12

Keypoints

1. The identification of key signaling networks involved in oncogenesis has led to the clinical development and subsequent regulatory approval of multiple molecularly targeted agents.
2. Drug resistance is almost inevitable due to different mechanisms, including the development of signaling crosstalk and the disruption of negative feedback loops. Mechanisms to overcome drug resistance include the development of novel molecularly targeted agents, optimization of trial designs and rational combinations of different therapies.
3. Features of successful early phase clinical trials include having a strong scientific rationale; robust data from preclinical model systems; incorporation of pharmacokinetic (PK) and pharmacodynamic (PD) proof-of-mechanism studies; use of optimal trial designs; and incorporation of predictive biomarkers of response to optimize patient selection to these trials.
4. Development of strategies focused on reversing drug resistance, e.g., through the use of rational combination therapies.

12.1 Introduction

Cancer formation and progression occur through a range of genetic and epigenetic alterations that affect the normal programs of cell growth, differentiation or migration as well as the tumor microenvironment, angiogenesis and inflamation [1–3]. A number of signaling pathways have been identified as key drivers of oncogenesis as a consequence of genetic alterations to cellular genes [4]. Few examples include the vascular endothelial growth factor (VEGF) [5] and fibroblast growth factor receptors (FGFR), [6] the RAF—MEK—mitogen-activated protein kinase (MAPK) [7] and the phosphatidylinositol 3-kinase (PIK3K)—AKT—mammalian target of rapamycin (mTOR) [8] pathways, the hepatocyte growth factor (HGF)—mesenchymal-epithelial transition factor (c-MET) axis [9], the Janus kinase (JAK)—signal transducers and activators of transcription (STAT) [10], Notch [11], Nuclear Factor kB (NF-kB) [12] and Wnt [13] signaling pathways, among many others (Fig. 12.1).

The identification of these drivers has led to the clinical development of specific therapies that specifically suppress these targets, with demonstrated efficacy over conventional chemotherapies in patients harboring the cognate genetic driver kinase [14]. The tyrosine kinase inhibitors osimertinib (epidermal growth factor receptor, EGFR) [15], imatinib (BCR-ABL) [16], larotrectinib (TRK) [17] and the small molecule vemurafenib (BRAF V600) [18] and antibody trastuzumab (human epidermal growth factor receptor 2, HER2) [19] are successful cases of this inhibition.

Importantly, in the context of genetic complexity of most human cancers, a single small molecule or antibody directed against an oncogenic target is rarely long-lasting and resistance develops. Thus, one strategy to improve the magnitude and

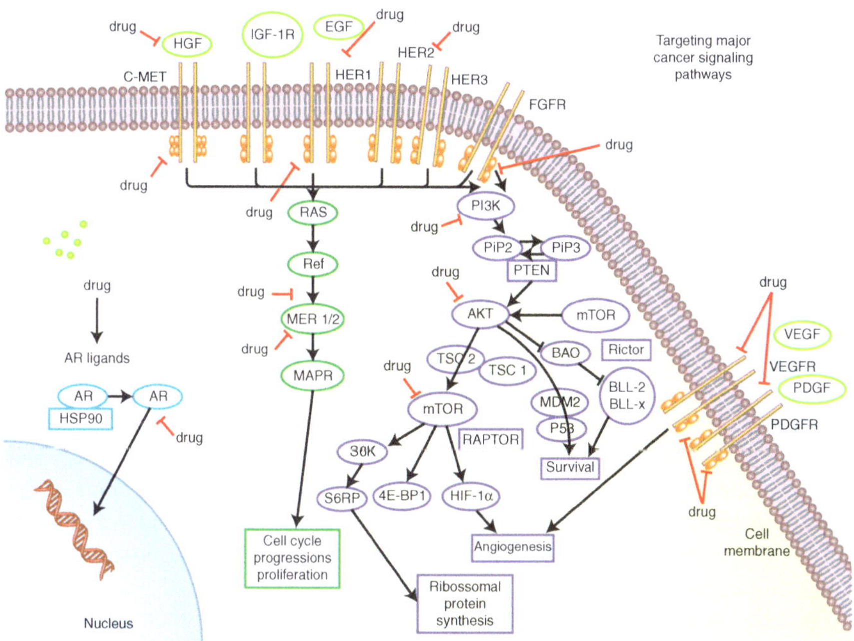

Fig. 12.1 Targeting the major cancer signaling pathways. A number of key transmembrane receptors, such as mesenchymal-epithelial transition factor (c-MET), insulin-like growth factor-1 receptor (IGF-1R), and the ErbB family of receptors, activate the RAS/RAF/MEK/mitogen-activated protein kinase (MAPK) and phosphatidylinositol 3-kinase (PI3K)/AKT signaling pathways. The vertical blockade of multiple targets with drugs that inhibit the same target but through alternative mechanisms or drugs that block different targets along the same molecular pathway; or compensatory blockade involving drugs that inhibit a primary target and the secondary signaling escape mechanism that develops as a result of adaptive resistance, such as targeting androgen receptor (AR) and PI3K/AKT pathways [1]. BCL-2 antagonist of cell death; *BCL* B-cell lymphoma; *EGFR* epidermal growth factor receptor; *HGF* hepatocyte growth factor; *FGFR* fibroblast growth factor receptor; *MDM2* mouse double minute 2 homolog; *mTOR* mammalian target of rapamycin; *mTORC* mTOR complex; *NFB* nuclear factor B; *PIP2* phosphatidylinositol (4,5)-bisphosphate; *PIP3* phosphatidylinositol (3,4,5)-trisphosphate; *PDGF(R)* Platelet-derived growth factor receptor; *RAPTOR* regulatory associated protein of mTOR; *Rheb* RAS homolog enriched in brain; *RICTOR* rapamycin-insensitive companion of mTOR; *TSC* tuberous sclerosis complex; *VEGF(R)* Vascular endothelial growth factor receptor

duration of therapeutic benefit may be achieved with the combination of molecularly targeted and/or cytotoxic drugs. However, the design of combinatorial studies presents specific challenges including but not limited to the predefined dose of each agent in a proposed combination, the optimal regimen schedule as well as the logistics and the regulatory aspects of that particular clinical study [20].

The present chapter summarizes the challenges and future directions for the development of novel targeted therapies and logical combinatorial studies in oncology.

12.2 Strategies for the Development of Molecularly Targeted Agents in Phase I Trials

Despite the advances in the understanding of the oncogenic process and the molecular characteristics of tumors, the drug attrition rate remains a concern in the drug development in oncology with most drugs tested in phase I trials failing to demonstrate a clinical benefit in confirmatory phase III studies [21, 22].

These highly unsuccessful rates of oncologic drugs compared with other therapeutic areas may be explained in part by their unique characteristics. They include diversity of targets and mechanisms of action, complex pharmacology, narrow therapeutic index, sparse pharmacokinetics and lack of data in healthy patients [23, 24]. Thus, it is essential to stay away from a one-size-fits-all model and develop a more efficient process, aiming to optimize the chances of success.

A number of solutions such as the incorporation of biomarkers in the early stages of development, use modern trial designs like adaptive trial designs, and Pharmacokinetic (PK) and Pharmacodynamic (PD) modeling. In this context, the Pharmacological Audit Trail (PhAT) framework was developed to address important questions relating to biomarkers during the drug development process and to make rational go/no-go drug development decisions [25–27].

The pharmacological audit trail (PhAT) comprises six important aspects: (1) definition of the target population through the use of predictive biomarkers of response (2) pharmacokinetics; (3) pharmacodynamics; (4) intermediate biomarkers of response; (5) tissue molecular analysis at resistance and (6) overcoming resistance through the use of predictive biomarkers of response and resistance [27].

Many novel targeted therapies aim to inhibit protein products of specific genomic alterations, such as EGFR mutations in lung cancer or HER2 amplification in breast cancer. When possible, before starting an early-phase study, it is helpful to define a biologically defined patient population to target. Frequently, however, this approach does not always identify those patients who are more likely to respond to treatment: for example, aberrations along the FGFR pathway do not robustly predict response to FGFR inhibitors in many solid tumors [28, 29].

With the availability of several next-generation sequencing (NGS) platforms in clinical practice, the number of basket studies including patients with a specific mutation irrespective of their tumor type, as well as the development of master protocols, has increased exponentially [30]. A good example is the NTRK inhibitor larotrectinib, which obtained the first tumor-agnostic approval in oncology for tumors expressing NTRK fusion, regardless of primary tumor [17].

PK and PD are essential in phase I drug development trials. PK data provide valuable information on drug exposures and plays an important role in go/no-go drug development decisions for investigational therapies. PK characterization, including its half-life, Cmax, and interaction with food and concomitant medications are critical aspects of early phase studies [31]. Similarly, the use of PD biomarkers such as proof-of-mechanism endpoints, is extremely valuable to demonstrate modulation of the target and pathway by the investigational drug [32]. In this regard, questions related to the optimal biomarker to measure, the best tissue to use (including normal vs tumor tissue) and the amount of target and pathway inhibition necessary are usually considered at this point [27]. Importantly, the inclusion of appropriate PD studies should be carefully considered given the effort and costs associated with developing such PD assays. For example, for molecularly targeted therapies expected to target a large number of kinases, the final activity may not be related with the PD biomarker studied [33].

Similarly, intermediate endpoint biomarkers of clinical response are gaining cumulative importance as they provide early insights as to whether patients will benefit (or not) from an investigational drug. As access to tumor tissue is not always feasible, circulating biomarkers, which may be either tumor-specific, such as prostate specific antigen (PSA) in prostate cancer or cancer antigen 125 (CA-125) in ovarian cancer; or circulating tumor DNA, have been incorporated into trials at different stages of drug development [34–37]. Functional imaging, such as with positron emission tomography (PET) scans, may provide early insights on antitumor responses to targeted therapies, as observed with FDG-PET during treatment with imatinib for the treatment of GIST [38].

The development of molecularly targeted therapies has been a successful approach in genomically-characterized tumors [15, 18, 39]. Nonetheless, acquired resistance invariably occurs. Reassessment of molecular characteristics at time of progression is therefore important in providing valuable information into mechanisms of resistance and to guide the switching or additional therapies with the potential to reverse tumor resistance. For example, *EGFR* T790M mutations found in patients with EGFR-mutant lung cancer progressing on first generation anti-EGFR therapies led to the development of novel third generation EGFR inhibitors, such as osimertinib, which has potent activity against *EGFR* T790M mutations [40]. The use of combinatorial regimens is another rational way to overcome tumor resistance.

12.3 Patient Selection and Predictive Biomarkers

Given the significant genetic and molecularly heterogeneity observed among tumors, biomarkers may potentially be used to establish a more homogeneous group of patients using the genetic profiling to inform the selection of rational treatments for each individual patient [41]. Many predictive biomarkers of response explore the concept of oncogene addiction, a molecular phenomenon where some tumors rely on a single dominant oncogene for growth and survival, thus inhibition of this specific oncogene is sufficient to achieve tumor control [42]. Several drug-predictive biomarker associations are now approved for specific genetic subtypes of tumors and include trastuzumab in HER2 positive metastatic breast cancer [43], crizotinib in echinoderm microtubule-associated protein-like 4 (EML4)-ALK rearranged non-small cell lung cancer [44], imatinib in chronic myelogenous leukemia targeting BCR-ABL [45], trametinib in V600E BRAF-mutated melanoma [46], and olaparib in *BRCA1/2*-mutated ovarian and breast cancer [47, 48].

However, considerable challenges exist with the incorporation of predictive biomarkers into clinical trials. Tumor heterogeneity between primary and metastatic lesions and the lack of longitudinal assessment of genetic and other alterations over time are major concerns for the successful treatment of advanced tumors [49]. Other issues include the absence of a clear cut-off to define the presence of a specific marker and the prime method of obtaining a tumor sample. These issues may help to explain why the presence or absence of a specific biomarker is not always a guarantee of clinical response. For example, not all *EGFR* mutant non-small cell lung cancers respond to EGFR inhibitors [50], while MEK and BRAF inhibitors have shown antitumor activity in non-small cell lung carcinoma (NSCLC), but not in colorectal carcinoma [51]. These differences may be explained by complex cellular networks or signaling crosstalk, or other feedback mechanisms that limit or bypass the oncoprotein blockade. Similarly, resistance to biomarker-based therapies may be multifactorial because of insufficient target inhibition, altered target by splice variant or mutation, modulation of the signaling pathway or other compensatory mechanisms [1].

12.4 Rationale for Combination Strategies

The full potential of molecularly targeted cancer therapeutics may be dependent on the selection of the best possible drug combinations. The rational design of therapeutic strategies is critical and relies on both tumor biology and the pharmacology of drugs tested *in vitro* using cultured cells, *in vivo* using animal models and in clinical studies, ultimately still with no guarantee of success [52–54]. Computational and bioinformatic approaches can inform this rational selection and may involve large biology high-throughput screening data [1, 52]. However, this is a complex process with several challenges, such as the (frequent) incomplete understanding of the underlying mechanism(s) of action of the growing number of new targets and agents under development, or the lack of standardized preclinical models to examine novel combinations of investigational agents [3].

Strategies focused on reverting drug resistance with rational combinatorial regimens may be successful pursued through the use of agents with different mechanisms of action [e.g. lenvatinib (VEGFR inhibitor) combined with everolimus (mTOR inhibitor) for renal cell carcinoma] [55]; or targeting the same target with two agents (e.g. combined with pertuzumab for HER2 positive breast cancer) [19], or through vertical blockade of signaling pathways (e.g. lapatinib combined with trastuzumab for HER2 positive breast cancer) [56]; or optimizing the inhibition of a specific target or pathway (e.g. trametinib combined with dabrafenib in melanoma) [57]. Between January 2012 and June 2018, nine different combinations that included targeted therapies were approved by the FDA for use in adult solid malignancies (Table 12.1) [58].

Given cancer heterogeneity and clonal evolution, prior therapies may impact the genomic phenotype of resistant clones upon progression, and the choice of the

Table 12.1 FDA regular approvals of targeted therapy combinations in adult solid tumors between January 2012 and June 2018 [58]

Year of approval	Tumor type	Combination	Biomarker
2012	Everolimus + exemestane[a]	Breast	HR positive, HER2 negative
2014	Trametinib + dabrafenib	Melanoma	BRAF V600 mutation
2015	Palbociclib + letrozole[a]	Breast	HR positive, HER2 negative
2015	Cobimetinib + vemurafenib	Melanoma	BRAF V600 mutation
2016	Palbociclib + fulvestrant[a]	Breast	HR positive, HER2 negative
2016	Lenvatinib + everolimus	RCC	
2017	Trametinib + dabrafenib	NSCLC	BRAF V600 mutation
2017	Pertuzumab + T	Breast	HER2 amplified/protein overexpression
2018	Trametinib + dabrafenib	Thyroid cancer	BRAF V600E mutation
2018	Abemaciclib + aromatase inhibitor[a]	Breast cancer	HR positive, HER2 negative
2018	Encorafenib + binimetinib	Melanoma	BRAF V600E or V600K mutation

HR hormone receptor, *NSCLC* non-small cell lung carcinoma, *RCC* renal cell carcinoma
[a]Targeted therapy-endocrine therapy

optimal targeted therapy is likely to be time-sensitive. For example, *EGFR* mutant non-small cell lung cancer may initially be responsive to EGFR tyrosine kinase inhibitors (TKIs) [59–61], but eventually progress and present frequently (60%) with a p.Thr790Met point mutation in the gene encoding *EGFR*. In these cases, the treatment with a third generation EGFR TKI, osimertinib (selective for both EGFR and T790M), has shown significantly greater efficacy than standard chemotherapy [40].

12.5 Trial Designs for Combination Regimens

Novel trial designs are required to optimize the investigation of anticancer drug combinations. The ideal design depends on several factors, including the characteristics of the individual drugs, potential toxicities and interactions, and the population of interest for that particular study [1]. Before testing, the biologically active dose and maximum tolerated dose (MTD) for both agents should ideally be defined, which should be based on available non-clinical data, such as PK, PD and toxicology studies [62]. As drug scheduling may have additive or synergistic effects on efficacy and/or toxicity, preclinical studies may explore alternate schedules that result in more consistent and optimal drug exposures [1].

There is no "one size fits all" approach for trial combination studies [2]. Nevertheless, there are in general three typical scenarios for two-drug combinations (drug A and B) [20]: when the combination of A plus B is active but both A and B as single agents are inactive (scenario 1), hence, the goal should be to optimize the ratio of A:B and the dose and schedule of the combination regimen. In scenario 2, drug B is inactive but modulates the activity of drug A; thus, the focus should be on evaluating the effect of the dose of drug B on the efficacy and toxicity of drug A. In scenario 3, drugs A and B are active, but the combination works better than single agents alone. In the latter case, the combination should be further evaluated in a suitably-powered randomized trial.

The design of combination phase I study should address the potential toxicities/dose-limiting toxicities (DLTs), the plausible mechanistic basis for pharmacodynamic interactions leading to DLTs, and the mechanistic basis for PK interactions between the combination partners [2]. Indeed, overlapping DLTs may limit escalation doses to levels required for optimal activity or may affect dose intensity due to dose reductions when the regimen is administered chronically. The PD interactions may result in toxicity and impact the combination dose achieved, e.g., the combination of bevacizumab and sorafenib or sunitinib resulted in proteinuria/thrombocytopenia [63]. By the same token, completion of an initial PK analysis of an individual drug prior to the drug combination is likely to increase the reliability of evidence for or against the interaction [64].

Classic DLT-driven studies, typically the "3 + 3" dose escalation designs or variations of, have been commonly used [65, 66]. However, for molecularly targeted agents, the biologically active dose may differ greatly from the MTD, which may pose significant challenges with regard to the optimal dose for future clinical trials. Newer designs have included targeted therapies and standard therapies, include several arms with different standard therapies in combination with targeted agents under investigation [67]. Bayesian adaptive models have been explored here and may prove useful as they incorporate the analysis of data from multiple doses and schedules, and use mathematic modelling to choose dose combinations optimizing efficacy and minimizing toxicity [1]. In general, these designs allow dose escalation and de-escalation, stop rules for toxicity, efficacy or futility, and adding or dropping new treatment arms and sample size re-estimation. They tend to be more efficient, flexible using fewer dose levels and treat more patients near the optimal biological dose [25]. On the other hand, the limitations related to the complex statistical analysis, scientific conclusions and logistics must also be considered [68].

12.6 Examples of Successful Combination Therapies in Oncology

In this section, we highlight a few key examples of successful combination regimens involving molecularly targeted agents.

1. Trastuzumab plus pertuzumab in breast cancer

The Epidermal Growth Factor (EGF) family comprises four receptors: epidermal growth factor receptor (HER1, erbB1), HER2 (erbB2), HER3 (erbB3), and HER4 (erbB4). Inside the human DNA, the HER2 gene is located on the long arm of chromosome 17 at q21 and encodes a 185-kDa transmembrane protein [69]. A low level of complement of HER2 membrane protein exists in normal tissues, however, an overexpression of the same is seen in 20–30% of breast cancers, and this has been shown to correlate with clinical aggressiveness and worse prognosis [43]. HER2 along with the estrogen receptor (ER) signaling pathways play a pivotal role in cell proliferation, differentiation and survival in majority of breast cancers. This pathway has led to an important milestone in the drug development history of breast cancer (Fig. 12.1).

Several randomized trials have demonstrated the efficacy of trastuzumab when used in combination with adjuvant chemotherapy for the treatment of early stage, HER2 positive breast cancer [70–73]. Similarly, multiple trials were conducted to test the efficacy of trastuzumab in the metastatic setting and all of them have shown that trastuzumab is effective in the treatment of HER2 positive breast cancer. The HERCULES trial [74] combined trastuzumab, cyclophosphamide and epirubicin for treatment of metastatic breast cancer. Tumor response rates were 57%, 60%, and 25% in the HEC-60, HEC-90, and EC-90 arms, respectively; while median time to progression was 12.5, 10.1, and 7.6 months, respectively. The M77001 trial [75] showed that trastuzumab when combined with docetaxel improves the overall survival, response rate, response duration, time to progression and time to treatment failure, with little additional toxicity. Similar results were seen in the HERTAX trial [76], when sequential testosterone followed by docetaxel was used as first line chemotherapy in patients with HER2 positive metastatic breast cancer. Other randomized studies such as HERNATA [77] and BCIRG 007 [78] have also shown similar results.

Pertuzumab binds to HER2 and subsequently, inhibits the dimerization of HER2 with other HER receptors (HER3, HER1 and HER4), especially with HER3, and reduces the percentage of heterodimers HER2-HER3, inhibiting the critical cell signaling [79]. Interestingly, pertuzumab, is more effective than trastuzumab in disrupting the HER receptor complexes. Pertuzumab acts by inhibiting the classical signaling pathways stimulated by active HER2, including receptor dimerization, receptor phosphorylation and the activation of signaling proteins downstream from HER receptors, including ERK and AKT. Trastuzumab acts mainly through other pathways than the classical HER2-signalling cascades, stimulates strong antibody dependent cell mediated cytotoxicity, and blocks the generation of active p95HER2 fragments by inhibiting the cleavage of HER2, and others [80]. The antitumor activity of these agents was tested on HER2 positive breast xenografts. Both trastuzumab and pertuzumab potently activate antibody-dependent cellular cytotoxicity *in vitro* assay [81].

The efficacy and safety of trastuzumab and pertuzumab were then investigated in patients with breast cancer, in the neoadjuvant, adjuvant as well as metastatic settings. After the positive results with this combination prior to surgery (NeoSphere study [82]) with a significant increase in complete responses (primary endpoint), FDA granted this regimen a breakthrough designation pending a confirmatory phase III study (APHINITY) in the adjuvant setting. Results from this study were recently presented and confirmed the improvement of the rates of invasive-disease–free survival among patients with HER2-positive early breast cancer [83]. Consequently, this regimen was granted regular approval by the Agency.

This combination was further tested in larger trials in the metastatic setting. The CLEOPATRA study [39], another phase 3 study, showed significantly longer median progression-free survival with pertuzumab, trastuzumab and docetaxel in patients with HER-positive metastatic breast cancer; and led to the approval of this regimen in the advanced setting as well.

Overall, this combination is very active and well tolerated, but cardiotoxicity was found to be one of the major adverse events related to this drug, requiring regular cardiac function monitoring. Otherwise, the safety profile is favorable.

Currently, trastuzumab and pertuzumab are the two most common HER2-targeted monoclonal antibodies to be used as standard of care for the treatment of HER2 positive breast cancer in different settings. In addition, this combination has been tested in different solid tumors in several basket trials that select patients based on the overexpression of HER2, such as the MyPathway (NCT01524978) and TAPUR (NCT02693535) studies.

2. BRAF inhibitor plus MEK inhibitor in melanoma

BRAF has been shown to play a crucial role in cancer and 50–60% of melanomas carry a *BRAF* mutation [84]. The most common mutations predominantly found in patients with melanoma are *BRAF* V600E (about 80%) and *BRAF* V600K (5–30%) [85]. BRAF belongs to the RAF family kinases, described almost 30 years ago, and acts primarily through the oncogenic RAS signaling pathway (Fig. 12.1). The catalytic activity of RAF depends on an allosteric mechanism driven by kinase domain dimerization [86]. RAF inhibitors unexpectedly induce ERK signaling by stimulating RAF dimerization [87]. Subsequently, BRAF inhibitors, such as vemurafenib and dabrafenib, were developed and tested in patients with melanoma.

After very promising early-phase data [88], vemurafenib (V600E mutated BRAF inhibition) was tested in the NCT01006980 BRIM-3 trial, which demonstrated improved median progression-free survival [PFS; hazard ratio (HR) 0.26; 95% confidence interval (CI) 0.20–0.33; $P < 0.001$] and overall survival (OS; HR 0.37; 95% CI 0.26–0.55; $P < 0.001$) compared with dacarbazine in patients with advanced melanoma [46]. This led to the regulatory approval of vemurafenib for the treatment of patients with *BRAF* V600 mutant metastatic melanoma.

Another BRAF inhibitor agent, dabrafenib (GSK2118436), which selectively inhibited *BRAF* V600E kinase was developed and tested in patients with advanced melanoma as well. In the phase III trial (BREAK-3) [89] enrolling 250 patients with metastatic melanoma with *BRAF* V600 mutation, there was a significantly longer PFS in the dabrafenib group compared with chemotherapy (HR 0.30; 95% confidence interval, 0.18–0.51; $P < 0.0001$).

From a safety perspective, these therapies showed mainly cutaneous toxicities, such as rash, hyperkeratosis, cutaneous squamous cell carcinoma, however the incidence of these were lesser with dabrafenib. Vemurafenib mostly led to photosensitivity and hepatitis, while dabrafenib caused pyrexia, that responded promptly to steroids.

The MAPK signaling pathway is downstream of BRAF, and MEK inhibitors were thus used to indirectly inhibit this target in *BRAF* mutant melanoma and other cancers. Trametinib is one of the best studied MEK inhibitors to date. A phase III study of trametinib [90] reported a response rate of 22% and a median PFS of 4.8 months, compared with an 8% responses and 1.4 months in PFS in the chemotherapy arm. The overall survival rate in the intention-to-treat population was 81% in the trametinib groups and 67% in the chemotherapy group. Toxicities observed were mild and included rash, hypertension, diarrhea, edema, transient mild cardiac dysfunction, rare ocular toxicity and also creatinine kinase elevation. Although trametinib showed its efficacy as a single agent, it was less effective than dabrafenib or vemurafenib, as single therapy. Furthermore, the reactivation of the MAPK pathway caused resistance to BRAF kinase inhibitors. Thus, the next logical step was to combine these two agents to create an effective strategy.

After promising results in early phase studies [91], one pivotal phase III study tested the combination of dabrafenib with trametinib in over 700 patients with metastatic melanoma with a *BRAF* V600 mutation to receive either the combination regimen or vemurafenib alone as first-line therapy [92]. At the preplanned interim OS analysis (the primary endpoint of this study), the OS rate at 12 months was 72% in the combination-therapy group versus 65% in the vemurafenib group (HR 0.69; 95% CI, 0.53–0.89, $p = 0.005$).

This combination of dabrafenib with trametinib was later tested in a different phase III trial (COMBI-AD) against placebo, enrolling 870 patients with stage III melanoma with *BRAF* V600K or V600K mutations [93]. The primary outcome of interest was the relapse-free survival (RFS) after 1 year of treatment. Patients who received the combination therapy had an improvement in recurrence-free survival compared to those receiving placebo (HR = 0.47; 95%ci = 0.39, 0.58; $P < 0.0001$). This combination was well tolerated, albeit associated with some adverse events, including pyrexia, fatigue, nausea, headache, chills, rash, diarrhea, vomiting, arthralgia, and myalgia. Pyrexia, decreased ejection fraction and chills was the most common adverse event with dabrafenib and trametinib that resulted in discontinuation, dose reduction, or dose interruption: dabrafenib (25%, 35%, and 66% of patients, respectively) and trametinib (24%, 23% and 54% of patients respectively).

The successful improvement in clinical outcomes in these studies led to FDA approval of dabrafenib plus trametinib for both the adjuvant and metastatic treatment of melanoma with *BRAF* V600E or V600K mutations. More recently, this same combination was also approved for the treatment of metastatic anaplastic thyroid cancer with *BRAF* V600E mutations, based on an open-label phase II study conducted in this patient population [94].

Of note, this combination is currently being investigated in other solid tumors in different basket studies for patients with solid tumors that express *BRAF* V600E or V600K mutations (NCT03668431, NCT02034110, NCT03091257).

3. Lenvatinib plus everolimus in renal cell carcinoma (RCC)

Genomic alterations in signaling pathways such as PI3K-AKT and angiogenesis, that control cell-cycle progression, apoptosis and cell growth are common hallmarks of cancer [95]. mTOR is activated through PI3K-AKT pathway signaling, and when activated, phosphorylates downstream proteins, including ribosomal S6 kinase 1 (S6K1) and eukaryotic initiation factor 4E binding protein 1 (4E-BP1), activating cell growth and protein synthesis (Fig. 12.1) [96]. Everolimus is an orally bioavailable mTOR inhibitor that acts by forming a complex with the immunophilin FK506-binding protein-12, which also binds mTOR with high affinity [97]. Everolimus has demonstrated antitumor activity in a variety of human solid tumors *in vitro* and *in vivo* [98–101]. Furthermore, in two phase I studies in both Caucasian and Asian patients, everolimus was well tolerated with predictable PK at 10 mg per day and also showed promising responses in different metastatic tumors, especially in RCC and esophago-gastric malignancies [102, 103]. In late-stage clinical studies, everolimus as a single-agent was compared with other targeted therapies (anti-angiogenesis) and immunotherapies, but showed limited clinical activity [104–106]. With the approval of other therapeutic options, the use of everolimus as monotherapy for metastatic RCC has declined in the last few years.

After the discovery of *VHL* mutations and the activation of VEGF, PDGF and other genes involved in angiogenesis, cell growth, and survival, several anti-angiogenic drugs have been successfully developed and shown to improve the clinical outcomes of patients with metastatic RCC [107]. Importantly, studies investigating the role of these therapies for patients who progress on prior anti-angiogenic drugs confirmed that these agents are valid options and remain active in the refractory setting [105, 108].

In this class of drugs, lenvatinib is a novel and potent small tyrosine kinase inhibitor that inhibits VEFGR1-3, fibroblast growth factor receptor (FGFR1-4), platelet derived growth factor receptor α (PDGFRα), stem cell factor receptor (KIT) and rearranged during transfection (RET) [109]. In a phase I study that assessed the safety and tolerability of lenvatinib as a single-agent in different advanced solid tumors, the MTD was defined as 25 mg with encouraging antitumor activity, especially in melanoma and renal cell carcinoma with objective responses and prolonged disease stabilization [110].

Preclinical data have demonstrated synergy between everolimus and different VEGFR inhibitors in several solid tumors [111–113]. Similarly, in human RCC xenograft models, the antitumor activity of lenvatinib and everolimus was greater than that of either agent alone, revealed by increased *in vitro* angiogenesis inhibition via VEGFR and FGF, microvessel density, proportion of proliferative cells, apoptosis and also the expression of proliferation-related genes and upregulation of hypoxia-related genes [114, 115].

This synergistic effect of anti-VEGF and mTOR inhibition has been tested in several early-phase studies combining everolimus with different anti-angiogenic agents, such as sunitinib [116], dovitinib [117], sorafenib [118] among others. While promising antitumor responses were observed across studies, significant toxicities limited the further development of several of these drug combinations. In one of these early studies, Molina and colleagues conducted a multicenter open-label phase Ib/II study investigating the safety and preliminary antitumor activity of lenvatinib plus everolimus in metastatic RCC [116]. In the phase Ib component, the most common treatment-emergent adverse events were consistent with those seen with individual agents and no new safety signals were observed. In addition, partial responses and stable disease were achieved in 33% and 50% of patients, respectively. The clinical activity and generally manageable toxicity led to further development of this combination. In the phase II portion of this study, a total of 153 patients with metastatic RCC who progressed on prior antiangiogenic therapy were allocated at a 1:1:1 to either everolimus 10 mg (n = 50), lenvatinib 24 mg (n = 52), or the combination of lenvatinib/everolimus 18 mg/5 mg (n = 51) [55, 119]. The investigator-assessed median PFS (the primary endpoint of the study) was 5.6 months in the everolimus arm compared with 9.0 months in the lenvatinib arm (HR 0.61; 95% CI, 0.38–0.98), and 12.8 months in the lenvatinib/everolimus arm (HR 0.40; 95% CI, 0.24–0.68). In light of the PFS benefit, the FDA approved this combination for the treatment of metastatic RCC following one prior anti-angiogenic therapy in May 2016 [58]. Of note, the toxicity signal observed in this phase II portion was in line with what was observed previously, with 71% of significant toxicities, including one toxic death (cerebral hemorrhage) observed in the combination arm, and 18% treatment discontinuation rates due to toxicities. A randomized trial comparing lenvatinib/everolimus at 14 mg/5 mg versus the standard dose 18 mg/5 mg is underway to assess if efficacy with an improved safety profile can be achieved (NCT03173560).

This combination is also being investigated in other adult solid tumors such as thyroid cancer (NCT03139747) and pediatric tumors (NCT03245151). In opposition to other approved combination regimens, there is yet no biomarker available to help select those patients who are more likely to benefit from this regimen. Understanding the importance of angiogenesis in RCC, there have been intense efforts to develop reliable markers for the seven antiangiogenic drugs approved by the FDA for RCC so far [120]. A number of markers, including serum VEGF levels [121], placental growth factor (PIGF) [122] or soluble carbonic anhydrase 9 [123]; clinical factors such as hypertension [124]; or imaging markers (e.g., targeted contrast-enhanced ultrasound) [125] have been tested, but data have been inconsistent [126–128].

The future of this combination is likely to include the identification of a better efficacy/toxicity ratio to allow a wider therapeutic index, and the testing of potential synergy with other agents such as immunotherapies. Future research may also expand the indication of this regimen to other cancers, and the development of robust predictive biomarkers of response to better select those patients who will derive greater benefit from these classes of drugs.

12.7 Regulatory Recommendations for Development of Combinatorial Studies

In contrast to the first-in-human testing of investigational new drugs, where preclinical evidence about its pharmacology (PK, PD and toxicology in at least two species) and efficacy is required prior to clinical testing, the same information, in general, is not necessary for many drug combinations by Regulatory Agencies

[129]. As it became clearer that combination studies needed special attention in particular when each drug has been investigated individually, the FDA's 21 CFR 300.50 "Combination Rule" addressed fixed-dose combinations and requiring the isolation of each compound through factorial trial designs (A vs. B vs A + B) [130]. However, unexpected but significant toxicities have been encountered, e.g., multiple severe cases of microangiopathic hemolytic anemia with bevacizumab-sunitinib combination which led to premature shut down of clinical trials testing these combinations [131]. To address these issues, a series of meetings and consultations among key players in drug development and resulted in the publication of a "Guidance for Industry Codevelopment of Two or More Unmarketed Investigational Drugs for Use in Combination" by the US Food and Drug Administration (FDA) in 2010, and later updated (2013) [132]. Similarly, the European agency European Medicines Agency (EMA) also provided guidance on the clinical development strategy for combination medicinal products [133]. Of note, the European and US agencies have also been working together and exchanging information through different collaborations, as the EMA-FDA Good Manufacturing Practice (GMP) and the Mutual Reliance initiative are few examples [134].

12.8 Specific Considerations for Combination of Immuno-Oncology (IO) Therapies

The treatment landscape of several cancers has recently changed when it was able to demonstrate that reactivating antitumor immune responses by blocking the immune checkpoints, can regress tumors. While cytotoxic antibodies against T-lymphocyte associated protein 4 (CTLA-4) and programed cell death 1 (PD-1/PD-L1) have shown remarkable clinical activity and favorable toxicity profile, their clinical benefit is limited to a fraction of patients. Thus, there has been an effort to further optimize the clinical benefit of immunotherapies by combining agents with synergistic mechanisms of action [135, 136]. The combination of ipilimumab (anti-CTLA4) and nivolumab (anti-PD-1) in melanoma and renal cell carcinoma or the combination of atezolizumab (anti-PD-L1) and bevacizumab (anti-VEGFR) are successful examples of these synergies with increase response rates including complete responses and prolonged survival compared with standard of care for each tumor [21, 137, 138]. In fact, the number of new clinical trials that combine checkpoint inhibitors with other therapies is soaring since 2011 increasing from 2 to 467 clinical studies. At the same time, the average planned enrolment for each trial is dropping, which is partially a consequence of more targeted study populations [139]. As more research data devoted to these combinations accumulate, factors like limited tumor immunogenicity, accelerated tumor growth extensive tumor, tumor metabolic competition and lack of biomarkers are emergent barriers to effective tumor eradication by reactivating the antitumor immune responses [136].

12.9 Future Directions

To adequately address the enormous complexity and heterogeneity of cancer, innovative studies assessing molecularly targeted agents will need to take into consideration the unique molecular and genomic profiles of patients in a contemporaneous fashion and have provisions to adapt therapies longitudinally to match evolving changes over time. There is now a burgeoning number of novel molecularly targeted therapeutics entering the clinic that will be helpful in dealing with such issues [67]. In addition, the use of rational combinations of novel molecules is likely to be of utmost importance to address some of these biological challenges temporally and spatially.

Despite the increasing number of molecular agents that target the major signaling pathways, significant insufficiencies remain with the existing framework of oncological drug development and trial design, resulting in substantial drug attrition and lengthy timelines to regulatory approval. One approach to improve the efficiency of combinatorial regimens is to strengthen the existing preclinical models to minimize the disconnect with the clinic, and to enable a more rational strategy to systematically evaluate different possible biomarker-driven drug combinations [140]. Ultimately, more translational research will be key to identifying more robust predictive biomarkers of response and resistance that can help better select patients and to predict their eventual response and resistance to specific therapies. In this search for predictive biomarkers, the ability to use circulating tumor DNA will enable the longitudinal evaluation of genomic changes that affect tumor pathogenesis, without the necessity for invasive biopsies. It also allows the analysis of molecular changes that occur secondary to treatment pressures and intra-patient tumor heterogeneity [1, 33]. Finally, the use of trial designs that shorten the testing time such as accelerated titration designs should be considered, especially where we have knowledge with other drugs in the same class, preclinical data in animal models, or other studies, that the drugs are safe at certain dose levels [67].

Key Expert Opinion Points

1. Our improved understanding of the key signaling networks involved in oncogenesis has led to the clinical development and subsequent regulatory approval of multiple molecularly targeted agents.
2. While multiple molecularly targeted agents have achieved regulatory approval as monotherapy strategies, drug resistance is almost inevitable due to different mechanisms.
3. Novel approaches to overcoming these different mechanisms of drug resistance include the development of novel molecularly targeted agents, optimization of trial designs and rational combinations of different therapies.
4. The key features of successful early phase clinical trials include having a strong scientific rationale; robust data from preclinical model systems; incorporation of pharmacokinetic (PK) and pharmacodynamic (PD) proof-of-mechanism studies;

use of optimal trial designs; and incorporation of predictive biomarkers of response to optimize patient selection to these trials.

5. The Pharmacological Audit Trail (PhAT) is a drug development framework, which addresses important questions relating to biomarkers during the drug development process and may be used to make rational go/no-go drug development decisions.

References

1. Yap TA, Omlin A, de Bono JS. Development of therapeutic combinations targeting major cancer signaling pathways. J Clin Oncol. 2013;31:1592–605.
2. Paller CJ, Bradbury PA, Ivy SP, et al. Design of phase I combination trials: recommendations of the clinical trial design task force of the NCI investigational drug steering committee. Clin Cancer Res. 2014;20:4210–7.
3. Kummar S, Chen HX, Wright J, et al. Utilizing targeted cancer therapeutic agents in combination: novel approaches and urgent requirements. Nat Rev Drug Discov. 2010;9:843–56.
4. Sever R, Brugge JS. Signal transduction in cancer. Cold Spring Harb Perspect Med. 2015;5:a006098.
5. Goel HL, Mercurio AM. VEGF targets the tumour cell. Nat Rev Cancer. 2013;13:871–82.
6. Porta R, Borea R, Coelho A, et al. FGFR a promising druggable target in cancer: molecular biology and new drugs. Crit Rev Oncol Hematol. 2017;113:256–67.
7. Roberts PJ, Der CJ. Targeting the Raf-MEK-ERK mitogen-activated protein kinase cascade for the treatment of cancer. Oncogene. 2007;26:3291–310.
8. Morgensztern D, McLeod HL. PI3K/Akt/mTOR pathway as a target for cancer therapy. Anti-Cancer Drugs. 2005;16:797–803.
9. Cecchi F, Rabe DC, Bottaro DP. Targeting the HGF/met signaling pathway in cancer. Eur J Cancer. 2010;46:1260–70.
10. Thomas SJ, Snowden JA, Zeidler MP, et al. The role of JAK/STAT signalling in the pathogenesis, prognosis and treatment of solid tumours. Br J Cancer. 2015;113:365–71.
11. Yuan X, Wu H, Xu H, et al. Notch signaling: an emerging therapeutic target for cancer treatment. Cancer Lett. 2015;369:20–7.
12. Xia Y, Shen S, Verma IM. NF-κB, an active player in human cancers. Cancer Immunol Res. 2014;2:823–30.
13. Zhan T, Rindtorff N, Boutros M. Wnt signaling in cancer. Oncogene. 2016;36:1461.
14. Neel DS, Bivona TG. Resistance is futile: overcoming resistance to targeted therapies in lung adenocarcinoma. Precis Oncol. 2017;1:3.
15. Soria J-C, Ohe Y, Vansteenkiste J, et al. Osimertinib in untreated EGFR-mutated advanced non–small-cell lung cancer. N Engl J Med. 2018;378:113–25.
16. Druker BJ, Guilhot F, O'Brien SG, et al. Five-year follow-up of patients receiving imatinib for chronic myeloid leukemia. N Engl J Med. 2006;355:2408–17.
17. Drilon A, Laetsch TW, Kummar S, et al. Efficacy of larotrectinib in TRK fusion-positive cancers in adults and children. N Engl J Med. 2018;378:731–9.
18. Hyman DM, Puzanov I, Subbiah V, et al. Vemurafenib in multiple nonmelanoma cancers with BRAF V600 mutations. N Engl J Med. 2015;373:726–36.
19. Swain SM, Baselga J, Kim S-B, et al. Pertuzumab, trastuzumab, and docetaxel in HER2-positive metastatic breast cancer. N Engl J Med. 2015;372:724–34.
20. Humphrey RW, Brockway-Lunardi LM, Bonk DT, et al. Opportunities and challenges in the development of experimental drug combinations for cancer. J Natl Cancer Inst. 2011;103:1222–6.

21. Motzer RJ, Tannir NM, McDermott DF, et al. Nivolumab plus Ipilimumab versus Sunitinib in advanced renal-cell carcinoma. N Engl J Med. 2018;378:1277–90.
22. Shih H-P, Zhang X, Aronov AM. Drug discovery effectiveness from the standpoint of therapeutic mechanisms and indications. Nat Rev Drug Discov. 2017;17:19.
23. Tuntland T, Ethell B, Kosaka T, et al. Implementation of pharmacokinetic and pharmacodynamic strategies in early research phases of drug discovery and development at Novartis Institute of Biomedical Research. Front Pharmacol. 2014;5:174.
24. Garralda E, Dienstmann R, Tabernero J. Pharmacokinetic/pharmacodynamic modeling for drug development in oncology. Am Soc Clin Oncol Educ Book. 2017:210–5.
25. Zang Y, Lee JJ. Adaptive clinical trial designs in oncology. Chin Clin Oncol. 2014;3:49.
26. Standing JF. Understanding and applying pharmacometric modelling and simulation in clinical practice and research. Br J Clin Pharmacol. 2017;83:247–54.
27. Banerji U, Workman P. Critical parameters in targeted drug development: the pharmacological audit trail. Semin Oncol. 2016;43:436–45.
28. Sweeney C, Percent IJ, Babu S, et al. Phase 1b/2 study of enzalutamide (ENZ) with LY3023414 (LY) or placebo (PL) in patients (pts) with metastatic castration-resistant prostate cancer (mCRPC) after progression on abiraterone. Proc Am Soc Clin Oncol. 2019;37:5009.
29. Baselga J, Campone M, Piccart M, et al. Everolimus in postmenopausal hormone-receptor–positive advanced breast cancer. N Engl J Med. 2011;366:520–9.
30. Hirakawa A, Asano J, Sato H, et al. Master protocol trials in oncology: review and new trial designs. Contemp Clin Trials Commun. 2018;12:1–8.
31. Cook N, Hansen AR, Siu LL, et al. Early phase clinical trials to identify optimal dosing and safety. Mol Oncol. 2015;9:997–1007.
32. Parchment RE, Doroshow JH. Pharmacodynamic endpoints as clinical trial objectives to answer important questions in oncology drug development. Semin Oncol. 2016;43:514–25.
33. Kurnit KC, Ileana Dumbrava EE, Litzenburger BC, et al. Precision oncology decision support: current approaches and strategies for the future. Clin Cancer Res. 2018;24:2719–31.
34. Yan W-T, Cui X, Chen Q, et al. Circulating tumor cell status monitors the treatment responses in breast cancer patients: a meta-analysis. Sci Rep. 2017;7:43464.
35. Araujo DV, Bratman SV, Siu LL. Designing circulating tumor DNA-based interventional clinical trials in oncology. Genome Med. 2019;11:22.
36. Scher HI, Morris MJ, Stadler WM, et al. Trial design and objectives for castration-resistant prostate cancer: updated recommendations from the prostate cancer clinical trials working group 3. J Clin Oncol. 2016;34:1402–18.
37. Rustin GJ, Vergote I, Eisenhauer E, et al. Definitions for response and progression in ovarian cancer clinical trials incorporating RECIST 1.1 and CA 125 agreed by the gynecological cancer intergroup (GCIG). Int J Gynecol Cancer. 2011;21:419–23.
38. Gayed I, Vu T, Iyer R, et al. The role of 18F-FDG PET in staging and early prediction of response to therapy of recurrent gastrointestinal stromal tumors. J Nucl Med. 2004;45:17–21.
39. Baselga J, Cortés J, Kim S-B, et al. Pertuzumab plus Trastuzumab plus Docetaxel for Metastatic Breast Cancer. N Engl J Med. 2012;366:109–19.
40. Mok TS, Wu Y-L, Ahn M-J, et al. Osimertinib or platinum–pemetrexed in EGFR T790M–positive lung cancer. N Engl J Med. 2017;376:629–40.
41. Wilhelm-Benartzi CS, Mt-Isa S, Fiorentino F, et al. Challenges and methodology in the incorporation of biomarkers in cancer clinical trials. Crit Rev Oncol Hematol. 2017;110:49–61.
42. Torti D, Trusolino L. Oncogene addiction as a foundational rationale for targeted anti-cancer therapy: promises and perils. EMBO Mol Med. 2011;3:623–36.
43. Slamon D, Eiermann W, Robert N, et al. Adjuvant trastuzumab in HER2-positive breast cancer. N Engl J Med. 2011;365:1273–83.
44. Solomon BJ, Mok T, Kim D-W, et al. First-line crizotinib versus chemotherapy in ALK-positive lung cancer. N Engl J Med. 2014;371:2167–77.
45. Hochhaus A, Larson RA, Guilhot F, et al. Long-term outcomes of imatinib treatment for chronic myeloid leukemia. N Engl J Med. 2017;376:917–27.

46. Chapman PB, Hauschild A, Robert C, et al. Improved survival with vemurafenib in melanoma with BRAF V600E mutation. N Engl J Med. 2011;364:2507–16.
47. Robson M, Im S-A, Senkus E, et al. Olaparib for metastatic breast cancer in patients with a germline BRCA mutation. N Engl J Med. 2017;377:523–33.
48. Ledermann J, Harter P, Gourley C, et al. Olaparib maintenance therapy in platinum-sensitive relapsed ovarian cancer. N Engl J Med. 2012;366:1382–92.
49. Kummar S, Williams PM, Lih CJ, et al. Application of molecular profiling in clinical trials for advanced metastatic cancers. J Natl Cancer Inst. 2015;107:djv003.
50. Mayo C, Bertran-Alamillo J, Molina-Vila MA, et al. Pharmacogenetics of EGFR in lung cancer: perspectives and clinical applications. Pharmacogenomics. 2012;13:789–802.
51. Tolcher AW, Baird RD, Patnaik A, et al. A phase I dose-escalation study of oral MK-2206 (allosteric AKT inhibitor) with oral selumetinib (AZD6244; MEK inhibitor) in patients with advanced or metastatic solid tumors. J Clin Oncol. 2011;29:–3004.
52. Al-Lazikani B, Banerji U, Workman P. Combinatorial drug therapy for cancer in the post-genomic era. Nat Biotechnol. 2012;30:679–92.
53. Garnett MJ, McDermott U. The evolving role of cancer cell line-based screens to define the impact of cancer genomes on drug response. Curr Opin Genet Dev. 2014;24:114–9.
54. Wong AHH, Li H, Jia Y, et al. Drug screening of cancer cell lines and human primary tumors using droplet microfluidics. Sci Rep. 2017;7:9109.
55. Motzer RJ, Hutson TE, Glen H, et al. Lenvatinib, everolimus, and the combination in patients with metastatic renal cell carcinoma: a randomised, phase 2, open-label, multicentre trial. Lancet Oncol. 2015;16:1473–82.
56. Baselga J, Bradbury I, Eidtmann H, et al. Lapatinib with trastuzumab for HER2-positive early breast cancer (NeoALTTO): a randomised, open-label, multicentre, phase 3 trial. Lancet. 2012;379:633–40.
57. Long GV, Stroyakovskiy D, Gogas H, et al. Combined BRAF and MEK inhibition versus BRAF inhibition alone in melanoma. N Engl J Med. 2014;371:1877–88.
58. US Food Drug Administration: US Food and Drug Administration Approved Drugs. 2018. www.fda.gov
59. Wu YL, Zhou C, Liam CK, et al. First-line erlotinib versus gemcitabine/cisplatin in patients with advanced EGFR mutation-positive non-small-cell lung cancer: analyses from the phase III, randomized, open-label, ENSURE study. Ann Oncol. 2015;26:1883–9.
60. Mok TS, Wu YL, Thongprasert S, et al. Gefitinib or carboplatin-paclitaxel in pulmonary adenocarcinoma. N Engl J Med. 2009;361:947–57.
61. Maemondo M, Inoue A, Kobayashi K, et al. Gefitinib or chemotherapy for non-small-cell lung cancer with mutated EGFR. N Engl J Med. 2010;362:2380–8.
62. Morrissey K, Yuraszeck T, Li CC, et al. Immunotherapy and novel combinations in oncology: current landscape, challenges, and opportunities. Clin Transl Sci. 2016;9:89–104.
63. Chou TC. Theoretical basis, experimental design, and computerized simulation of synergism and antagonism in drug combination studies. Pharmacol Rev. 2006;58:621–81.
64. Hamberg P, Verweij J. Phase I drug combination trial design: walking the tightrope. J Clin Oncol. 2009;27:4441–3.
65. Storer BE. Design and analysis of phase I clinical trials. Biometrics. 1989;45:925–37.
66. Le Tourneau C, Lee JJ, Siu LL. Dose escalation methods in phase I cancer clinical trials. J Natl Cancer Inst. 2009;101:708–20.
67. LoRusso PM, Boerner SA, Seymour L. An overview of the optimal planning, design, and conduct of phase I studies of new therapeutics. Clin Cancer Res. 2010;16:1710–8.
68. Cook T, DeMets DL. Review of draft FDA adaptive design guidance. J Biopharm Stat. 2010;20:1132–42.
69. Fukushige S, Matsubara K, Yoshida M, et al. Localization of a novel v-erbB-related gene, c-erbB-2, on human chromosome 17 and its amplification in a gastric cancer cell line. Mol Cell Biol. 1986;6:955–8.

70. Madarnas Y, Trudeau M, Franek JA, et al. Adjuvant/neoadjuvant trastuzumab therapy in women with HER-2/neu-overexpressing breast cancer: a systematic review. Cancer Treat Rev. 2008;34:539–57.
71. Mariani G, Fasolo A, De Benedictis E, et al. Trastuzumab as adjuvant systemic therapy for HER2-positive breast cancer. Nat Clin Pract Oncol. 2009;6:93–104.
72. Piccart-Gebhart MJ, Procter M, Leyland-Jones B, et al. Trastuzumab after adjuvant chemotherapy in HER2-positive breast cancer. N Engl J Med. 2005;353:1659–72.
73. Romond EH, Perez EA, Bryant J, et al. Trastuzumab plus adjuvant chemotherapy for operable HER2-positive breast cancer. N Engl J Med. 2005;353:1673–84.
74. Untch M, Muscholl M, Tjulandin S, et al. First-line trastuzumab plus epirubicin and cyclophosphamide therapy in patients with human epidermal growth factor receptor 2-positive metastatic breast cancer: cardiac safety and efficacy data from the herceptin, cyclophosphamide, and epirubicin (HERCULES) trial. J Clin Oncol. 2010;28:1473–80.
75. Marty M, Cognetti F, Maraninchi D, et al. Randomized phase II trial of the efficacy and safety of trastuzumab combined with docetaxel in patients with human epidermal growth factor receptor 2–positive metastatic breast cancer administered as first-line treatment: the M77001 study group. J Clin Oncol. 2005;23:4265–74.
76. Hamberg P, Bos MMEM, Braun HJJ, et al. Randomized phase II study comparing efficacy and safety of combination-therapy trastuzumab and docetaxel vs. sequential therapy of trastuzumab followed by docetaxel alone at progression as first-line chemotherapy in patients with HER2+ metastatic breast cancer: HERTAX trial. Clin Breast Cancer. 2011;11:103–13.
77. Andersson M, Lidbrink E, Bjerre K, et al. Phase III randomized study comparing docetaxel plus trastuzumab with vinorelbine plus trastuzumab as first-line therapy of metastatic or locally advanced human epidermal growth factor receptor 2–positive breast cancer: the HERNATA study. J Clin Oncol. 2011;29:264–71.
78. Valero V, Forbes J, Pegram MD, et al. Multicenter phase III randomized trial comparing docetaxel and trastuzumab with docetaxel, carboplatin, and trastuzumab as first-line chemotherapy for patients with HER2-gene-amplified metastatic breast cancer (BCIRG 007 study): two highly active therapeutic regimens. J Clin Oncol. 2011;29:149–56.
79. Franklin MC, Carey KD, Vajdos FF, et al. Insights into ErbB signaling from the structure of the ErbB2-pertuzumab complex. Cancer Cell. 2004;5:317–28.
80. Nami B, Maadi H, Wang Z. Mechanisms underlying the action and synergism of trastuzumab and pertuzumab in targeting HER2-positive breast cancer. Cancers. 2018;10:342.
81. Scheuer W, Friess T, Burtscher H, et al. Strongly enhanced antitumor activity of trastuzumab and pertuzumab combination treatment on HER2-positive human xenograft tumor models. Cancer Res. 2009;69:9330–6.
82. Gianni L, Pienkowski T, Im YH, et al. Efficacy and safety of neoadjuvant pertuzumab and trastuzumab in women with locally advanced, inflammatory, or early HER2-positive breast cancer (NeoSphere): a randomised multicentre, open-label, phase 2 trial. Lancet Oncol. 2012;13:25–32.
83. von Minckwitz G, Procter M, de Azambuja E, et al. Adjuvant pertuzumab and trastuzumab in early HER2-positive breast cancer. N Engl J Med. 2017;377:122–31.
84. Colombino M, Capone M, Lissia A, et al. BRAF/NRAS mutation frequencies among primary tumors and metastases in patients with melanoma. J Clin Oncol. 2012;30:2522–9.
85. Menzies AM, Haydu LE, Visintin L, et al. Distinguishing clinicopathologic features of patients with V600E and V600K BRAF-mutant metastatic melanoma. Clin Cancer Res. 2012;18:3242–9.
86. Yuan J, Ng WH, Lam PYP, et al. The dimer-dependent catalytic activity of RAF family kinases is revealed through characterizing their oncogenic mutants. Oncogene. 2018;37:5719–34.
87. Lavoie H, Therrien M. Regulation of RAF protein kinases in ERK signalling. Nat Rev Mol Cell Biol. 2015;16:281–98.

88. Sosman JA, Kim KB, Schuchter L, et al. Survival in BRAF V600-mutant advanced melanoma treated with vemurafenib. N Engl J Med. 2012;366:707–14.
89. Hauschild A, Grob JJ, Demidov LV, et al. Dabrafenib in BRAF-mutated metastatic melanoma: a multicentre, open-label, phase 3 randomised controlled trial. Lancet. 2012;380:358–65.
90. Flaherty KT, Robert C, Hersey P, et al. Improved survival with MEK inhibition in BRAF-mutated melanoma. N Engl J Med. 2012;367:107–14.
91. Flaherty KT, Infante JR, Daud A, et al. Combined BRAF and MEK inhibition in melanoma with BRAF V600 mutations. N Engl J Med. 2012;367:1694–703.
92. Robert C, Karaszewska B, Schachter J, et al. Improved overall survival in melanoma with combined dabrafenib and trametinib. N Engl J Med. 2015;372:30–9.
93. Long GV, Hauschild A, Santinami M, et al. Adjuvant dabrafenib plus trametinib in stage III BRAF-mutated melanoma. N Engl J Med. 2017;377:1813–23.
94. Subbiah V, Kreitman RJ, Wainberg ZA, et al. Dabrafenib and trametinib treatment in patients with locally advanced or metastatic BRAF V600-mutant anaplastic thyroid cancer. J Clin Oncol. 2018;36:7–13.
95. Sanchez-Vega F, Mina M, Armenia J, et al. Oncogenic signaling pathways in the cancer genome atlas. Cell. 2018;173:321–37.
96. Huang Z, Wu Y, Zhou X, et al. Clinical efficacy of mTOR inhibitors in solid tumors: a systematic review. Future Oncol. 2015;11:1687–99.
97. Seeliger H, Guba M, Kleespies A, et al. Role of mTOR in solid tumor systems: a therapeutical target against primary tumor growth, metastases, and angiogenesis. Cancer Metastasis Rev. 2007;26:611–21.
98. O'Reilly T, McSheehy PMJ, Brueggen J, et al. *In vivo* antitumor activity of RAD001 (everolimus) in 58 specialized human tumor xenograft models. Cancer Res. 2008;68:–2917.
99. Lane H, Tanaka C, Kovarik J, et al. Preclinical and clinical pharmacokinetic/pharmacodynamic (PK/PD) modeling to help define an optimal biological dose for the oral mTOR inhibitor, RAD001, in oncology. Proc Am Soc Clin Oncol. 2003;22:237.
100. Mabuchi S, Altomare DA, Cheung M, et al. RAD001 inhibits human ovarian cancer cell proliferation, enhances cisplatin-induced apoptosis, and prolongs survival in an ovarian cancer model. Clin Cancer Res. 2007;13:4261–70.
101. Boulay A, Rudloff J, Ye J, et al. Dual inhibition of mTOR and estrogen receptor signaling in vitro induces cell death in models of breast cancer. Clin Cancer Res. 2005;11:5319–28.
102. O'Donnell A, Faivre S, Burris HA 3rd, et al. Phase I pharmacokinetic and pharmacodynamic study of the oral mammalian target of rapamycin inhibitor everolimus in patients with advanced solid tumors. J Clin Oncol. 2008;26:1588–95.
103. Okamoto I, Doi T, Ohtsu A, et al. Phase I clinical and pharmacokinetic study of RAD001 (everolimus) administered daily to Japanese patients with advanced solid tumors. Jpn J Clin Oncol. 2010;40:17–23.
104. Motzer RJ, Escudier B, Oudard S, et al. Efficacy of everolimus in advanced renal cell carcinoma: a double-blind, randomised, placebo-controlled phase III trial. Lancet. 2008;372:449–56.
105. Choueiri TK, Escudier B, Powles T, et al. Cabozantinib versus everolimus in advanced renal-cell carcinoma. N Engl J Med. 2015;373:1814–23.
106. Motzer RJ, Escudier B, McDermott DF, et al. Nivolumab versus everolimus in advanced renal-cell carcinoma. N Engl J Med. 2015;373:1803–13.
107. Choueiri TK, Motzer RJ. Systemic therapy for metastatic renal-cell carcinoma. N Engl J Med. 2017;376:354–66.
108. Rini BI, Escudier B, Tomczak P, et al. Comparative effectiveness of axitinib versus sorafenib in advanced renal cell carcinoma (AXIS): a randomised phase 3 trial. Lancet. 2011;378:1931–9.
109. Matsui J, Yamamoto Y, Funahashi Y, et al. E7080, a novel inhibitor that targets multiple kinases, has potent antitumor activities against stem cell factor producing human small cell lung cancer H146, based on angiogenesis inhibition. Int J Cancer. 2008;122:664–71.
110. Boss DS, Glen H, Beijnen JH, et al. A phase I study of E7080, a multitargeted tyrosine kinase inhibitor, in patients with advanced solid tumours. Br J Cancer. 2012;106:1598–604.

111. Fuereder T, Jaeger-Lansky A, Hoeflmayer D, et al. mTOR inhibition by everolimus counteracts VEGF induction by sunitinib and improves anti-tumor activity against gastric cancer in vivo. Cancer Lett. 2010;296:249–56.
112. Mariniello B, Rosato A, Zuccolotto G, et al. Combination of sorafenib and everolimus impacts therapeutically on adrenocortical tumor models. Endocr Relat Cancer. 2012;19:527–39.
113. Wang Z, Zhou J, Fan J, et al. Effect of rapamycin alone and in combination with sorafenib in an orthotopic model of human hepatocellular carcinoma. Clin Cancer Res. 2008;14:5124–30.
114. Adachi Y, Matsuki M, Yamaguchi A, et al. Abstract 3264: Lenvatinib in combination with everolimus demonstrated enhanced antiangiogenesis and antitumor activity in human RCC xenograft models. Cancer Res. 2016;76:–3264.
115. Kimura T, Adachi Y, Matsuki M, et al. The antitumor activity of lenvatinib (LEN) in combination with everolimus (EVE) in human renal cell carcinoma (RCC) xenograft models is dependent on VEGFR and FGFR signaling. Ann Oncol. 2016;27:vi2.
116. Molina AM, Feldman DR, Voss MH, et al. Phase 1 trial of everolimus plus sunitinib in patients with metastatic renal cell carcinoma. Cancer. 2012;118:1868–76.
117. Powles T, Foreshew S-JS, Shamash J, et al. A phase Ib study investigating the combination of everolimus and dovitinib in vascular endothelial growth factor refractory clear cell renal cancer. Eur J Cancer. 2014;50:2057–64.
118. Harzstark AL, Small EJ, Weinberg VK, et al. A phase 1 study of everolimus and sorafenib for metastatic clear cell renal cell carcinoma. Cancer. 2011;117:4194–200.
119. Leonetti A, Leonardi F, Bersanelli M, et al. Clinical use of lenvatinib in combination with everolimus for the treatment of advanced renal cell carcinoma. Ther Clin Risk Manag. 2017;13:799–806.
120. Barata PC, Rini BI. Treatment of renal cell carcinoma: current status and future directions. CA Cancer J Clin. 2017;67:507–24.
121. Escudier B, Eisen T, Stadler WM, et al. Sorafenib for treatment of renal cell carcinoma: final efficacy and safety results of the phase III treatment approaches in renal cancer global evaluation trial. J Clin Oncol. 2009;27:3312–8.
122. Rini BI, Michaelson MD, Rosenberg JE, et al. Antitumor activity and biomarker analysis of sunitinib in patients with bevacizumab-refractory metastatic renal cell carcinoma. J Clin Oncol. 2008;26:3743–8.
123. Zurita AJ, Jonasch E, Wang X, et al. A cytokine and angiogenic factor (CAF) analysis in plasma for selection of sorafenib therapy in patients with metastatic renal cell carcinoma. Ann Oncol. 2012;23:46–52.
124. Rini BI, Quinn DI, Baum M, et al. Hypertension among patients with renal cell carcinoma receiving axitinib or sorafenib: analysis from the randomized phase III AXIS trial. Target Oncol. 2015;10:45–53.
125. Wei S, Fu N, Sun Y, et al. Targeted contrast-enhanced ultrasound imaging of angiogenesis in an orthotopic mouse tumor model of renal carcinoma. Ultrasound Med Biol. 2014;40:1250–9.
126. Farber NJ, Kim CJ, Modi PK, et al. Renal cell carcinoma: the search for a reliable biomarker. Transl Cancer Res. 2017;6:620–32.
127. Duda DG, Munn LL, Jain RK. Can we identify predictive biomarkers for antiangiogenic therapy of cancer using mathematical modeling? J Natl Cancer Inst. 2013;105:762–5.
128. Jain RK, Duda DG, Willett CG, et al. Biomarkers of response and resistance to antiangiogenic therapy. Nat Rev Clin Oncol. 2009;6:327–38.
129. Tsimberidou A-M, Kurzrock R, Anderson KC, et al. Targeted therapy in translational cancer research: John Wiley & Sons; 2015.
130. US Food Drug Administration: CFR-code of federal regulations title 21. Current good manufacturing practice for finished pharmaceuticals Part 211, 2015.
131. Feldman DR, Baum MS, Ginsberg MS, et al. Phase I trial of bevacizumab plus escalated doses of sunitinib in patients with metastatic renal cell carcinoma. J Clin Oncol. 2009;27:1432–9.

132. US Food Drug Administration: Codevelopment of two or more unmarketed investigational drugs for use in combination. www.fda.gov, 2015.
133. US Food Drug Administration: Guideline on clinical development of fixed combination medicinal products. www.ema.europa.eu, 2017.
134. US Food Drug Administration: Center for Biologics Evaluation and Research (CBER) Foreign Inspectional Collaborations. www.fda.gov, 2018.
135. Ott PA, Hodi FS, Kaufman HL, et al. Combination immunotherapy: a road map. J Immunother Cancer. 2017;5:16.
136. Zappasodi R, Merghoub T, Wolchok JD. Emerging concepts for immune checkpoint blockade-based combination therapies. Cancer Cell. 2018;33:581–98.
137. Wolchok JD, Chiarion-Sileni V, Gonzalez R, et al. Overall survival with combined nivolumab and ipilimumab in advanced melanoma. N Engl J Med. 2017;377:1345–56.
138. Motzer RJ, Powles T, Atkins MB, et al. IMmotion151: a randomized phase III study of atezolizumab plus bevacizumab vs sunitinib in untreated metastatic renal cell carcinoma (mRCC). J Clin Oncol. 2018;36:578.
139. Schmidt C. The benefits of immunotherapy combinations. Nature. 2017;552:S67–s69.
140. Klauschen F, Andreeff M, Keilholz U, et al. The combinatorial complexity of cancer precision medicine. Onco Targets Ther. 2014;1:504–9.

Chapter 13
Incorporating Precision Medicine into Phase I Clinical Trials

Funda Meric-Bernstam

Abstract There has been growing interest in molecular profiling of tumors in order to identify actionable alterations and offer molecularly matched therapies. Given the rapid incorporation of next generation sequencing into clinical care, genomic profiling has led the way with transcriptional profiling and immune profiling closely following. Increasing numbers of Phase I trials are biomarker-selected, and there are large number of biomarker-selected Phase II basket trials or signal-seeking expansions. Although there have been several recent successes, genomically-informed therapy has several challenges. In this chapter we will review the pros and cons of biomarker-selected early phase therapies and review strategies for patient screening. We will also review challenges in genomically-informed therapy including need for functional annotation and determining decision support, tumor heterogeneity, genomic evolution, and management of incidental results.

Keywords Precision oncology · Personalized cancer therapy · Biomarker Genomics · Next generation sequencing · Tumor heterogeneity · Phase I trials Incidental results

Key Points

- Increasing numbers of Phase I and Phase II studies are exploring molecular specific populations.
- Biomarker based selection studies allow for increased efficacy, earlier line of patient but may slow accrual and require increased sites who have biomarker capability.
- Biomarker selection marker trials need decision support in order to succeed.
- Even in earlier trials there is increasing use of research biopsies and biomarker analysis.
- Trial design strategies in biomarker selected trials can increase feasibility and enrollment.

F. Meric-Bernstam (✉)
Department of Investigational Cancer Therapeutics, The University of Texas MD Anderson Cancer Center, Houston, TX, USA
e-mail: fmeric@mdanderson.org

T. A. Yap et al. (eds.), *Phase I Oncology Drug Development*,
https://doi.org/10.1007/978-3-030-47682-3_13

13.1 Considerations for Biomarker Selected Trials

13.1.1 Design of Biomarker Selected Trial

Biomarker selected trials can be designed in several ways. In most cases trials are genomically-selected, enrolling patients with a specific alteration or a class of alterations to be enrolled, for treatment with matching therapy. Trials can be ongoing in a selected tumor type, allocating patients with different alterations to different matching therapies, often referred to as "umbrella trials". Other trials maybe open to multiple tumor types, enrolling patients with specific alterations to get a specific treatment, often referred to a "Basket trials". In the context of a Phase I trials that are genotype-selected enrollment is often across a variety of tumor types, with either biomarker-selected histology specific expansions (e.g. BRAF V600E mutant lung cancer, BRAF V600E mutant melanoma etc.) or can be a biomarker-selected tumor agnostic "basket" expansion (e.g. BRAFV600E mutant solid tumors).

13.1.2 Advantages and Disadvantages of Using Genomic Markers for Patient Selection for Phase I trials

Increasingly drugs are developed targeting known genomic alterations within a tumor. If there is strong scientific rationale as to efficacy in a specific genotype, there is rationale in introducing biomarkers selection early. The advantages of early biomarker selection include (a) increasing likelihood of efficacy signal early in the drug development by enrolling matched patients, (b) decreasing likelihood of treating patients that are less likely to respond, (c) potential of referral of molecularly matched patients earlier in their treatment course. However, there are also disadvantages of biomarker selection in a Phase I trial: (1) slowing down accrual, (2) need for more sites, (3) need to engage centers that do biomarker testing already or support screening (4) miss the opportunity to identify efficacy signal beyond indications that were considered initially. Thus given advantages and disadvantages, Phase I trials need to be designed balancing different needs to identify recommended phase 2 dose (RP2D) efficiently while treating the most relevant patient population. Strategies to balance this can be also implemented at the level of enrollment, such as accruing "allcomers" in dose escalation to facilitate rapid identification of RP2D, but allowing for additional "backfill" slots for patients with desired genotypes as they are identified. Backfill slots can also be utilized to build out patients who are able to undergo pre-treatment and on-treatment biopsies for pharmacodynamic analysis in genomically matched patients.

13.1.3 Patient Screening for Biomarker-Selected Trials

Feasibility of enrolling to genomically-selected trials is expedited by the fact that many major centers as well as community practices are increasingly performing genomic testing for tumor characterization and treatment selection. Thus genomic characterization of mutations, copy number changes, and in some cases fusions, may be already available and will facilitate enrollment of patients with actionable alterations.

Other clinical trials may be using patient selection with nonstandard of care tests. This may be an RNA based assay to look at expression levels, or immunohistochemistry assay looking for targets of a therapeutic agent, such as targeted therapy or antibody drug conjugate, or alternatively looking at more complex markers, such as immune infiltration or expression of a protein on selected cell, such as PDL1 expression on tumor infiltrating immune cells. These assays, if not standard of care for that tumor type, need to be specifically offered to patients for patient accrual. This could be done using two strategies, either by consenting a patient for prescreening upon progression of next line of therapy, or by offering prescreening on patients already on another therapy with the intent of offering them a trial participation upon progression. Each approach has advantages and disadvantages. The first approach has the advantage of only offering prescreening to patients who are ready for trial enrollment and committed to getting treated on the trial, but has the disadvantage of delays in archival tissue at recruitment and biomarker testing with a potential of decline in patient performance status in the interim or progression. The ultimate strategy of prescreening while another line of therapy is often favored by investigators and patients alike, as it allows for patients to receive treatment while getting prescreening. The disadvantage is that there will be a significant drop off in the number of patients prescreened to those who have undergone treatment because the patient may either progress with the decline of performance not being available and eligible for treatment, or may have worsening or may continue to benefit from ongoing treatment, and not require another treatment, or alternatively may elect to pursue another treatment upon progression. Finally, some biomarkers are expected to be static and therefore can be tested on archival tissue while some other biomarkers, such as immune microenvironment changes, may be modulated by last line of treatment and there may be a competitive advantage of fresh biopsy and biomarker assessment of the new tissue. Therefore these are important considerations in clinical trial design.

13.2 Interpreting Biomarker Reports for Patient Selection

13.2.1 Need for Decision Support

A critical part of success for precision oncology clinical trials is to have the infrastructure in place for decision support. This includes having ready access to a knowledge base and a mechanism for clinical trial matching. There are several approaches being developed commercially as well as public resources being developed. In addition, many major cancer centers have established institutional efforts including knowledgebases, decision support teams, automatic clinical trial alert systems or automatic clinical trial matching systems.

13.2.2 Determination of Actionability

A key step in precision oncology is determining if a patient has an actionable alteration upon molecular profiling. With increasing understanding in genomics, several genetic alterations are increasingly recognized as drivers of cancer development and progression. Such a genomic alteration can be considered actionable therapeutically if it predicts therapeutic response either sensitive or resistant, affects the cancer related gene, can be targeted directly or indirectly with an approved investigational agent, or it is specific to eligible criteria for enrollment in genotype selected trials. Additionally, an actionable alteration can be actionable if it assists in establishing diagnosis or prognosis, modulates drug metabolism and/or adverse events, or may predict future risk of cancer or other diseases.

In the context of genomic testing, the first step includes assessment of the quality of the genomic report and ensuring that testing was performed in a CLIA platform. Then, assessment focuses on identifying whether the patient has mutations, copy number changes, or fusions in a gene that is considered actionable. Next step is to determine the functional consequence of the alteration determining whether there is clinical data or any preclinical information suggesting that the alteration affects the function in the gene which would drive oncogenesis or affect sensitivity to therapeutic strategy. There are also a large number of computational tools being developed to assess likelihood an alteration affects function, or that it is a driver [1, 2]. Although such computational functional predictions can also be utilized in the assessment of variants of unknown significance (VUS), their predicted ability has not been confirmed enough to warrant their use in clinical application in many cases. Putting all this information together, the clinician decides whether there is a functional alteration in the driver gene and whether there are any relevant targeting drugs, whether direct or indirect. In the context of an alteration that has Level 1 evidence, treatment with that therapeutic agent would be construed to be standard of care. However, in the absence of level of evidence, clinical trial enrollment with genotype relevant trials can considered, but one would expect informed consent to provide information to the patient regarding what is known about the alteration and what is the known therapeutic efficacy in targeting that alteration.

Whether enrollment genomically selected trials should be limited to patients with known functional alterations or those with any alteration (functional as well as VUSs) has been controversial. Although allowing for patients with VUSs can speed up accrual, it is likely to dilute the efficacy signal to be seen and expose patients less likely to be benefiting from targeted therapy from an investigational agent. Thus, for alterations that are more common, there is an advantage of limiting enrollment to functional alterations, even in phase I trials, and especially so in the expansion phase where there is a definite signal seeking intent for efficacy.

13.2.3 Treatment Selection in the Setting of Multiple Alterations

A common concern is how to handle treatment selection in patients who have more than one alteration. In patients with more than one actionable alteration, an important consideration is whether the co-alterations alterations will be expected to affect the efficacy of the target. In the absence of such information, decision is based on the level of evidence of actionable alteration as well as mutant allelic frequency or extent of copy number changes in making the decision.

When co-alterations may affect the sensitivity of targeted therapy, important considerations is whether the alteration is clonal, and if the level of evidence that the coalteration may limit therapeutic efficacy, and to what extent. For example, while *PIK3CA* mutations have been associated relative resistance with decreased sensitivity to HER2 inhibitors, this is a difference in relative sensitivity and not an absolute resistance marker. In contrast, *KRAS* mutations in the context of EGFR targeting are known to make therapy ineffective, and therefore are considered absolute resistance markers. These nuances are important in deciding whether co-alterations indeed are strong enough resistance marker to change therapeutic plan or whether a patient can cautiously be treated with planned targeted therapy or whether it is possible to pursue clinical trials that would target both alterations or treat with a strategy that would not be limited by either marker.

13.3 Tumor Heterogeneity and Genomic Evolution

Another limitation of precision oncology is that there may be substantial tumor heterogeneity in biomarkers of response including differences between the primary tumor metastasis, between different metastases, and even with different areas of the same tumor [3]. Although in some scenarios there has been shown to be convergent evolution, with heterogeneity within a tumor but with different alterations in different areas within the tumor, but with common pathways getting activated [4]. However, differences between primary and metastasis have also been to affect actionable genes [5], including demonstration of acquired resistance mutations, such as *ESR1* mutations [6] seen in breast cancer patients after treatment with endocrine therapy in the adjuvant or metastatic setting. Thus therapeutic choices, and potentially therapeutic sensitivity, may differ based on what was sequenced. Tumor heterogeneity is genuine concern in drug development, and may play a role in early resistance development or mechanism acquired resistance. Upon treatment with targeted therapy, patients may lose a target or develop acquired resistance mechanisms with the enrichment of new genomic alterations driving the same pathway or an alternate survival pathway. Although truncal alterations found in the primary tumor (as well as the metastasis) are likely to be the most effective strategy therapeutically, in patients who have had targeted therapy with progression after initial response or stable disease, repeat biopsy or assessment of the genomic profile with liquid biopsies may be a consideration to ensure the patients have not had genomic evolution with mechanism acquired resistance. For the purpose of clinical trials it would be reasonable to enroll patients based on testing of archival tissue; however, pretreatment biopsy with central testing at the completion the study may be able to give insights the differential efficacy seen between patients. For targets that are known to have significant genomic evolution such as *HER2* especially in diseases where there is great heterogeneity already, such as in gastric cancer, there may be an advantage for pretreatment biopsy and repeat testing to ensure that patients who are truly still HER2 positive are enrolled in trials to enhance efficacy signals seen even in early phase clinical trials. The advantages of biopsies for confirmation of drivers of course is to be balanced with the cost of the biopsy and risk of adverse events associated with the biopsy as well the concerns about delays of treatment with repeat testing.

13.4 Biomarker Discovery and Validation in Biomarker-Selected Trials

Even in Phase I trials, there is increasing utilization of research biopsies and biomarker analysis. Thus the following can be incorporated for biomarker analysis (Fig. 13.1):

1. Pre-treatment biopsies: Obtaining pre-treatment biopsies can facilitate assessment of the biomarker that was used for selection in the archival tissue to confirm concordance. It will also allow for whole exome sequencing, RNA sequencing, immunohistochemistry for putative predictive markers to better characterize biomarkers associated with response or clinical benefit
2. On-treatment biopsies: On treatment biopsies can help determine target engagement, pathway inhibition, adaptive responses and effects on microenvironment

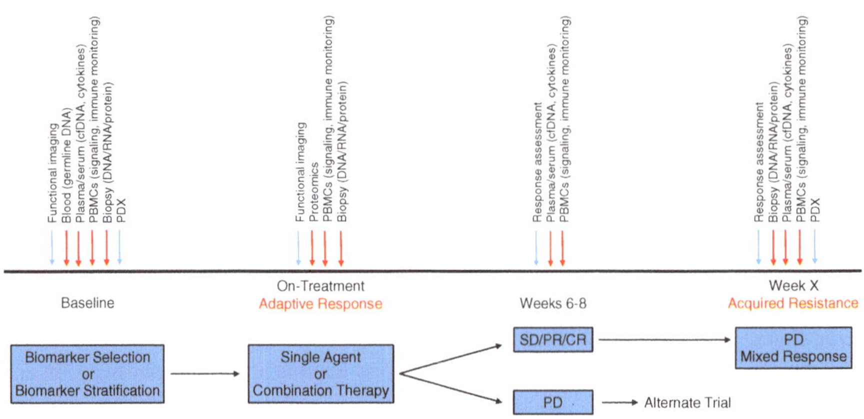

Fig. 13.1 Incorporating biomarkers into clinical trials. Pre-treatment, on-treatment and post-progression biopsies with tumor and liquid biopsies

and immune environment. These can help determine if biologically relevant doses are achieved, of the expected biological effect are obtained and can help design future combination therapy trials. Timing of on-treatment biopsies can be a bit more complicated to determine,
3. Post-progression biopsies: In patients with initial response or prolonged stable disease, a post-progression biopsy can be invaluable to determine mechanism of acquired resistance. Further, molecular characterization in the CLIA environment can also help provide guidance for selection of next line of therapy.
4. Liquid biopsies: There is increasing interest in using circulating free DNA for use in clinical decision-making as well as research. Liquid biopsies pre-treatment can give insight into predictive markers. On-treatment longitudinal sampling can give insight into cfDNA dynamics as an early response marker. Post-progression sampling can help with discovery of resistance markers. There is also interest in exosomal DNA and RNA, circulating tumor cells and other markers.
5. Other surrogate markers: Other surrogate tissue such as skin, hair follicles, platelet rich plasma or peripheral blood mononuclear cells are all of interest to assess target inhibition or other pharmacodynamic effects. Similarly longitudinal serum /plasma can be used to look at tumor markers (such as CEA), surrogate markers of target inhibition (such as macrophage inhibitor cytokine-1 for MDM2 inhibition) [7], or cytokines (such as IL-6).

13.5 Strategies for Patient Identification and Enhancing Accrual to Genomically-Selected Trials

Although the genomic testing holds much promise, in initial genomic characterization efforts within MD Anderson, only 11% of patients with mutations in actionable genes were found to undergo treatment on genotype matched trials, representing only 5% of the entire population who underwent genomic testing. However with the implementation of institution-wide Precision Oncology Decision Support efforts, including establishing a knowledge base, and personalized decision support reports, it was found that 27% of patients with actionable or potentially actionable alterations went on a genomically matched trial, and there was a statistically significant difference ($P = 0.00004$) in likelihood of being treated with genomically matched therapy if a patient had an actionable or potentially actionable alteration vs unknown alteration or not actionable alteration [8]. This suggests that implementing Precision Oncology Services can help with trial accrual and also offer patients molecularly matched therapy.

Overall several strategies can be implemented either using local tools or emerging commercial tools to enhance clinical trial accrual to genomically selected early phase trials.

1. Trial Design and Feasibility

   Establishment of molecularly annotated clinical databases can help with clinical trials even at the design level or at determining feasibility, by assessing the frequency of alteration within a tumor type or across tumor types, and number of patients with specific alterations seen at center yearly.

2. Cohort Identification

   Upon activation of a genomically-selected trial, identifying active patients with appropriate stage/disease with that alteration/biomarker can help rapid accrual from the time of trial activation. Patients can be simply tracked until progression or be made aware of the trial in advance, so that patients to be familiar with the trial as a future treatment option.

3. Patient identification

   Establishment of alerts to study PI or study team when patients have an appropriate alteration upon testing can help with accrual by focusing patient screening efforts on patients with eligible alterations.

4. Trial identification

   Notifying treating oncologist of potential trial options, either through careful annotation of genomic reports or by trial alerts to the clinical care team can help ensure team is aware of the fact that genomic testing results are back and that the results are actionable, with potential clinical trials. There has been also interest in patient notification tools as well as giving patients direct access to genomic reports as well as even research testing results. The best practices to share data with patients to make genomic testing most informative and clinical impactful has not yet been determined.

5. Trial matching search engines

   There are many parallel efforts for clinical trial matching. Many simply leverage disease type and study title, while others provide more detailed matching taking clinical characteristics and eligibility criteria into consideration as well as more molecularly oriented biomarker-drug matching algorithms [9]. Some rely on patient or clinicians to enter data into an interface. Further, many commercial systems are exploring use of natural language processing for patient characteristics matching, as well as gene-drug associations.

13.6 Experience with Genomically Informed Early Phase Clinical Trials

Recently there has been a large number of clinical trials that were genomically selected, several showing signal efficacy in phase I clinical trials, as well as in phase II basket trials. These strategies can be easily deployed as histology specific clinical trials when the target is a common alteration in a relatively common tumor, such as *PIK3CA* mutation in hormone receptor positive breast cancer. Design and accrual to clinical trials such as this are more complicated when the alteration is relatively rare in a common tumor, such as *BRAF* mutation in lung cancer and becomes exceedingly more complex as the alteration becomes even rarer across common tumors or found commonly in rare tumors, such in the case of *TRK* fusions. For clinical trial design, one strategy enrolling patients with such trials in a histology independent fashion, therefore patients with the same alteration regardless of histology, are enrolled and analyzed together. The advantage of this is to be able to determine whether the biomarker has predictive value for targeted therapy, independent of histology with a potential of even pursuing a tumor agnostic registration approach. Alternately, many targeted therapies may have variable efficacy depending on histology or other co-alterations. This has led to several clinical trials where in the phase II component the targeted therapy efficacy was assessed in histology specific expansion cohorts. Examples of this include demonstration of efficacy of vemurafenib in a basket trial for BRAF V600+ mutant tumors, with ultimate registration of BRAF V600 vemurafenib for Erdheim-Chester Disease and Langerhans cell histiocytosis [10]. Another example is a basket trial for dabrafenib and trametinib for BRAF anaplastic thyroid carcinoma,.leading to approval of these agents for anaplastic thyroid carcinoma [11]. In contrast, TRK fusions regardless of histology having shown to have sensitivity to larotrectinib, thus the phase I trial was quickly followed up with a phase II trial and the combined data from these three trials, conducted in adults and pediatric populations led to registration of larotrectinib in a histology agonist fashion [12].

13.7 Return of Incidental or Secondary Results

It is notable that genomic testing is likely to also identify incidental or secondary finding of germline pathogenic mutations. For example, in the MD Anderson series, 3% of patients who underwent targeted genome sequencing in a research environment were found to have a germline alteration that was pathogenic or likely pathogenic in highly actionable genes. Many of these alterations were not previously known by the provider. Thus, it is important when patients undergoing tumor only testing that there is recognition that the alterations reported may be germline, and when patients are undergoing paired tumor versus normal testing that efforts be made to identify germline alterations that are pathogenic. It is especially important as many pathogenic germline alterations, especially alterations in the DNA damage repair pathways, are increasing becoming actionable themselves with many therapeutic agents such PARP inhibitors, ATR inhibitors, platinum agents and other DNA damage repair modulators. Furthermore, although the focus in patients with advanced disease is often on the care of the patient, when a germline pathogenic variant is found, there are also implications for the family; support for genetic counseling of family members and cascade testing should be offered.

Key Expert Opinion Points

It is critical to try to identify biomarkers of response during early drug development.

When an agent is thought to be likely to only be effective in biomarker positive patients, performing trials in a biomarker-selected fashion can ensure each patient counts and each patient gets drugs they are most likely to benefit from.

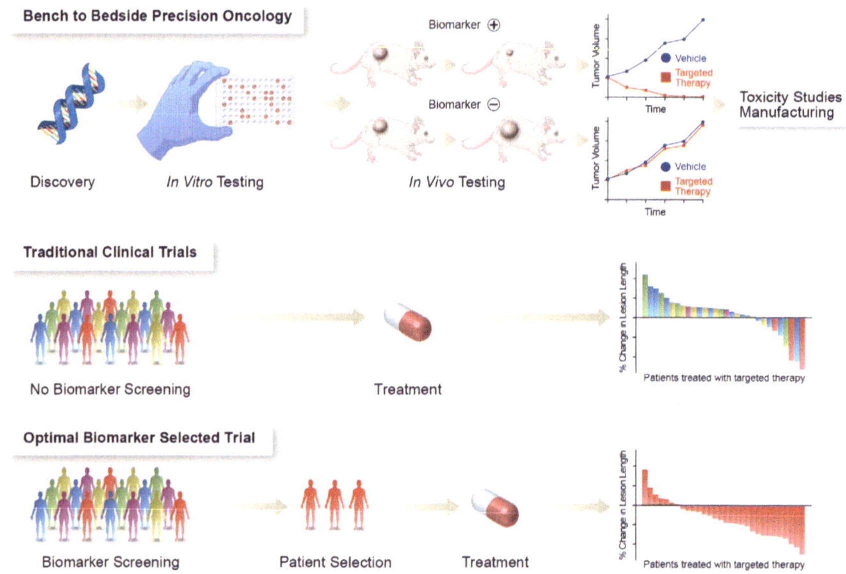

Fig. 13.2 Bench to bedside precision oncology

Determining actionability of individual alterations can ensure only patients with actionable variants are enrolled on genotype-matched trials, increasing the likelihood for success for trial and the patient.

Carefully designed biomarker discovery efforts during Phase I development can give important insights into target engagement and impact on tumor microenvironment including immunologic effects.

There is increasing interest in precision medicine, with a focus on identifying unique vulnerabilities in tumors that can be exploited for therapy. This drug development approach represents a bench to bedside continuum, from target discovery to development of a lead compound that hits the target, to preclinical studies demonstrating efficacy of the new molecular entity in target-positive models *in vitro* and *in vivo* followed by safety studies and proof of concept Phase I clinical trials (Fig. 13.2). It is expected by limiting enrollment of early phase trials to patients with relevant biomarkers, or at least by enriching trials with patients with relevant markers, we can enhance the signal of clinical efficacy in Phase I trials.

With the growing portfolio of targeted therapies, molecular profiling is increasingly used in the clinic in order to identify actionable alterations and offer molecularly matched approved or investigational therapies. Given the rapid incorporation of next generation sequencing into clinical care, genomic profiling has led the way in this case. However, transcriptional profiling is now increasingly being explored as a tool as well, while methylomics and metabolomics remain areas of extensive research. In addition, there is interest in immune profiling given the success of immune-therapeutics, and emerging biomarkers for immune-oncology as well, thus immune-profiling through combination of immunohistochemistry of other multiplex testing for immune biomarkers as well as RNA based diagnostics to better decipher the immune environment also are being increasingly explored for precision oncology and are likely to be incorporated further in early clinical trials.

References

1. Wang Z, Ng KS, Chen T, Kim TB, Wang F, Shaw K, et al. Cancer driver mutation prediction through Bayesian integration of multi-omic data. PLoS One. 2018;13(5):e0196939.
2. Bailey MH, Tokheim C, Porta-Pardo E, Sengupta S, Bertrand D, Weerasinghe A, et al. Comprehensive characterization of Cancer driver genes and mutations. Cell. 2018;174(4):1034–5.
3. Meric-Bernstam F, Mills GB. Overcoming implementation challenges of personalized cancer therapy. Nat Rev Clin Oncol. 2012;9:542–8.
4. Gerlinger M, Rowan AJ, Horswell S, Math M, Larkin J, Endesfelder D, et al. Intratumor heterogeneity and branched evolution revealed by multiregion sequencing. N Engl J Med. 2012;366(10):883–92.
5. Meric-Bernstam F, Frampton GM, Ferrer-Lozano J, Yelensky R, Perez-Fidalgo JA, Wang Y, et al. Concordance of genomic alterations between primary and recurrent breast cancer. Mol Cancer Ther. 2014;13(5):1382–9.
6. Jeselsohn R, Yelensky R, Buchwalter G, Frampton G, Meric-Bernstam F, Gonzalez-Angulo AM, et al. Emergence of constitutively active estrogen receptor-alpha mutations in pretreated advanced estrogen receptor-positive breast cancer. Clin Cancer Res. 2014;20(7):1757–67.
7. Andreeff M, Kelly KR, Yee K, Assouline S, Strair R, Popplewell L, et al. Results of the phase I trial of RG7112, a small-molecule MDM2 antagonist in leukemia. Clin Cancer Res. 2016;22(4):868–76.
8. Johnson A, Khotskaya YB, Brusco L, Zeng J, Holla V, Bailey AM, et al. Clinical use of precision oncology decision support. JCO Precis Oncol. 2017;1:1–12.
9. Zeng J, Shufean MA, Khotskaya Y, Yang D, Kahle M, Johnson A, et al. OCTANE: oncology clinical trial annotation engine. J Clin Oncol. 2019;3:1–11.
10. Diamond EL, Subbiah V, Lockhart AC, Blay JY, Puzanov I, Chau I, et al. Vemurafenib for BRAF V600-mutant Erdheim-Chester disease and langerhans cell histiocytosis: analysis of data from the histology-independent, phase 2, open-label VE-BASKET study. JAMA Oncol. 2018;4(3):384–8.
11. Subbiah V, Kreitman RJ, Wainberg ZA, Cho JY, Schellens JHM, Soria JC, et al. Dabrafenib and trametinib treatment in patients with locally advanced or metastatic BRAF V600-mutant anaplastic thyroid cancer. J Clin Oncol. 2018;36(1):7–13.
12. Drilon A, Laetsch TW, Kummar S, DuBois SG, Lassen UN, Demetri GD, et al. Efficacy of larotrectinib in TRK fusion–positive cancers in adults and children. N Engl J Med. 2018;378(8):731–9.

Chapter 14
Incorporating Circulating Biomarkers into Clinical Trials

Filip Janku

Abstract Knowing the cancer genomic profile with underlying druggable molecular alterations is important for the optimal choice of cancer therapy. However, molecular analysis of tumor DNA can be limited by the availability of the cancer tissue, which has to be obtained from therapeutic or diagnostic procedures. Molecular analysis of liquid biopsies utilizing the circulating tumor cell-free DNA offers a minimally invasive and low-risk method that can be performed at multiple time points for molecular analysis. Molecular testing of cell-free DNA can be used in multiple clinically useful applications, such as identification of molecular targets for cancer therapy, assessment of cancer prognosis, monitoring of response to cancer therapy, monitoring of tumor molecular profiles in real time, and study target engagement when developing new therapies.

Keyword Liquid biopsy · Cell-free DNA · Molecular testing · Cancer · Treatment

Key Points

- Liquid biopsies are minimally invasive and can provide tumor DNA for molecular testing.
- Molecular testing of cell-free DNA can help to determine cancer prognosis.
- Molecular testing of cell-free DNA isolated from blood or other body fluids can identify targets for cancer therapy.
- Serial molecular testing of cell-free DNA has potential as a tool for assessment of therapeutic response to cancer therapy.
- Serial molecular testing of cell-free DNA can be used to study clonal evolution and mechanisms of therapeutic resistance.
- Liquid biopsies have potential to be used in pharmacodynamic studies in clinical trials.

F. Janku (✉)
Department of Investigational Cancer Therapeutics (Phase I Clinical Trials Program), The University of Texas MD Anderson Cancer Center, Houston, TX, USA
e-mail: FJanku@mdanderson.org

T. A. Yap et al. (eds.), *Phase I Oncology Drug Development*,
https://doi.org/10.1007/978-3-030-47682-3_14

14.1 Introduction

Selection of an optimal treatment strategy requires detailed analysis of the cancer genome and identification of molecular targets for cancer therapy in each individual patient [1, 2]. Molecular testing of tumor samples obtained from diagnostic or therapeutic procedures remains the current standard of care. However, this approach has significant limitations because of tumor heterogeneity and the dynamic nature of tumor genotypes, which would mandate multiple biopsies from primary and metastatic sites at multiple time points [3, 4]. This is hardly feasible because of medical, ethical, financial and logistic considerations. To overcome these limitations, novel minimally invasive methods to detect pertinent molecular alterations in tumor DNA associated with less risk to the patient and lower cost are being developed. Mandel and Métais in 1948 noted the presence of cell-free nucleic acids (cfNA) in human blood [5, 6]. However, it took about six decades before reports were published on detection of oncogenic aberrations in blood-derived cell-free DNA (cfDNA) in patients with cancer [7]. Fragments of cfDNA can be detected in plasma, urine, cerebrospinal fluid (CSF), and other body fluids [5, 8–20]. These cfDNA fragments can be used for detection of underlying cancer-related molecular abnormalities, and such approach has become known as a liquid biopsy [12, 19, 21, 22]. In clinical trials, liquid biopsies can be used to identify targets for cancer therapy, to assess cancer prognosis, to assess efficacy of cancer therapy, to monitor cancer molecular profiles in real time and for assessment of target engagement. DNA or its fragments can enter the circulation by several distinct mechanisms, including release of nuclear and mitochondrial DNA from dying cells during either apoptosis or necrosis (Fig. 14.1). Other mechanisms of DNA release include autophagy and necroptosis [5, 23]. Fragments of cfDNA can vary in size substantially based on their mechanism of release. For instance, fragments of DNA released from apoptotic cells average around

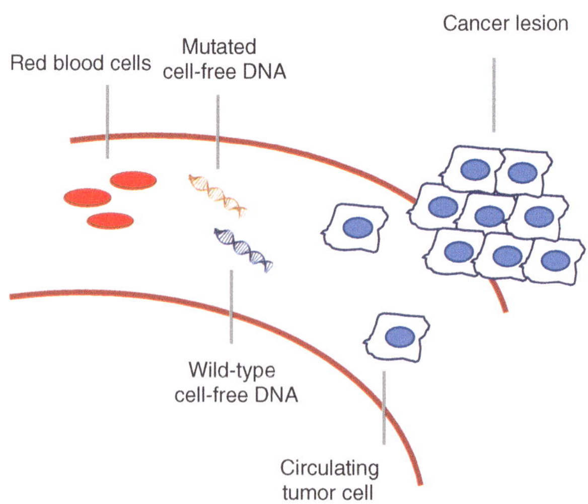

Fig. 14.1 Fragments of cell-free DNA and other sources of cancer DNA in the circulation

160–180 bp in length, while the fragments of DNA from necrotic cells are usually longer. The average lengths of cfDNA fragments from apoptotic and necrotic processes, and their ratio, may be assessed as an important element of the DNA integrity index, which may have prognostic implications [24]. The cfDNA fragments are cleared from the circulation with half-lives ranging from 15 min to a few hours [21].

14.2 Methods for Molecular Testing of cfDNA

Sample collection and processing times can impact DNA integrity and accuracy of cfDNA assessment [5, 25]. Plasma is the most frequent source of circulating cfDNA, which is preferred to serum due to lower level of high molecular contamination by non-cancerous cfDNA from lysis of normal leukocytes. Because timely processing is among the most important factors to maintain cfDNA integrity, cell-stabilizing blood collection tubes, which allow sample processing to be delayed for several days, have become increasingly popular for collection of blood samples intended for cfDNA analysis [5, 26, 27]. Other materials, such urine, CSF or other body fluids are less cellular and arguably less prone to DNA degradation [10, 12, 18–20, 28].

The tumor-specific fraction also called circulating tumor DNA (ctDNA) of the total cfDNA can be identified by the presence of cancer-specific alterations, such as hot spot mutations, or through detection of cancer-specific epigenetic modifications such as methylation patterns [5, 9]. The tumor-specific fraction in plasma can vary from 0.01% to more than 90% [5]. Lower-stage tumors have lower levels of cfDNA shedding compared to advanced disease [29]. Therefore, highly sensitive methods are required for detection of cfDNA in early disease [29, 30].

Polymerase chain reaction (PCR) approaches, or next-generation sequencing (NGS), has dominated molecular testing of cfDNA [5]. PCR methods include ARMS-Scorpion PCR (amplification refractory mutation system), PCR-SSCP (single-strand conformation polymorphism), ME-PCR (mutant enriched), MASA-PCR (mutant allele–specific amplification), PAP-A amplification (pyrophosphorolysis-activated polymerization allele-specific amplification), or RFLP-PCR (restriction fragment length polymorphism) or similar (Table 14.1) [31–36]. However, molecular testing of

Table 14.1 Examples of methods for molecular testing of cell-free DNA

Methods for cell-free DNA testing	
PCR	Next generation gequencing
Digital PCR	*Amplicon-based NGS*
Droplet digital PCR	Tam-Seq
BEAMing	***Capture-based NGS***
Quantitative PCR	CAPP-Seq
ARMS-qPCR	Safe-seq
ICE-COLD PCR	Ultra-deep NGS
Idylla	Digital sequencing

Table 14.2 Possible applications for PCR vs. NGS

PCR	NGS
Limited number of well-defined markers	Broad molecular diagnostics
Serial monitoring of a limited number of known alterations	Detection of copy number variations and fusions
Detection of alterations causing adaptive resistance in scenarios when these mechanisms are well-understood and limited in number	Detection of adaptive resistance in scenarios when these mechanisms are either poorly understood or investigated or include a large number of scenarios

cfDNA requires very high sensitivity to detect specific alterations with very low allele fractions. Therefore, novel methods using digital PCR such as droplet-based systems or the use of beads, emulsions, amplification, and magnetics (BEAMing), or microfluidic assays, are increasingly used [17, 21, 37–44]. The most significant limitation of PCR is its inability to simultaneously detect a large spectrum of aberrations.

Unlike PCR, NGS allows detection of multiple alterations across wider regions of the cancer genome. The specific regions of cfDNA can be analyzed by using targeted deep-sequencing techniques such as TAm-Seq (tagged amplicon deep sequencing), Ion AmpliSeq, Safe-Seq (safe-sequencing system), CAPP-seq (cancer personalized profiling by deep sequencing), digital sequencing or other methods [8, 14, 45–49]. The most comprehensive techniques include whole-exome and whole-genome sequencing of plasma samples; however, these approaches are less reliable in samples with lower content of ctDNA [5, 45, 50, 51]. The advantages of PCR-based and NGS-based approaches are summarized in Table 14.2.

14.3 Identification of Molecular Targets for Treatment

The feasibility of molecular testing of cfDNA was tested by comparing its concordance with molecular testing of tumor tissue. In a pilot study of 18 patients with metastatic colorectal cancer who were candidates for surgical resection or radiofrequency ablation, oncogenic mutations (*APC*, *TP53*, *PIK3CA*, and *KRAS*) were assessed by direct sequencing in tumor tissue, and at least one mutation was identified in each unique tumor [21]. Subsequently, cfDNA isolated from plasma was tested with BEAMing digital PCR. The study demonstrated oncogenic mutations can be detected in cfDNA isolated from plasma in cancer patients.

Interesting insight about factors influencing concordance was offered by a study testing a cohort of patients with advanced breast cancer. First, there was 100% concordance (34 of 34 cases) between BEAMing-detected *PIK3CA* mutations in plasma cfDNA and in tumor tissues in a cohort with simultaneous plasma and tumor collection; however, the concordance decreased to 79% in the second cohort of 60 patients when tumor samples and plasma cfDNA were obtained at different time points [39]. The relationship between concordance and time between specimen collection has been demonstrated by other studies. For instance, results of a single institution study in 168 patients with advanced cancers demonstrated that targeted digital NGS of plasma cfDNA misses known mutations in 4 major oncogenes (*TP53*, *EGFR*, *PIK3CA* and *ERBB2*) in 22–33% if the interval between tumor tissue and plasma acquisition is 6 months or less compared to 31% to 39% if the interval between tumor tissue and plasma acquisition is more than 6 months [52]. In a study of 157 patients with advanced cancer that progressed on systemic therapy who were referred for treatment with experimental targeted therapies, a panel of 21 oncogenic mutations in the *BRAF*, *EGFR*, *KRAS*, and *PIK3CA* genes was assessed in plasma cfDNA by BEAMing technology. The results demonstrated acceptable concordance (*BRAF*, 91%; *EGFR*, 99%; *KRAS*, 83%; *PIK3CA*, 91%) with results of standard-of-care mutation analysis of primary or metastatic tumor tissue obtained during clinical care [38].

Thierry et al. tested *KRAS* and *BRAF* mutations in plasma-derived cfDNA from 106 patients with metastatic colorectal cancer using allele-specific quantitative PCR and compared results to standard-of-care testing of tumor tissue and demonstrated for plasma testing 100% specificity and sensitivity for the *BRAF V600E* mutation and 98% specificity and 92% sensitivity for the common *KRAS* mutations [53].

Forshew et al. [49] tested the TAm-Seq method for identification and monitoring of oncogenic mutations in plasma cfDNA. Investigators screened 5995 genomic bases in coding regions of *TP53* and *PTEN*, and selected regions of *EGFR*, *BRAF*, *KRAS*, and *PIK3CA* for low-frequency mutations. The assay was able to detect mutations in cfDNA with sensitivity and specificity of >97%. Moreover, in one patient with synchronous primary cancers of the bowel and ovary, disease relapse was identified as being derived from the original ovarian tumor. A plasma sample collected at relapse revealed the *TP53* mutation originally found in the ovarian primary tumor, whereas the colorectal cancer-associated mutations were not detected.

Newman et al. [48] developed CAPP-Seq, an ultrasensitive NGS-based method for quantifying tumor-derived plasma cfDNA by targeting recurrently mutated regions in the cancer of interest. In patients with non-small cell lung cancer, the CAPP-Seq method was able to detect cfDNA in 100% of patients with stage II–IV disease and 50% of patients with stage I disease. The method specificity was 96% for mutant allele fractions as low as 0.02%.

In addition, we performed a series of comparative studies, which demonstrated that concordance for plasma and tumor tissue samples collected non-synchronously in common metastatic cancers ranges from 80% to >90% for digital PCR technologies and from about 70% to 80% for NGS [8, 37, 38].

In a prospective study published by Sacher et al. [17] in metastatic non-small cell lung cancer (NSCLC) it was demonstrated that ddPCR testing for *KRAS* and *EGFR* mutations has high sensitivity (64%–86%) and specificity (100%) for initiating mutations. In addition, molecular testing of plasma-derived cfDNA was associated with shorter processing timelines compared to simultaneous molecular testing of tumor tissue.

Another study in patients with *EGFR*-mutated NSCLC previously treated with first generation EGFR tyrosine kinase inhibitors demonstrated that molecular testing of plasma cfDNA before starting on third generation EGFR inhibitor

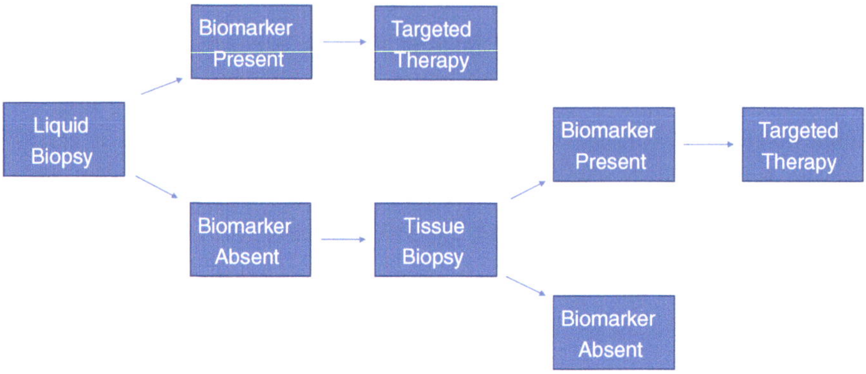

Fig. 14.2 Possible algorithm for integrating cell-free DNA-based liquid biopsy in the molecular testing

osimertinib reliably detects patients with *EGFR*^{T790M} mutations who benefit from therapy with an objective response rate (ORR) of 63% [54]. However, in patients lacking plasma *EGFR*^{T790M} mutations, the reported ORR to osimertinib was 46%, and the majority of patients with tumor shrinkage had *EGFR*^{T790M} mutations detected in tumor tissue. These data suggest that molecular testing of cfDNA might be acceptable as an initial test; however, negative results for mutations of therapeutic interest may warrant tissue confirmation (Fig. 14.2).

Finally, novel targeted NGS approaches covering a larger portion of the genome expanded ctDNA molecular diagnostics to include tumor mutation burden (TMB) testing in order to predict efficacy of PD-L1-based immune checkpoint inhibitors [55]. Early data suggest that high TMB in plasma cfDNA is an actionable marker predicting favorable outcomes for immune checkpoint inhibitors in NSCLC.

14.4 Assessment of Prognosis

The quantification of total and/or mutant cfDNA has been studied for prognosis assessment in various tumor types. Some studies demonstrated that, in cancer patients, higher levels of cfDNA are associated with higher risk of disease recurrence and progression [8, 21, 37, 38, 47, 52, 56–59]. In a study by Diehl et al. [21] in 18 colorectal cancer patients, the absence of cfDNA in plasma during the first follow-up visit after surgical resection was associated with 100% recurrence-free survival.

Early limited data suggested that persistence of *TP53* mutations in plasma cfDNA of patients with stage II or III breast cancer that were in remission was associated with higher likelihood of disease recurrence; however, the small sample size precluded any definitive conclusion [32]. In a very preliminary study in 11 colorectal cancer patients who underwent surgery, primary tumors and corresponding plasma samples were screened for *KRAS* mutations and *p16INK4a* promoter hypermethylation [34]. On follow up, these alterations were identified in plasma cfDNA only from patients with disease recurrence.

The amount of mutant cfDNA has been found to be of prognostic significance. Spindler et al. [58] demonstrated the prognostic value of the amount of total cfDNA and *KRAS* mutant cfDNA in a study of 108 patients with metastatic colorectal cancer treated with third-line cetuximab and irinotecan. Patients with higher cfDNA levels had shorter progression-free survival (PFS; 2.1 vs. 4.4 months; P = 0.0015) and overall survival (OS; 3.6 vs. 10.4 months; P < 0.0001) than patients with lower cfDNA levels. Similarly, patients with higher levels of *KRAS*-mutant cfDNA had shorter PFS (1.8 vs. 2.3 months; P = 0.008) and OS (2.1 vs. 5 months; P = 0.0005) than patients with lower levels of *KRAS*-mutant cfDNA.

The previously mentioned study, which evaluated BEAMing for the detection of 21 mutations in *BRAF*, *EGFR*, *KRAS*, and *PIK3CA* in plasma cfDNA of 157 patients with advanced cancer, also examined the prognostic impact of the amount of mutated plasma cfDNA [38]. A higher percentage of mutant cfDNA (>1% [n = 67 patients] vs. ≤1% [n = 33 patients]), irrespective of mutation type, was associated with a shorter OS (5.5 vs. 9.8 months; P = 0.001), which was confirmed in a multivariable analysis. Similarly, 41 patients with >1% of *KRAS* mutant (codon 12 or 13) cfDNA had a shorter median OS than 20 patients with ≤1% of *KRAS* mutant cfDNA (4.8 vs. 7.3 months; P = 0.008). Significant differences in OS were not observed for mutations in other examined genes, likely due to the small sample size.

In another study of 246 patients with advanced non-small-cell lung carcinoma (NSCLC) treated with platinum and vinorelbine chemotherapy, the patients with detectable plasma *KRAS* mutant (codon 12 or 13) cfDNA had a shorter median OS (4.8 vs 9.5 months; P = 0.0002) and shorter median PFS (3.0 vs 5.6 months; P = 0.0043) than patients whose cancer expressed wild-type *KRAS* [59]. A multivariate analysis confirmed the independent prognostic value of *KRAS* mutant cfDNA in OS but not in PFS. Wang et al. [60] showed the negative prognostic effect of *KRAS* mutations (codon 12 or 13) in plasma cfDNA of 273 patients with advanced NSCLC. The median PFS of patients with a plasma *KRAS* mutation was 2.5 months, while that of patients with wild-type *KRAS* was 8.8 months (P < 0.001).

In a study of 44 pancreatic cancer patients, the 1-year survival rate was 0% in those with *KRAS* codon-12 mutations in cfDNA, and 24% in those with *KRAS* wild-type in cfDNA (P < 0.005), and plasma *KRAS* mutation status was the only independent prognostic factor (odds ratio, 1.51; 95% confidence interval [CI], 1.02–2.23) [36]. In 103 patients with melanoma receiving biochemotherapy, those with a *BRAF* mutation in serum cfDNA had significantly shorter OS than those that did not have the *BRAF* mutation in serum cfDNA (13 vs. 30.6 months, P = 0.039) [61].

The negative prognostic impact of increased levels of mutant cfDNA was supported by other studies in breast cancer, colorectal cancer, ovarian cancer, and other tumor types [62–65]. Furthermore, the presence of other tumor-related genomic cfDNA aberrations was associated with poor prognosis. Detection of loss of heterozygosity and microsatellite instability in cfDNA was associated with worse prognosis for patients with breast cancer, ovarian cancer, melanoma, lung cancer, or other tumor types [66–69].

14.5 Efficacy Assessment and Monitoring

The liquid biopsy could be used as a minimally invasive way to predict and monitor therapy response in real time (Fig. 14.3) [5]. Arguably, because of the relatively short half-life of cfDNA, its changes might indicate therapeutic response, or lack of there of, earlier than conventional imaging, which is typically done after several weeks or even months of therapy [70]. In addition, early data suggest that molecular testing of dynamic changes in ctDNA can help to differentiate progression from pseudo-progression in patients treated with immunotherapy [71].

In a study of 1060 patients with advanced NSCLC treated with gefitinib, *EGFR* mutations were detected in primary tumors and corresponding plasma samples [72]. ORR were 76.9% (95% CI, 65.4–85.5) for patients with detected mutations in both tumor and plasma and 59.5% (95% CI, 43.5–73.7) for patients with mutation in the tumor but not in plasma, which demonstrated that *EGFR* mutation status could be assessed in cfDNA and serve as a positive predictive biomarker for targeted therapy.

In contrast, another study assessed *BRAF* mutations in plasma cfDNA from 160 patients with advanced cancer and known *BRAF* status from archival tumor samples [57]. Patients whose archival tumor samples had a $BRAF^{V600}$ mutation (n = 51) received therapy with a BRAF and/or MEK inhibitor. The time to treatment failure (TTF) of 13 patients with a $BRAF^{V600}$ mutations in the tumor but not in plasma obtained before therapy was significantly longer than that of 38 patients whose baseline plasma cfDNA had a $BRAF^{V600}$ mutation (13.1 vs. 3.0 months; P = 0.001).

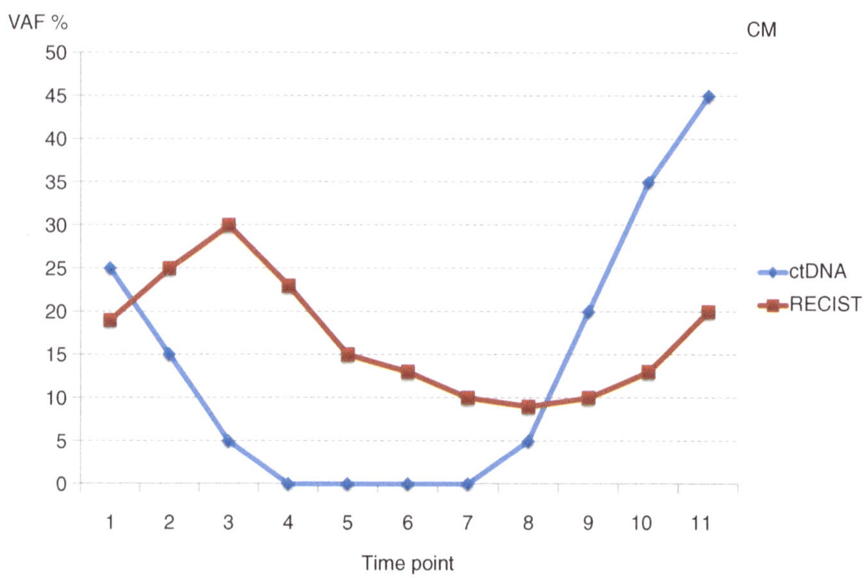

Fig. 14.3 Concept of dynamic tracking of circulating tumor DNA (ctDNA) to assess response to therapy. Blue line indicates % variant allele frequency (VAF) in the circulation and red line the sum of target lesions per RECIST criteria (please note that increase at time points 2 and 3 indicate pseudoprogression)

The absence of *BRAF*^{V600}–mutant cfDNA also was associated with longer TTF (HR, 0.31; P = 0.004) in multivariate analysis.

Dynamic tracking of ctDNA was investigated in a prospective study of 52 patients with metastatic breast cancer [40]. The plasma cfDNA was monitored to qualitatively and quantitatively assess disease progression and treatment response and compare with levels of circulating tumor cells (CTC), tumor marker cancer antigen 15-3 (CA15-3), and computed tomography (CT) imaging. The cfDNA was detected by identification of the same *PIK3CA* and *TP53* mutations and structural variations as were found in the tumor tissues. The levels of cfDNA in plasma generally correlated well with the treatment response assessed by CT imaging (as defined by Response Evaluation Criteria in Solid Tumors) [73, 74]. However, two patients in this study had discordant correlations. In 10 of the 19 patients who experienced disease progression, the cfDNA levels increased at one or more consecutive time points, on average 5 months before progressive disease was observed on imaging. Moreover, the cfDNA was found to be a more accurate biomarker for monitoring metastatic disease than CTCs, CA 15-3, or CT imaging.

Another study with 72 patients with advanced NSCLC examined the dynamic changes in cfDNA *EGFR* mutations as a predictor of response to EGFR tyrosine-kinase inhibitor targeted therapy [75]. Failure to clear plasma *EGFR* mutations after EGFR tyrosine kinase inhibitors (TKIs) was an independent predictor for shorter PFS (hazard ratio [HR] 1.97, P = 0.001) and OS (HR 1.82, P = 0.036). The *EGFR* mutations were detected by ddPCR in serial plasma samples of non-small cell lung cancer patients treated with erlotinib [76]. The study demonstrated the disappearance of *EGFR* mutations in exon 19 and 21 and the emergence of *EGFR*^{T790M} resistance mutations several weeks before radiographic disease progression.

Other studies showed that patients with advanced cancers and decrease in ctDNA on therapy compared to those with no change or increase have favorable therapeutic outcomes such as TTF [8, 9, 19]. However, it remains unclear how to translate these findings to the individualized treatment of cancer patients.

Overall, dynamic tracking of ctDNA appears to be reliable in scenarios where the cancer is heavily dependent on the alterations included in ctDNA assays (e.g. testing for *BRAF* mutation in non-Langerhans malignant histiocytosis); however, ctDNA efficacy monitoring seems to be more complicated in tumors with more heterogeneous molecular profiles [18, 37].

14.5.1 Molecular Profiling in Real-Time and Assessment of Target Engagement

Implementing principles of personalized medicine and targeted therapy into routine oncology practice provides an important shift in the treatment of advanced cancers. In metastatic disease, a chronic course is no longer unusual, and patients can survive for many years [77]. However, despite the significant initial therapeutic effect of targeted therapy, the vast majority of patients eventually develop resistance and experience tumor progression. The tumor adaptive resistance results from acquisition of mutations in the targeted genes or signaling pathways of cancer cells under therapeutic selective pressure. The mutations causing resistance also can be present in the infrequent subclones of pretreatment tumor cells and can predict the further failure of targeted therapy [3, 5, 78, 79].

The mechanisms of resistance are often known; however, since routine multiple sequential biopsies are not performed, we have no tools to describe these mechanisms at the level of an individual patient. Both intrinsic and adaptive resistance can occur because of pre-existing or acquired molecular abnormalities, such as emergence of *KRAS* mutations on treatment with EGFR monoclonal antibodies in metastatic colorectal cancer, or emergence of *EGFR*^{T790M} mutations which cause resistance to EGFR TKIs in non-small cell lung cancer [42, 54]. Lastly, *ALK* mutations L1196M or C1156Y mediates adaptive resistance to crizotinib in NSCLC with *ALK* rearrangement, and mutations in *NRAS*, *MEK,* and *BRAF* amplification indicate resistance to *BRAF* inhibitor vemurafenib in *BRAF*-mutant melanoma [80–82]. Because liquid biopsies can be obtained at low cost at multiple time points, they offer a useful tool for monitoring molecular changes associated with resistance to certain cancer therapies.

An example of emerging resistance mutations in response to targeted therapy is the acquisition of tumor *KRAS* mutations in codons 12, 13, or 61 in patients with advanced colorectal cancer treated with anti-EGFR monoclonal antibodies cetuximab or panitumumab [42, 43]. Two landmark studies have shown the possibility of detecting and monitoring these emerging *KRAS* mutations in patients with colorectal cancer in cfDNA by using BEAMing technology [42, 43]. Testing of serum cfDNA from 28 colorectal cancer patients receiving panitumumab showed that 9 of 24 patients whose tumor and cfDNA were initially *KRAS* wild-type had developed detectable cfDNA *KRAS* mutations [43]. Interestingly, multiple *KRAS* cfDNA mutations were detected in three individuals. The appearance of mutations generally occurred between 5 and 6 months following initiation of treatment. In the second study, emergence of *KRAS* aberrations was found in tumor tissue samples from metastatic sites obtained after initiation of therapy [42]. Corresponding plasma samples also showed emergence of *KRAS* mutations in cfDNA, which may have occurred as early as 10 months before radiographic progression [42]. Furthermore, our group at MD Anderson Cancer Center, using BEAMing technology, reported acquired *KRAS* and/or *EGFR* ectodomain mutations in 44% (27/62) and 8% (5/62) of plasma samples from patients with advanced colorectal cancer treated with cetuximab or panitumumab, respectively [83]. *KRAS* codon 61 and 146 mutations were predominant (33% and 11%, respectively).

Even if the candidate-gene techniques to monitor emerging resistance mutations to various targeted therapeutics provide promising results, such approaches have substantial drawbacks, most notably the requirement for prior knowledge of mechanisms of resistance and corresponding mutations. Application of unbiased approaches for detecting emergence of resistant cancer cell subclones using NGS technologies directly on the plasma samples could overcome these limitations. A proof-of-principle study by Murtaza et al. [45] monitored cancer clonal evolution and the acquisition of secondary resistance mutations to various anticancer treatments in serial plasma samples from six patients with advanced breast, ovarian, or lung cancer using unbiased whole-exome sequencing. Follow-up intervals were 1–2 years, and the exome sequencing was performed on two to five plasma samples in each patient. The results revealed emergence of distinct secondary mutations, such as an activating mutation in *PIK3CA* after paclitaxel, a truncating mutation in *RB1* after cisplatin, a truncating mutation in *MED1* after tamoxifen and trastuzumab and a splicing mutation in *GAS6* after subsequent treatment with lapatinib in the same patient, and an *EGFR* ^{T790M} mutation after treatment with gefitinib. The results of this study established that exome-wide analysis of cfDNA could complement standard biopsy to detect mutations associated with acquired resistance to therapeutic agents in advanced cancers. However, it should be noted that the detected mutant allele fractions for the aberrations were rather high (3%–45%), which can limit the applicability of such an approach to a limited subset of patients.

Recently, molecular testing of cfDNA was tested as a tool to assess pharmacodynamic endpoints in clinical trials. One of the examples was an early phase development of a novel switch pocket KIT and PDGFR inhibitor ripretinib [84]. Serial collections of blood samples from patients treated with ripretinib showed significant decrease in *KIT*-mutated ctDNA confirming on-target effects of therapy.

14.6 Conclusions

Liquid biopsy offers an attractive tool for identification of molecular targets for cancer therapy, determination of prognosis, assessment of response to anticancer therapy, real-time monitoring of cancer molecular profiles, and assessment of target engagement. Liquid biopsies are increasingly accepted as a clinical tool to detect molecular targets for cancer therapy; however, the clinical utility of other applications, such as dynamic tracking during therapy, remain to be proven in prospective studies. Furthermore, cfDNA consists of both nonmalignant and tumor DNA, and the tumor DNA fraction can be relatively small. This issue increases the demand for higher sensitivity testing, which is associated with higher cost and often prevents some more comprehensive approaches such as whole-genome or -exome NGS.

Key Expert Opinion Points

- Knowing the cancer genomic profile with underlying druggable molecular alterations is important for the optimal choice of cancer therapy.
- Molecular analysis of tumor DNA can be limited by the availability of the cancer tissue, which has to be obtained from therapeutic or diagnostic procedures.
- Molecular analysis of liquid biopsies utilizing the circulating tumor cell-free DNA offers a minimally invasive and low-risk method that can be performed at multiple time-points for molecular analysis.
- Molecular testing of cell-free DNA can be used in multiple clinically useful applications, such as identification of molecular targets for cancer therapy, assessment of cancer prognosis, monitoring of response to cancer therapy, monitoring of tumor molecular profile in real time and study target engagement when developing new therapies.

References

1. Rodon J, Soria JC, Berger R, et al. Genomic and transcriptomic profiling expands precision cancer medicine: the WINTHER trial. Nat Med. 2019;25:751–8.
2. Meric-Bernstam F, Brusco L, Shaw K, et al. Feasibility of large-scale genomic testing to facilitate enrollment onto genomically matched clinical trials. J Clin Oncol. 2015;33:2753–62.
3. Gerlinger M, Rowan AJ, Horswell S, et al. Intratumor heterogeneity and branched evolution revealed by multiregion sequencing. N Engl J Med. 2012;366:883–92.
4. Janku F. Tumor heterogeneity in the clinic: is it a real problem? Ther Adv Med Oncol. 2014;6:43–51.
5. Polivka J Jr, Pesta M, Janku F. Testing for oncogenic molecular aberrations in cell-free DNA-based liquid biopsies in the clinic: are we there yet? Expert Rev Mol Diagn. 2015;15:1631–44.
6. Mandel P, Metais P. Les Acides Nucleiques Du Plasma Sanguin Chez Lhomme. Cr Soc Biol. 1948;142:241–3.
7. Diehl F, Li M, Dressman D, et al. Detection and quantification of mutations in the plasma of patients with colorectal tumors. Proc Natl Acad Sci U S A. 2005;102:16368–73.
8. Janku F, Zhang S, Waters J, et al. Development and validation of an ultra-deep next-generation sequencing assay for testing of plasma cell-free DNA from patients with advanced cancer. Clin Cancer Res. 2017;23(18):5648–56.
9. Liu L, Toung JM, Jassowicz AF, et al. Targeted methylation sequencing of plasma cell-free DNA for cancer detection and classification. Ann Oncol. 2018;29(6):1445–53.
10. Pan W, Gu W, Nagpal S, Gephart MH, Quake SR. Brain tumor mutations detected in cerebral spinal fluid. Clin Chem. 2015;61:514–22.
11. Shi W, Lv C, Qi J, et al. Prognostic value of free DNA quantification in serum and cerebrospinal fluid in glioma patients. J Mol Neurosci. 2012;46:470–5.
12. Wang Y, Springer S, Zhang M, et al. Detection of tumor-derived DNA in cerebrospinal fluid of patients with primary tumors of the brain and spinal cord. Proc Natl Acad Sci U S A. 2015;112:9704–9.
13. Lanman RB, Mortimer SA, Zill OA, et al. Analytical and clinical validation of a digital sequencing panel for quantitative, highly accurate evaluation of cell-free circulating tumor DNA. PLoS One. 2015;10:e0140712.
14. Odegaard JI, Vincent JJ, Mortimer S, et al. Validation of a plasma-based comprehensive cancer genotyping assay utilizing orthogonal tissue- and plasma-based methodologies. Clin Cancer Res. 2018;24(15):3539–49.
15. Zill OA, Banks KC, Fairclough SR, et al. The landscape of actionable genomic alterations in cell-free circulating tumor DNA from 21,807 advanced cancer patients. Clin Cancer Res. 2018;24:3528–38.
16. Zill OA, Greene C, Sebisanovic D, et al. Cell-free DNA next-generation sequencing in pancreatobiliary carcinomas. Cancer Discov. 2015;5(10):1040–8.
17. Sacher AG, Paweletz C, Dahlberg SE, et al. Prospective validation of rapid plasma genotyping for the detection of EGFR and KRAS mutations in advanced lung cancer. JAMA Oncol. 2016;2(8):1014–22.
18. Hyman DM, Diamond EL, Vibat CR, et al. Prospective blinded study of BRAFV600E mutation detection in cell-free DNA of patients with systemic histiocytic disorders. Cancer Discov. 2015;5:64–71.
19. Fujii T, Barzi A, Sartore-Bianchi A, et al. Mutation-enrichment next-generation sequencing for quantitative detection of KRAS mutations in urine cell-free DNA from patients with advanced cancers. Clin Cancer Res. 2017;23:3657–66.
20. Husain H, Nykin D, Bui N, et al. Cell-free DNA from ascites and pleural effusions: molecular insights into genomic aberrations and disease biology. Mol Cancer Ther. 2017;16:948–55.
21. Diehl F, Schmidt K, Choti MA, et al. Circulating mutant DNA to assess tumor dynamics. Nat Med. 2008;14:985–90.

22. Mouliere F, Robert B, Arnau Peyrotte E, et al. High fragmentation characterizes tumour-derived circulating DNA. PLoS One. 2011;6:e23418.
23. Jahr S, Hentze H, Englisch S, et al. DNA fragments in the blood plasma of cancer patients: quantitations and evidence for their origin from apoptotic and necrotic cells. Cancer Res. 2001;61:1659–65.
24. Lapin M, Oltedal S, Tjensvoll K, et al. Fragment size and level of cell-free DNA provide prognostic information in patients with advanced pancreatic cancer. J Transl Med. 2018;16:300.
25. El Messaoudi S, Rolet F, Mouliere F, Thierry AR. Circulating cell free DNA: preanalytical considerations. Clin Chim Acta. 2013;424:222–30.
26. Warton K, Yuwono NL, Cowley MJ, McCabe MJ, So A, Ford CE. Evaluation of streck BCT and PAXgene stabilised blood collection tubes for cell-free circulating DNA studies in plasma. Mol Diagn Ther. 2017;21:563–70.
27. Wong D, Moturi S, Angkachatchai V, et al. Optimizing blood collection, transport and storage conditions for cell free DNA increases access to prenatal testing. Clin Biochem. 2013;46:1099–104.
28. Janku F, Vibat CR, Kosco K, et al. BRAF V600E mutations in urine and plasma cell-free DNA from patients with Erdheim-Chester disease. Oncotarget. 2014;5:3607–10.
29. Cohen JD, Li L, Wang Y, et al. Detection and localization of surgically resectable cancers with a multi-analyte blood test. Science. 2018;359:926–30.
30. Chan KCA, Woo JKS, King A, et al. Analysis of plasma Epstein-Barr virus DNA to screen for nasopharyngeal cancer. New Engl J Med. 2017;377:513–22.
31. Board RE, Wardley AM, Dixon JM, et al. Detection of PIK3CA mutations in circulating free DNA in patients with breast cancer. Breast Cancer Res Treat. 2010;120:461–7.
32. Chen Z, Feng J, Buzin CH, et al. Analysis of cancer mutation signatures in blood by a novel ultra-sensitive assay: monitoring of therapy or recurrence in non-metastatic breast cancer. PLoS One. 2009;4:e7220.
33. Wang JY, Hsieh JS, Chang MY, et al. Molecular detection of APC, K-ras, and p53 mutations in the serum of colorectal cancer patients as circulating biomarkers. World J Surg. 2004;28:721–6.
34. Frattini M, Gallino G, Signoroni S, et al. Quantitative and qualitative characterization of plasma DNA identifies primary and recurrent colorectal cancer. Cancer Lett. 2008;263:170–81.
35. Yamada T, Nakamori S, Ohzato H, et al. Detection of K-ras gene mutations in plasma DNA of patients with pancreatic adenocarcinoma: correlation with clinicopathological features. Clin Cancer Res. 1998;4:1527–32.
36. Castells A, Puig P, Mora J, et al. K-ras mutations in DNA extracted from the plasma of patients with pancreatic carcinoma: diagnostic utility and prognostic significance. J Clin Oncol. 1999;17:578–84.
37. Janku F, Huang HJ, Fujii T, et al. Multiplex KRASG12/G13 mutation testing of unamplified cell-free DNA from the plasma of patients with advanced cancers using droplet digital polymerase chain reaction. Ann Oncol. 2017;28:642–50.
38. Janku F, Angenendt P, Tsimberidou AM, et al. Actionable mutations in plasma cell-free DNA in patients with advanced cancers referred for experimental targeted therapies. Oncotarget. 2015;6:12809–21.
39. Higgins MJ, Jelovac D, Barnathan E, et al. Detection of tumor PIK3CA status in metastatic breast cancer using peripheral blood. Clin Cancer Res. 2012;18:3462–9.
40. Dawson SJ, Tsui DW, Murtaza M, et al. Analysis of circulating tumor DNA to monitor metastatic breast cancer. N Engl J Med. 2013;368:1199–209.
41. Mohrmann L, Huang H, Hong DS, et al. Liquid biopsies using plasma exosomal nucleic acids and plasma cell-free DNA compared with clinical outcomes of patients with advanced cancers. Clin Cancer Res. 2017;24(1):181–8.
42. Misale S, Yaeger R, Hobor S, et al. Emergence of KRAS mutations and acquired resistance to anti-EGFR therapy in colorectal cancer. Nature. 2012;486:532–6.
43. Diaz LA Jr, Williams RT, Wu J, et al. The molecular evolution of acquired resistance to targeted EGFR blockade in colorectal cancers. Nature. 2012;486:537–40.

44. Cai X, Janku F, Zhan Q, Fan JB. Accessing genetic information with liquid biopsies. Trends Genet. 2015;31:564–75.
45. Murtaza M, Dawson SJ, Tsui DW, et al. Non-invasive analysis of acquired resistance to cancer therapy by sequencing of plasma DNA. Nature. 2013;497:108–12.
46. Carreira S, Romanel A, Goodall J, et al. Tumor clone dynamics in lethal prostate cancer. Sci Transl Med. 2014;6:254ra125.
47. Bettegowda C, Sausen M, Leary RJ, et al. Detection of circulating tumor DNA in early- and late-stage human malignancies. Sci Transl Med. 2014;6:224ra24.
48. Newman AM, Bratman SV, To J, et al. An ultrasensitive method for quantitating circulating tumor DNA with broad patient coverage. Nat Med. 2014;20:548–54.
49. Forshew T, Murtaza M, Parkinson C, et al. Noninvasive identification and monitoring of cancer mutations by targeted deep sequencing of plasma DNA. Sci Transl Med. 2012;4:136ra68.
50. Chan KC, Jiang P, Zheng YW, et al. Cancer genome scanning in plasma: detection of tumor-associated copy number aberrations, single-nucleotide variants, and tumoral heterogeneity by massively parallel sequencing. Clin Chem. 2013;59:211–24.
51. Heitzer E, Ulz P, Belic J, et al. Tumor-associated copy number changes in the circulation of patients with prostate cancer identified through whole-genome sequencing. Genome Med. 2013;5:30.
52. Schwaederle M, Husain H, Fanta PT, et al. Use of liquid biopsies in clinical oncology: pilot experience in 168 patients. Clin Cancer Res. 2016;22:5497–505.
53. Thierry AR, Mouliere F, El Messaoudi S, et al. Clinical validation of the detection of KRAS and BRAF mutations from circulating tumor DNA. Nat Med. 2014;20:430–5.
54. Oxnard GR, Thress KS, Alden RS, et al. Association between plasma genotyping and outcomes of treatment with osimertinib (AZD9291) in advanced non-small-cell lung cancer. J Clin Oncol. 2016;34:3375–82.
55. Gandara DR, Paul SM, Kowanetz M, et al. Blood-based tumor mutational burden as a predictor of clinical benefit in non-small-cell lung cancer patients treated with atezolizumab. Nat Med. 2018;24:1441–8.
56. Hashad D, Sorour A, Ghazal A, Talaat I. Free circulating tumor DNA as a diagnostic marker for breast cancer. J Clin Lab Anal. 2012;26:467–72.
57. Janku F, Huang HJ, Claes B, et al. BRAF mutation testing in cell-free DNA from the plasma of patients with advanced cancers using a rapid, automated molecular diagnostics system. Mol Cancer Ther. 2016;15:1397–404.
58. Spindler KL, Pallisgaard N, Vogelius I, Jakobsen A. Quantitative cell-free DNA, KRAS, and BRAF mutations in plasma from patients with metastatic colorectal cancer during treatment with cetuximab and irinotecan. Clin Cancer Res. 2012;18:1177–85.
59. Nygaard AD, Garm Spindler KL, Pallisgaard N, Andersen RF, Jakobsen A. The prognostic value of KRAS mutated plasma DNA in advanced non-small cell lung cancer. Lung Cancer. 2013;79:312–7.
60. Wang S, An T, Wang J, et al. Potential clinical significance of a plasma-based KRAS mutation analysis in patients with advanced non-small cell lung cancer. Clin Cancer Res. 2010;16:1324–30.
61. Shinozaki M, O'Day SJ, Kitago M, et al. Utility of circulating B-RAF DNA mutation in serum for monitoring melanoma patients receiving biochemotherapy. Clin Cancer Res. 2007;13:2068–74.
62. Silva JM, Silva J, Sanchez A, et al. Tumor DNA in plasma at diagnosis of breast cancer patients is a valuable predictor of disease-free survival. Clin Cancer Res. 2002;8:3761–6.
63. Lefebure B, Charbonnier F, Di Fiore F, et al. Prognostic value of circulating mutant DNA in unresectable metastatic colorectal cancer. Ann Surg. 2010;251:275–80.
64. Trevisiol C, Di Fabio F, Nascimbeni R, et al. Prognostic value of circulating KRAS2 gene mutations in colorectal cancer with distant metastases. Int J Biol Markers. 2006;21:223–8.
65. Swisher EM, Wollan M, Mahtani SM, et al. Tumor-specific p53 sequences in blood and peritoneal fluid of women with epithelial ovarian cancer. Am J Obstet Gynecol. 2005;193:662–7.

66. Schwarzenbach H, Eichelser C, Kropidlowski J, Janni W, Rack B, Pantel K. Loss of heterozygosity at tumor suppressor genes detectable on fractionated circulating cell-free tumor DNA as indicator of breast cancer progression. Clin Cancer Res. 2012;18:5719–30.
67. Kuhlmann JD, Schwarzenbach H, Wimberger P, Poetsch M, Kimmig R, Kasimir-Bauer S. LOH at 6q and 10q in fractionated circulating DNA of ovarian cancer patients is predictive for tumor cell spread and overall survival. BMC Cancer. 2012;12:325.
68. Fujimoto A, O'Day SJ, Taback B, Elashoff D, Hoon DS. Allelic imbalance on 12q22-23 in serum circulating DNA of melanoma patients predicts disease outcome. Cancer Res. 2004;64:4085–8.
69. Sozzi G, Conte D, Mariani L, et al. Analysis of circulating tumor DNA in plasma at diagnosis and during follow-up of lung cancer patients. Cancer Res. 2001;61:4675–8.
70. Husain H, Melnikova VO, Kosco K, et al. Monitoring daily dynamics of early tumor response to targeted therapy by detecting circulating tumor DNA in urine. Clin Cancer Res. 2017;23:4716–23.
71. Lee JH, Long GV, Menzies AM, et al. Association between circulating tumor DNA and pseudoprogression in patients with metastatic melanoma treated with anti-programmed cell death 1 antibodies. JAMA Oncol. 2018;4:717–21.
72. Douillard JY, Ostoros G, Cobo M, et al. Gefitinib treatment in EGFR mutated caucasian NSCLC: circulating-free tumor DNA as a surrogate for determination of EGFR status. J Thorac Oncol. 2014;9:1345–53.
73. Eisenhauer EA, Therasse P, Bogaerts J, et al. New response evaluation criteria in solid tumours: revised RECIST guideline (version 1.1). Eur J Cancer. 2009;45:228–47.
74. Therasse P, Arbuck SG, Eisenhauer EA, et al. New guidelines to evaluate the response to treatment in solid tumors. European Organization for Research and Treatment of Cancer, National Cancer Institute of the United States, National Cancer Institute of Canada. J Natl Cancer Inst. 2000;92:205–16.
75. Tseng JS, Yang TY, Tsai CR, et al. Dynamic plasma EGFR mutation status as a predictor of EGFR-TKI efficacy in patients with EGFR-mutant lung adenocarcinoma. J Thorac Oncol. 2015;10:603–10.
76. Oxnard GR, Paweletz CP, Kuang Y, et al. Noninvasive detection of response and resistance in EGFR-mutant lung cancer using quantitative next-generation genotyping of cell-free plasma DNA. Clin Cancer Res. 2014;20:1698–705.
77. Normanno N, Rachiglio AM, Roma C, et al. Molecular diagnostics and personalized medicine in oncology: challenges and opportunities. J Cell Biochem. 2013;114:514–24.
78. Crowley E, Di Nicolantonio F, Loupakis F, Bardelli A. Liquid biopsy: monitoring cancer-genetics in the blood. Nat Rev Clin Oncol. 2013;10:472–84.
79. Ramos P, Bentires-Alj M. Mechanism-based cancer therapy: resistance to therapy, therapy for resistance. Oncogene. 2015;34:3617–26.
80. Choi YL, Soda M, Yamashita Y, et al. EML4-ALK mutations in lung cancer that confer resistance to ALK inhibitors. N Engl J Med. 2010;363:1734–9.
81. Long GV, Fung C, Menzies AM, et al. Increased MAPK reactivation in early resistance to dabrafenib/trametinib combination therapy of BRAF-mutant metastatic melanoma. Nat Commun. 2014;5:5694.
82. Mao M, Tian F, Mariadason JM, et al. Resistance to BRAF inhibition in BRAF-mutant colon cancer can be overcome with PI3K inhibition or demethylating agents. Clin Cancer Res. 2013;19:657–67.
83. Morelli MP, Overman MJ, Dasari A, et al. Characterizing the patterns of clonal selection in circulating tumor DNA from patients with colorectal cancer refractory to anti-EGFR treatment. Ann Oncol. 2015;26:731–6.
84. Smith BD, Kaufman MD, Lu WP, et al. Ripretinib (DCC-2618) is a switch control kinase inhibitor of a broad spectrum of oncogenic and drug-resistant KIT and PDGFRA variants. Cancer Cell. 2019;35:738–51.

Chapter 15
Development of Immunotherapeutic Strategies for Early Phase Clinical Trials

Patricia Martin-Romano, Roman Chabanon, Adrien Procureur, Sandrine Aspeslagh, and Sophie Postel-Vinay

Abstract Immunotherapy has revolutionized cancer therapy and outcomes over the past 5 years. Following the initial successes of anti-PD-(L)1 and anti-CTLA-4 agents, a huge wave of novel agents and novel combinations has entered early phase trials, leading to an unprecedented exponential increase in phase 1 trials. These agents, which display different characteristics from conventional cytotoxic therapy and targeted therapies, have deeply challenged many paradigms of traditional phase 1 studies, including dose-determination, safety, pharmacokinetics and pharmacodynamics, efficacy evaluation, patient selection, routes of administration, trial design and endpoints. The historical "safety" phase 1 trials have been transformed to "phase 1 registration" trials, using seamless designs, enrolling several hundreds of patients and sometimes leading to drug approval. However, severe unexpected toxicities have also been observed, especially in combination trials, calling for cautious, rationale and measured drug development. In this chapter, we present the different types of immunotherapy agents currently being evaluated in phase 1 trials,

P. Martin-Romano · A. Procureur
Drug Development Department (DITEP), Gustave Roussy Cancer Campus, Paris-Saclay University, Villejuif, France
e-mail: Patricia.MARTIN-ROMANO@gustaveroussy.fr

R. Chabanon
INSERM, UMR981, ATIP-Avenir Group, Villejuif, France
e-mail: roman.chabanon@icr.ac.uk

S. Aspeslagh
Universitair Ziekenhuis, Brussel, Belgium
e-mail: Sandrine.aspeslagh@uzbrussel.be

S. Postel-Vinay (✉)
Drug Development Department (DITEP), Gustave Roussy Cancer Campus, Paris-Saclay University, Villejuif, France

INSERM, UMR981, ATIP-Avenir Group, Villejuif, France
e-mail: SOPHIE.POSTEL-VINAY@gustaveroussy.fr

T. A. Yap et al. (eds.), *Phase I Oncology Drug Development*,
https://doi.org/10.1007/978-3-030-47682-3_15

detail the major transformations in phase 1 trial designs, and discuss challenges that will need to be tackled to rationally optimize immunotherapy development.

Keywords Immunotherapy · Immune-related adverse event · Non-monotonous dose-efficacy relationship · Patient selection · Seamless design

Keypoints
- Immunotherapies comprise a myriad of different agents which all have specific characteristics
- The number of early phase trials evaluating immunotherapies is increasing exponentially
- Novel immunotherapies bring novel challenges in phase 1 studies: specific trial designs, toxicity management, drug administration routes, patient selection and tumor evaluation criteria are required
- Phase 1 immunotherapy trials are increasingly searching for efficacy
- Immunotherapy combination trials lead to unpredictable toxicities

15.1 Introduction

Over the last few years, immunotherapy has revolutionized cancer treatment, leading to unprecedented antitumor responses and long-term survival benefit in some histologies. Immunotherapy has consequently become the standard of care in several histologies, such as melanoma, non-small cell lung cancer (NSCLC), head and neck squamous cell carcinoma (HNSCC) and renal cell carcinoma (RCC).

The number of phase 1 trials assessing immunotherapies has been increasing exponentially over the last few years, with currently more than 3300 immuno-oncology (IO) therapies in development, corresponding to a 67% increase between 2017 and 2018 [1]. Phase 1 trials traditionally aim at assessing the safety profile of a novel drug, establishing a recommended phase 2 dose (RP2D) and searching for preliminary signs of activity. Phase 1 trial designs and drug development have been deeply challenged by novel immunotherapies, which present peculiar toxicity profiles, pharmacokinetic/pharmacodynamic characteristics, routes of administration and evaluation criteria [2]. In parallel, Phase 1 trial designs have evolved to bring forward efficacy criteria, which were previously traditionally assessed in Phase 2 trials [2].

Here, we present the different forms of immunotherapies currently evaluated in phase 1 immuno-oncology (IO) trials and will discuss how these have transformed phase 1 trials from being mostly toxicity-focused studies to efficacy-searching studies that potentially lead to drug approval. We will finally present the current and future challenges of immunotherapy early drug development, including combination therapy and patient selection.

15.2 The Many Faces of Immunotherapy

"Immunotherapy" gathers a myriad of approaches that all use immune-related effectors to either directly counteract tumor development or indirectly enhance antitumor immune responses through modulation of immune effectors. These approaches are classically categorized into two major classes: (i) passive immunotherapy, which uses effectors of the immune system (antibodies, immune cells) or pathogens as direct antitumor agents to trigger a short-term anticancer immune response and (ii) active immunotherapy, which exploits immune-based systems to activate the patient's antitumor immunity and establish a durable memory antitumor immune response. Immunotherapeutic approaches can further be sub-divided according to their ability to engage an antigen-specific immunity (Fig. 15.1).

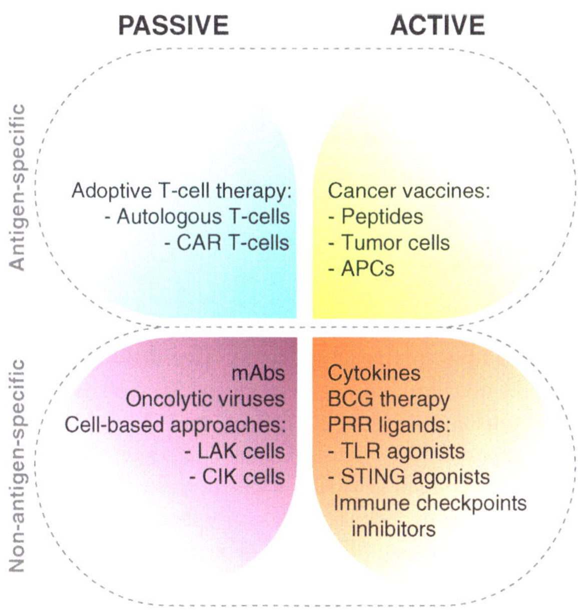

Fig. 15.1 Classification of current immunotherapy approaches. Current immunotherapy approaches can be classified in four main categories according to (i) the concept on which they are based (passive vs. active immunotherapy), and (ii) the antigen-specificity of the approach (antigen-specific vs. non-antigen-specific approaches). Passive immunotherapy refers to therapeutic approaches that use effectors of the immune system to substitute an immune response against cancer. Active immunotherapy refers to therapeutic approaches that aim to stimulate or reactivate an established host antitumor immune response. Antigen-specific approaches aim to enhance the immune response to a particular tumor-derived antigen or set of closely associated antigens. Non-antigen-specific approaches aim to stimulate the antitumor immune response without necessarily targeting a particular tumor-derived antigen. *APCs* antigen-presenting cells, *CAR T-cells* chimeric antigen receptor T-cells, *CIK cells* cytokine-induced killer cells, *LAK cells* lymphokine-activated killer cells, *mAbs* monoclonal antibodies, *TLR* Toll-like receptors, *STING* stimulator of interferon genes

15.2.1 Passive Immunotherapy Approaches

15.2.1.1 Monoclonal Antibodies

Monoclonal antibodies (mAbs) exert cytotoxic effects against tumor cells through various mechanisms that include (i) direct trigger of apoptotic signals through binding to their target; (ii) complement-dependent cytotoxicity (CDC); and (iii) antibody-dependent cellular cytotoxicity (ADCC), which mediates tumor cells phagocytosis through the recruitment of immune effectors whose membrane-surface antigens have been bound to the antibody. Not all mAbs have such properties, and the relative importance of each of these mechanisms in determining the clinical response of mAbs remains partly unclear. For example, the anti-CD20 rituximab triggers both CDC and ADCC [3]; the anti-HER2 trastuzumab induces CDC and potentially innate and adaptive immune responses [4].

Novel IO mAb include bispecific mAbs, which recognize two different epitopes and can, for example, bind both tumor cells and T-cells, thereby facilitating their interaction. Such bispecific mAb include catumaxomab (CD3 x EpCam), which has shown efficacy in the treatment of epithelial cancer-related ascites [5], and blinatumomab (CD3 x CD19), which was recently approved for the treatment of relapsed ALL [6, 7].

15.2.1.2 Oncolytic Viruses

This therapeutic approach utilizes native or genetically-modified viruses, which can selectively replicate within malignant cells [8]. Two distinct and potentially concomitant mechanisms of action have been proposed: (i) selective replication in cancer cells, which results in a direct lytic effect, and (ii) induction of a systemic antitumor immune response through production of pathogen- and damage-associated molecular patterns (PAMPs and DAMPs). Despite the early discovery of oncolytic viruses [9], their therapeutic efficacy has only been evidenced recently [10]. Imlygic®, a modified herpes simplex virus type 1 encoding granulocyte–macrophage colony-stimulating factor (GM-CSF), was the first oncolytic virus approved in patients with advanced melanoma [11].

15.2.1.3 Non-Antigen-Specific Cell-Based Approaches

Lymphokine-activated killer (LAK) cells and cytokine-induced killer (CIK) cells are immune cells cultured *ex vivo* that are subsequently re-inoculated to patients to elicit non-MHC-dependent cytotoxicity [12, 13]. Few clinical successes have been obtained with such approach so far.

15.2.1.4 Antigen-Specific Cell-Based Approaches

Adoptive T-cell transfer involves the inoculation of autologous T lymphocytes to mediate antitumor effects. Chimeric Antigen Receptor (CAR) T-cells are T lymphocytes from patients that have been genetically engineered *in vitro* to express genes encoding receptors that recognize tumor-specific antigens [14]. The first demonstration of CAR T-cells efficacy was made in 2013 in a pilot study evaluating a CD19-specific CD28/CD3ζ second-generation dual-signaling CAR in B cell ALL patients [15] and the first-in-class CAR T-cell therapy was approved in 2017 for the treatment of relapsed B-cell ALL [16].

15.2.2 Active Immunotherapy Approaches

15.2.2.1 Cancer Vaccines

Cancer vaccines are cells- or peptides-containing solutions capable of inducing T-cell- and B cell-mediated anticancer immune responses. The first cancer vaccine, GVAX, was composed of irradiated tumor cells genetically modified to express GM-CSF [17]. Peptide vaccines were subsequently developed, including the antigen glycoprotein 100 (gp100) and MAGE-A3 cancer-testis antigen vaccines. The only autologous cell-based vaccine currently licensed is Sipuleucel-T, which has efficacy in metastatic castration-resistant prostate cancer (mCRPC) [18].

15.2.2.2 Immune Checkpoint Inhibitors

Immune checkpoint Inhibitors (ICI) are mAbs that target co-inhibitory (or co-stimulatory) immune checkpoints to reactivate antitumor immunity. To date, two major classes of ICI have been registered (anti-CTLA-4 and anti-PD(L)1) and many others are in clinical development. Anti-CTLA4 block the CTLA4-CD80/CD86 interaction on APCs, thus allowing preferential binding to their co-activator CD28 and stimulation of T-cell priming [19]. The PD-1/PD-L1 immune checkpoint is a central signaling axis within the tumor microenvironment, which promotes immune evasion by inhibiting the recognition of tumor cells by PD-1-expressing CD8^{+} T-cells [19]. Anti-PD(L)1 mAbs block the PD-1/PD-L1 interaction and restore the ability of T-cells to eliminate antigen-expressing tumor cells. The first ICI to enter clinical development was the anti-CTLA4 ipilimumab (Yervoy®, Bristol-Myers Squibb), which rapidly demonstrated efficacy in patients with metastatic melanoma [20, 21]. Other anti-CTLA4 are being developed, such as tremelimumab [22]. In 2012, anti-PD-(L)1 therapies including the anti-PD-1 pembrolizumab (Keytruda®, Merck) and nivolumab (Opdivo®, Bristol-Myers Squibb), and the anti-PD-L1 atezolizumab (Tecentriq®, Genentech/Roche), durvalumab (Imfinzi®, AstraZeneca/MedImmune), and avelumab (Bavencio®, Pfizer) entered clinical development. Significant benefit in overall response rate (ORR), progression-free survival and subsequently overall survival in malignant melanoma, RCC, and NSCLC [23], led to their accelerated approval in 2014–2015; their outstanding activity in several histologies awarded them "drugs of the year" in 2013 [24]. Further reflecting the significance of these advances, the Nobel Prize in Physiology and Medicine 2018 was awarded jointly to James P. Allison and Tasuku Honjo, for their discovery of cancer therapy by inhibition of immune checkpoints.

15.2.2.3 Non-Antigen-Specific Approaches

Non-antigen specific approaches include the historical BCG instillations for prophylaxis of primary recurrence in papillary urothelial bladder carcinoma (UBC) following transurethral resection [25]. More recently, Toll-like receptors (TLR) agonists, which exploit a similar principle by providing danger signals to immune cells [26], and Stimulator of interferon genes (STING) agonists [27], which aim to trigger interferon responses in cancer or immune cells, have been developed. Intratumoral administration of these agents was shown to result in remarkable therapeutic activity in various mouse models of cancer [28] and clinical implementation and results will be discussed below. Finally, cytokines have also been used as active immunotherapy in immunogenic tumors such as RCC [29].

Because of their specific mechanisms of action, these therapies require specific drug development processes. The most innovative approaches that are currently evaluated in early phase trials will be presented below.

15.3 Phase 1 Trials in the Immunotherapy Era—Novel Designs, Toxicity Profiles, Routes of Administration and Evaluation Criteria

15.3.1 Dose-Limiting Toxicities and MTD Definition

Historically, phase 1 trials evaluate toxicity and safety of a novel drug (or drug combination) using dose-escalation schemes aimed at: (i) treating a limited number of patients at low, potentially inefficacious doses; (ii) performing an efficient dose-escalation to rapidly determine the maximal tolerated dose (MTD) and recommended phase 2 dose (RP2D), i.e. the dose presenting the optimal efficacy/safety profile (iii) establishing the pharmacodynamic and pharmacokinetic characteristics of a novel drug in humans. The determination of the MTD is based on the number of pre-defined dose-limiting toxicities (DLTs). Traditionally, these consist of severe toxicities (Grade 3 and beyond) classified according to the National Cancer Institute—Common Terminology Criteria for Adverse Events (NCI-CTCAE).

Timing for detecting and recording these toxicities is classically the first therapy cycle (3–4 weeks). Phase 1 trials aim at escalating doses until reaching a toxicity rate of 17%–33% of patients, with a MTD defined as the dose level at which one or less than one out of 6 patients present a DLT. The RP2D is traditionally equal to the MTD, with the assumption that highest doses correlate with better antitumor effects. Several dose-escalation methods exist: the most commonly used is the 3 + 3 dose-escalation method, but alternative designs—such as adaptive designs including Bayesian and Continuous Reassessment Methods—are now used more frequently; by making statistical modeling on the anticipated toxicity rate which takes into account toxicities observed in patients treated at previous dose levels, these allow reaching the RP2D faster, while limiting the number of patients treated at potentially inefficacious dose levels [2].

Contrary to cytotoxic therapies, toxicities related to immune therapies, also called immune-related Adverse Events (irAEs) rarely occur during the first cycle but can start at any time on trial, usually after week 4 and within the first 3 months for ICI (with the exception of infusion-related reactions) [30]. Consequently and similar to what has been observed with targeted therapies [31], a DLT definition that only takes into account toxicities observed during the first cycle is inappropriate, as it does not capture most of the potentially dose-limiting toxicities. Therefore, toxicities observed over the entire trial should be accurately reported, together with their cycle of occurrence, duration and impact on treatment administration and dose-intensity (temporary or definitive treatment interruption; dose modification) [32]. As an illustration, among phase 1 trials evaluating anti-CTLA4, anti-PD1 or anti-PD-L1 ICI as monotherapy, only one trial identified per-protocol-defined DLTs [2]. To address this, some phase 1 trials (e.g. BMS-936559 [33] and MEDI4736 [34]) have chosen to lengthened the DLT period to two cycles, which better takes into account immune-related toxicities. Interestingly, late onset irAEs have also been described after treatment cessation, suggesting that a longer follow-up than the traditional 1-month period may be needed [35].

15.3.2 Safety Profile and Specificities of Immune-Related Adverse Events

Several adverse events (AEs) are independently reported in Phase 1 trials of immunotherapies: treatment-related AEs (trAEs), immune-related AEs (irAEs) and AE of specific interest (AESI).

15.3.2.1 Dose-Toxicity Relationship

No relationship between dose and toxicity has been established in most phase 1 trials of ICI—with the exception of the anti-CTLA4 ipilimumab. For example, the safety profile of nivolumab was similar at doses ranging from 0.1 to 10 mg/kg in all phase 1/1b trials; although initial dose of 3 or 10 mg/kg q2 or q3 weeks were initially recommended, nivolumab is currently prescribed at a flat dose of 240 mg IV q2 weeks or 480 mg IV q4 weeks that is neither adjusted on body weight nor on body surface area [36]. This is currently the case for most approved anti-PD(L)1 therapies, whose frequency of administration is also most often dictated by the associated chemotherapy or targeted therapy [37]. Because no MTD has been established in most IO trials, the recommended phase 2 dose (RP2D) has most often been determined as the maximum feasible dose (MFD)—which could accordingly be called a "treatment-based limiting dose".

Contrary to ICI, other forms of immune therapies still display early dose-dependent toxicities (e.g. CAR T-cells or bi-specific antibodies such as blinatomumab), calling for customized protocol designs, DLT and MTD definitions according to the evaluated agent [38].

15.3.2.2 Toxicity Profile

Toxicities of immune therapies can be drug-dependent (i.e. shared within a drug family) or patient-dependent, when they are for example favored by specific genetic polymorphisms (e.g. HLA-A status) or microbiota. Although any organ can be affected by irAEs, these most commonly involve endocrine functions, gastrointestinal tract, skin, and liver (Fig. 15.2). Meta-analyses have reported an overall incidence irAEs of any grade in 30% and 70% of patients receiving anti-PD-1 and anti-CTLA-4 in monotherapy, respectively [39], with severe irAEs observed in 5–8% and 24% of patients, respectively [40, 41]. In phase 1 trials, investigators should distinguish irAEs that are drug-specific (e.g. anti-CLTA4-related skin and GI toxicities, or anti-PD-L1-related dysthyroiditis and pneumonitis) from infusion-related reactions (IRR), which are not typically deemed to be DLTs [39]. Although most IRR are mild and manageable with paracetamol (tylenol) and anti-histamines, severe IRR should be treated in intensive care units (ICUs) and may require immunosuppressive agents, such as anti-TNF and anti-IL-6. Specific life-threatening neurologic toxicities are also observed in 4–6% of patients treated with immune therapies, and up to 70% of patients receiving CAR-T-cells (see corresponding section) [42]. Specific toxicity challenges brought by IO combination trials will be presented in the corresponding section.

15.3.2.3 Toxicity Management

Because irAEs can affect any organ and may rapidly become life-threatening, these should be managed by multi-disciplinary teams and require rapid access to ICUs [43]. Most protocols recommend stopping the investigational agent as soon as irAEs reach G2, introducing steroids and referring patients to specialized organ specialists [44];

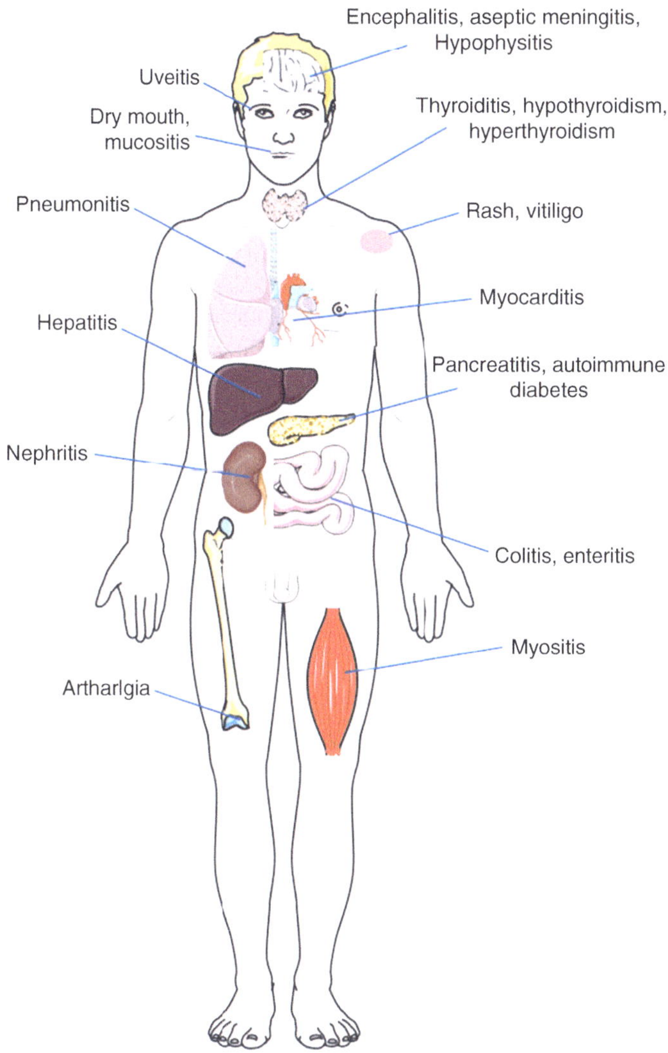

Fig. 15.2 Main organs affected by immune-related adverse events. Frequency may vary according to the type of immunotherapy (Champiat et al., Ann Oncol 2016)

severe irAEs require high-dose steroids, anti-TNF and anti-IL6 (tocilizumab) and transfer to ICU [43]. Exhaustive management guidelines are available in Phase 1 protocols, which are either drug-specific or which follow ASCO guidelines [45]. Importantly, all signs and symptoms of irAEs should be carefully described in patient medical records and a biopsy of the organ displaying toxicity should be performed whenever feasible, in order to investigate the physiopathology.

15.3.3 Pharmacokinetics

Mechanism of absorption, distribution, metabolism and elimination are highly variable according to the type of agent [46]. Most ICIs developed so far are monoclonal antibodies that harbor different half-lives according to the Fc IgG isotype, ranging from 27 days for nivolumab and pembrolizumab (IgG4), to 17 days for durvalumab (Fc-mutated IgG1) and 6 days for avelumab (IgG1). Although these were initially developed at different doses and schedules, most of them are currently prescribed at a flat dose Q2 or Q4weeks—although the safety of such regimens has formally been assessed in equivalence trials only for some of them [47]. The pharmacokinetic profile of antibodies is complex and may be influenced by multiple parameters, including body weight, inflammatory parameters (such as high CRP that associates with faster clearance), IgG subtype (IgG1 and IgG3 cause NK-cell mediated ADCC whereas IgG4 which rather activate the alternative complement pathway), and other factors, including a variable concentration-dependent half-life, the ability of the Fc region to bind to the salvage receptor (FcRn) [48], or the presence of circulating soluble forms of the ligand. Nivolumab clearance has also been reported to increase with worse PS, male gender and anti-drug antibodies (ADA) generation, and to decrease with tumor shrinkage (up to 40%) [49]. All this introduces important variability and complexity in the assessment of pharmacokinetic characteristics of ICI and support a thorough interpretation of PK data obtained in Phase 1 trials, in light of both patient and drug specificities. Contrary to anti-PD(L)1 agents, ipilimumab presents linear PK, dose-efficacy and dose-toxicity relationship, suggesting that this ICI may not purely work as an antagonistic checkpoint inhibitor, but which also has ADCC-related dose-dependent depleting properties [50]. The anti-CTLA4 IgG2 tremelimumab represents another interesting example of ICI development: following results of the phase 1/2 study, a dose schedule of 15 mg/kg every 3 months was selected [51]; this was subsequently changed to 10 mg/kg Q4weeks, following negative results of a phase 3 trial in patients with melanoma—although overall survival curves were similar to the ones observed with ipilimumab [22, 52]. Whether ICI dosing needs to be adjusted on a case-by-case basis to a target trough concentration (i.e. lowest concentration reached before the next dose is administered) warrants consideration, especially as recent results suggest an exposure-efficacy relationship approach may be best evaluated in dedicated pharmacokinetic expansion cohorts [53].

By contrast, bi-specific antibodies lacking an Fc region traditionally have a very short half-life, which can be advantageous, notably with regards to the duration of irAEs and the development of cytokine release syndrome ADAs [54, 55]. The bi-specific T-cell engaging (BiTE®) antibody anti-CD19 x CD3 blinatumomab (Blincyto®), for example, has a half-life of approximately 2 h [56].

Finally, novel routes of administration, such as intratumor administration, lead to novel challenges with a maximum administrable volume and the requirement to assess pharmacokinetics not only in the peripheral blood but also locally.

15.3.4 Pharmacodynamics

The difficulty in designing appropriate pharmacodynamic assays for ICI resides in the highly variable level and pattern of expression of the target. For example, PD-1 is mostly expressed on T-cell surface, while CTLA-4 only displays transient expression, and biomarker expression can both be constitutive or inducible [57]. Thus, flow cytometry methods assessing receptor occupancy on circulating T-cells are feasible and relevant only for a fraction of molecules. Such techniques could successfully be used for a phase 1 trial evaluating nivolumab [58], where receptor occupancy appeared to rapidly reach a plateau at 0.1 mg/kg q2weeks (3% of the recommended dose) and above [49]. The scenario is different for PD-L1, for which a 10-fold higher dose is needed to saturate the receptor because of higher expression in the body. In any case, because these molecules are antagonistic antibodies, the level of receptor occupancy that should be achieved to trigger the optimal immune modulation is unknown, and findings observed in circulating lymphocytes may not appropriately reflect what is happening in the tumor bed. The recent developments of metabolic tracers, such as ^{18}F-BMS-986192 or ^{89}Zr-nivolumab, may bring additional data on target modulation; their implementation as early as phase 1 trials—notably for trials evaluating drug combinations using an anti-PD(L)1 backbone—could be envisioned [59].

Immunomonitoring, i.e. assessing the levels of cytokines, chemokines, and immunophenotyping in peripheral blood, represents another attractive pharmacodynamic biomarker for immunotherapies. Although most trials currently perform such analyses (which have the advantage of being dynamic and repeatable in a longitudinal fashion in a single patient), results obtained in peripheral blood infrequently correspond to what happens within the tumor. For example, in the phase 1 trial assessing the 9B12 anti-OX40 monoclonal antibody, the comparison of OX40 surface expression on T_{reg} from the peripheral blood and on tumor infiltrating T_{regs} in three patients for which tumor tissue was available, revealed that less than 20% of circulating T_{reg} expressed this marker, whereas more than 50% of infiltrating T_{regs} were OX40 positive [60]. Because immunophenotyping is costly and needs to be performed on fresh material, the added value of such analysis should be cautiously considered prior to implementation in Phase 1 trials.

15.3.5 Dose-Efficacy Relationship and Dose Selection

Perhaps because most immune checkpoints developed so far are monoclonal antibodies, no clear correlation has been found between dose, toxicity and efficacy—again with the exception of anti-CTLA4 agents—and most immunotherapies display non-monotonous dose-response curves [2]. For example, a plateau in efficacy was observed with nivolumab at doses above 1 mg/kg [36]. This may be related both to the pharmaceutical characteristics of ICI and to their mechanism of action, as prolonged memory responses can be observed once an antitumor immune response has been triggered. Novel small molecules that are currently developed to inhibit the PD-1/PD-L1 checkpoint (e.g. BMS-1166) should bring interesting data in this regard, as these will disrupt the same target, and therefore theoretically have similar pharmacodynamic characteristic, but display completely different pharmacokinetics [61].

Preclinical data suggest that other immunotherapies—such as STING agonists, agents acting on the interferon response and CD40 agonists—may display a bell-shaped dose-response curves [62]. In this case, higher doses may not only be more toxic, but also be detrimental to antitumor efficacy.

Overall, aiming at administering the highest tolerable dose is not relevant for some immunotherapies and their potential for efficacy at lower dose levels should be systematically explored. In this context, innovative designs, allowing to dose-escalate rapidly (accelerated titration designs or modified toxicity probability interval designs [63]) and to expand at low dose levels as soon as satisfactory pharmacokinetic and pharmacodynamics parameters have been obtained should be prioritized (Fig. 15.3); efficacy signals may otherwise be missed.

15.3.6 Response and Efficacy Assessment

IO agents have displayed novel patterns of response that had not previously been observed with conventional chemotherapy and targeted therapies. These new response patterns are inherent to the mechanism of action of immunotherapies, which do not directly target the tumor cell but act on immune cells or the microenvironment: responses may thus be delayed and even sometimes occur after an initial phase of pseudo-progression; conversely, immune therapies can be detrimental to a subset of patients and lead to hyper-progression. In this context, novel criteria have been developed, e.g. the immune iRECIST criteria [64]; these are now implemented in phase 1 trials evaluating immunotherapies and allow the avoidance of premature treatment discontinuation in patients who may benefit from the drug. Briefly, iRECIST criteria are based on the standard RECIST terminology (immune complete response iCR, partial response iPR or stable disease iSD) but include two novel progression patterns: unconfirmed PD (iUPD) or confirmed PD (iCPD). iUPD corresponds to a progressive disease according to traditional RECIST criteria, but must be confirmed by a new imaging assessment at least 4 weeks after the first assessment. If PD is confirmed on that subsequent imaging (appearance of additional new lesions, increase in size of target lesions >20%, progression of non-target lesions or increase in new target lesions >5 mm), the patient is considered as presenting iCPD and should discontinue the study. If PD is not confirmed, the patient may be considered as displaying pseudo-progression, delayed response or dissociated response, and be permitted to continue treatment. Because of the implementation of these

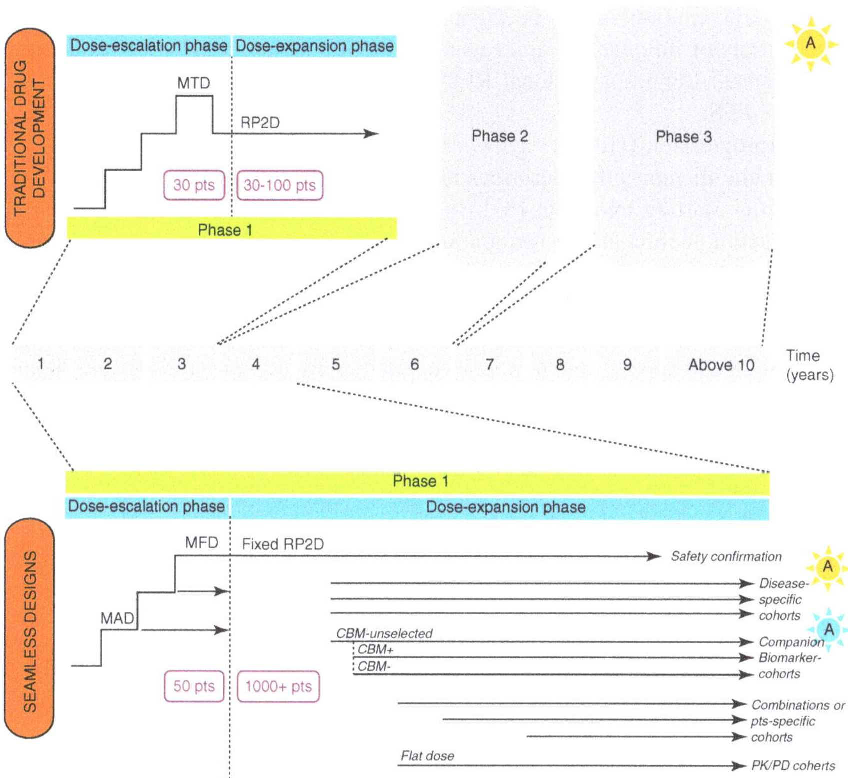

Fig. 15.3 Novel phase 1 designs in the era of immuno-oncology. The traditional drug development process (top panel) includes three separate phase 1, 2, and 3 studies prior to reaching drug approval (depicted by "A" in the sun-shape). Classical phase 1 associates a dose-escalation phase followed by a single-cohort dose-expansion phase primarily looking for safety and confirmation of the recommended phase 2 dose. This 3 years-long phase 1 is, in case of data supporting preliminary activity, followed by subsequent phase 2 and 3 trials, for a total drug development duration of more than 10 years. Novel seamless designs include "drug registration phase 1 trials", in which expansion cohorts do not only look for safety, but also activity in disease-specific cohorts that are adequately powered to do so. During the dose-escalation phase additional patients could also be enrolled at dose levels that have proven to be safe and are above the Minimum Active Dose; this allows enriching for safety, PK, PD and efficacy data at several dose levels, while increasing the number of patients who will potentially benefit from the drug, without any delay in dose-escalation. This may be particularly relevant when the drug displays a bell-shaped dose-activity relationship. In the expansion phase, multiple cohorts can be launched as a part of the original phase 1 trial (pending protocol amendment) to confirm efficacy in specific tumor types, to develop a companion biomarker that would concomitantly be registered, to evaluate the safety in specific patient populations or in various combinations, or to assess the equivalence of a flat dose. These multiple parallel cohorts can include several hundreds of patients and lead to breakthrough designation, conditional or accelerated approval, thereby significantly shortening the drug development process. *CBM* Companion Biomarker, *MAD* Minimum Active Dose, *MFD* Maximum Feasible Dose, *MTD* Maximum Tolerated Dose, *RP2D* Recommended Phase 2 Dose

novel criteria, caution should be recommended when comparing median PFS in phase 1 trials of immune therapies using iRECIST with phase 1 trials evaluating non-IO agents using conventional RECIST criteria, as iRECIST may artificially increase mPFS.

Hyperprogression (HPD) is a specific pattern of disease progression observed with immune therapies that describes an acceleration of the natural course of the disease after starting treatment [65]. In this case, immunotherapy is detrimental. Any suspicion of clinical hyperprogression justifies an anticipated imaging evaluation. Multiple criteria for defining HPD have been proposed, including increases in tumor sizes of 20% or 100% at various timepoints or evaluation of tumor growth rate [66]. With reported rates of HPD ranging from 4% to 29% according to studies, this phenomenon appears much more frequent than pseudo-progression and should be identified early. The biological rationale for HPD is still unknown and the role of *MDM2/MDM4* amplifications, *EGFR* alterations or tumor-associated macrophages has been suggested [67]. Even if phase 1 trials are performed on a more heterogeneous population than later phase trials, these represent the first opportunity to detect and explore thoroughly such unusual cases, from a biological and dose-relationship point of view. Also, scores based on copy number instability in cfDNA that have been proposed for early detection of HPD may be implemented in phase 1 trials of immune therapies to allow identification of drugs that may be detrimental to some patients. A simpler way to control for HPD would be to systematically perform a CT-scan 4-weeks prior to starting treatment, in order to be able to calculate a tumor growth rate. Indeed, other methods that also allow capturing the various profiles of response observed with immune therapies, such as tumor growth rate or metabolic imaging, may deserve more frequent implementation in IO phase 1 trials.

Finally, some Phase 1/2 trials now request the collection of overall survival data. Although this is sensible considering the mechanism of action of immune therapies, phase 1 trials are ultimately not the relevant place to assess overall survival for multiple reasons: (i) they do not contain any control arm and are not powered to do so; (ii) subsequent therapies will represent confounding factors; (iii) challenges associated with patient follow-up since most phase 1 patients are referred from outside centers and will return to their local hospital after trial completion; and (iv) phase 1 studies are increasingly conducted earlier in the patient's treatment setting, such data may never be communicated as events will be available several years after trial completion.

15.3.7 Patient Eligibility

Patients participating in phase 1 trials are required to have a life expectancy of at least 12 weeks. Several objective scores had been developed in the era of cytotoxic and targeted therapies, such as the Royal Marsden Score based on LDH, albumin and number of metastatic sites [68]. These have been refined to better consider additional parameters that are specifically important for immune therapies. For example, the GRIm Score (Gustave Roussy Immune Score), based on albumin, LDH, and neutrophil-to-lymphocyte ratio, allows a better patient selection for IO phase 1 trials and can help in assessing patient eligibility [69].

Because of the mechanism of action of immunotherapies and their potential for triggering auto-immune toxicities or favoring the reactivation of viral infections, patients with a history of auto-immune or inflammatory diseases, severe allergic reactions, or chronic viral infections have been excluded from phase 1 trials evaluating ICI. This is a sound and safe approach in view of the potential harm (vs benefit) such immunotherapies may cause. Such criteria should however be gradually lifted in dedicated cohorts of the phase 1 trial expansion phase once investigators are familiar with the safety profile of the drug. This will enable the inclusion of patient populations that are more representative of advanced cancer patients who are be treated in later phase trials. In addition, other commonly implemented exclusion criteria, such as the presence of brain metastases, ECOG performance status of 2 or elevated LDH should also be reconsidered: clinical benefit has been observed in patients with elevated LDH receiving tremelimumab [51], in patients with ECOG performance status of 2 treated with the anti-PD-L1 BMS-936559 [33], and in patients with brain metastases [70, 71] with no additional toxicity. Finally, although high-dose steroids at the start of a clinical trial may be detrimental to the outcome of immunotherapy, it is currently estimated that the administration of steroids for drug-induced irAEs has no deleterious effect; therefore, patients taking low-dose steroids ($\leq$10 mg/kg) should still be eligible for phase 1 immunotherapy trials [72]. Because Phase 1 trials of immunotherapies are increasingly becoming phase 1 registration trials, the opportunity of opening expansion cohorts with less restrictive eligibility criteria should be systematically considered.

Finally, one major current limiting factor for enrolling patients in phase 1 trials of immunotherapies is the pre-requisite of being "immune-naïve" patients and having received a maximum of 1 or 2 previous antitumor treatment lines. Although it Is widely recognized that immunotherapies bring substantial benefit especially when administered early, this brings practical limitations and significantly restricts eligible patients, thereby slowing down trial recruitment. Further, in the case of combinations that have proven to be more toxic than the active drug in monotherapy (e.g. anti-PD-(L)1), this is deleterious for the patient. Therefore, such criteria should ideally not be implemented as early as the dose-escalation phase and, when implemented, should be thoroughly justified.

15.3.8 Patient Selection for Personalized Immunotherapy

Analogous to the implementation of patient selection biomarkers in Phase 1 trials of targeted therapies, predictive biomarkers of response are increasingly included in the expansion phase of different phase 1 immunotherapy trials. For example, the Keynote-001 study used a elegant seamless design and conducted dedicated biomarker-selected or -unselected cohorts (i.e. PD-L1-positive vs PD-L1 unselected) in parallel, in which several doses of pembrolizumab were also compared [73]. Because biomarkers of response to immune therapies are incredibly variable—ranging from tumor mutational load, immune (notably interferon) signatures, checkpoint expression, to microbiota characteristics—their implementation in phase 1 trials may be challenging. Further, some markers can be expressed on the tumor and/or immune cells, or display dynamic expression profiles [19]. Therefore, although their implementation should be encouraged in trials, several important considerations need to be highlighted. First, phase 1 trials need to be designed to enroll patients quickly and efficiently. Therefore, careful consideration should be given to the inclusion of molecular selection during the dose-escalation phase, where the primary objective must remain the determination of the DLTs and recommended phase 2 dose (RP2D)/MTD. Second, molecular enrichment should ideally be performed in a dose-expansion dedicated "companion biomarker" cohort—as illustrated by successful development and approval of the 22C3 IHC PD-L1 PharmDx test, together with pembrolizumab [73]. Third, because none of the current selection biomarkers used with immunotherapies has a sufficient negative predictive value to completely exclude patients from receiving the drug, stringent selection should not be implemented too early; this may otherwise prevent the detection of signals of efficacy in patient populations that may ultimately benefit from the drug, e.g. PD-L1 negative populations [74, 75], or tumors with very low mutational load such as Hodgkin lymphomas or *SMARCA4*-deficient small cell carcinoma of the ovary [76, 77]. Fourth, exceptional responders or hyperprogressive patients should be extensively explored from a biological and molecular angle, as these may be extremely informative on predictive biomarkers and drug mechanism of action in humans.

15.3.9 Specific Therapeutic Agents and Novel Routes of Administration

15.3.9.1 Intratumor Delivery

Intratumoral immunotherapy (ITI) aims at modulating both innate and adaptive immune responses by triggering immunogenic cell death, inducing tumor antigen release, enhancing tumor antigen presentation, activating immune effector cells and depleting immunosuppressive cells locally, in order to subsequently inducing a systemic antitumor immune response following antigen cross-presentation in the draining lymph node [78]. Phase 1 trials of ITI should therefore distinguish between toxicities, PK/PD and responses occurring in injected (enestic) lesions from toxicity, PK/PD and responses occurring in non-injected (anenestic) lesions, which result from systemic immune effects. Similarly, DLT definition should distinguish between systemic toxicities (cytokine release syndrome, pyrexia etc.), local toxicities (injection site pain, tumor pain) and limitations in dose escalation due to feasibility (injected volume).

Several anticancer therapies have been reported to cause immunogenic cell death or increase tumor immunogenicity through the above-described mechanisms and could be used as ITI [79]. The main advantage of ITI is to allow an improved therapeutic window and enhanced biodistribution within the tumor, while sparing normal cells from toxicity induced by systemic administration—thereby avoiding uncontrolled activation of the immune system, e.g. by STING or TLR agonists. Also, local injections allow the achievement of higher drug concentrations and, in some cases, a sustained release of the drug within a few days following injection. A major limitation of ITI is the accessibility of the lesion: small or deep tumor lesions are not eligible to this approach, and novel strategies are being developed to improve drug delivery or to allow injecting deeper lesions [80]. However, ITI can now be performed routinely at the patient bed in day care, either for subcutaneous injections or ultrasound-guided injection in liver metastases.

Currently, different immunostimulatory ITI are evaluated in monotherapy in combination with other local and/or systemic agents, including STING and TLR agonists.

Stimulator of Interferon Genes (STING) Agonist

Stimulator of interferon genes (STING) pathway is a cytosolic DNA sensing pathway that activates innate immune signaling. STING agonists can therefore act as adjuvants to trigger T-cell priming, following the induction of a type 1 IFN response and production of pro-inflammatory cytokines by the tumor cell and/or immune cells [81]. Clinical compounds are mostly modifier cyclic dinucleotides that are developed as ITI in Phase 1 trials, though a recent publication reported the ability of symmetry-related amidobenzimidazole (ABZI)-based compounds to bind and activate STING intratumorally following systemic administration in mice [82].

The intratumoral injection of STING agonists has been reported to induce local tumor regression and generate systemic immune responses, mediating the rejection of distant metastases and providing immunologic T-cell memory [28]. Several clinical trials are currently assessing the safety and efficacy of ITI with STING agonists in monotherapy or in combination with anti-PD(L)1 agents (NCT03010176, NCT03843359, NCT03172936). Antitumor efficacy has been reported with both monotherapy and combination strategies, especially in PD-(L)1-naïve patients. Interestingly, although no MTD could be reached in the trial evaluating MK-1454, PK/PD data as well as the profile of responses suggested that STING agonists may display a bell-shaped efficacy curve, similar to what was recently suggested in preclinical models.

Toll-Like Receptors (TLR) Agonists

TLRs are both expressed by tumor cells, where they exert direct cytotoxic effects upon stimulation, and antigen presenting cells, where TLR stimulation induces MHC II, CD80 and CD86 upregulation, resulting in the conversion of APCs from tolerogenic to immunogenic. TLR agonists have been used for more than 10 years in skin cancers, inducing antitumor responses as topical agents (e.g. TLR7-8 agonist imiquimod) in basal cell carcinoma and cutaneous melanoma [83].

Several TLR agonists are currently evaluated in phase 1 trials and successes have been limited in monotherapy. More promising results have been obtained in combination, notably with radiotherapy hematological malignancies, suggesting that local immune priming by TLR agonist along may be insufficient to induce a systemic anticancer immune response. Similarly, an overall response rate of 38% has recently been reported in a phase 1/2 study evaluating intratumoral tilsotolimod (TLR9 agonist) and ipilimumab in anti-PD1 inhibitor refractory melanoma patients [84]. No MTD could be identified in the corresponding dose-escalation study, where the possibility of a non-monotonal dose-response was not reported. Combinations of TLR agonists with other ITI, anticancer vaccines, or systemic IO agents are ongoing (NCT00960752, NCT01421017, NCT02431559, NCT02643303, NCT03301896, NCT02556463).

15.3.9.2 CAR-T-Cell Therapy

Because each CAR T-cell is dedicated to a specific patient, the early development of this novel class of immunotherapy differs considerably from other therapies and has brought new safety and organizational challenges [85].

Multiplicity of Treatment Modalities and Trial Designs

The variety of CAR T-cells engineering methods, administration routes, schedules and dosing make each CAR T-cell trial unique [85]. For example, cells can come from an autologous or allogenic source, can be dosed per kg or per m^2, have various single chain variable fragments (scFv), are generated through variable engineering methods and can harbor different co-stimulatory signals; finally, patient conditioning prior to CAR T-cell infusion can also vary. Contrary to other immunotherapy trials, the number of patients enrolled in CAR T-cell trials is very limited, ranging from 3 to 30 patients [86].

Specific Logistical Requirement

The implementation of CAR T-cell therapies in early drug development centers is limited by the requirement for highly specialized structures and expertise, including an appropriate leukapheresis platform, specialized CAR-T-cell preparation pharmacy, dedicated neurologist and ICU [86]. CAR T-cell production is patient-specific and involves many complex steps and quality controls, for a median manufacturing period of 2 weeks. ZUMA-1 was the first trial that organized a centralized streamline process compatible with large-scale production and an approximately 8 days production period. Because CAR-T cell production takes on average 2 weeks, patients usually receive their infusion 4 weeks after starting screening, which may be incompatible with advanced cancers. Most studies report a 90% infusion rate, which would need to be increased thanks to faster production [87].

Specific Toxicity Management

More than any other phase 1 trial, CAR T-cell administration is unavoidably associated with severe toxicities that can be life-threatening. Specific patient information has to be delivered accordingly. Schematically, toxicities can be distinguished as follows (Fig. 15.4):

On-target, on-tumor toxicity: Cytokine Release Syndrome (CRS) is the most frequently observed serious AE, which is experienced by 50–100% of patients. It is mediated by the activation of T-cells upon target engagement, followed by endothelial cells and macrophage activation, leading to massive cytokine release, including IL2, INFγ, GM-CSF, TNFα and IL6. CRS is characterized by fever, flu-like symptoms and sometimes nausea. Severe CRS includes capillary leak syndrome (leading to refractory hypotension, hypoxia and possibly multi-organ dysfunction) and macrophage activation syndrome; it requires management in an ICU. The grade and severity of CRS are associated with the level of CAR-T cell expansion, the increase of soluble IL-2R levels and the peak of IL6, ferritin and C-reactive protein. CRS occurs mainly in the first week post-infusion [88].

CRS severity can be graded using dedicated scales (CARTOX, Lee's scale) [88]. The management of grade 2 CRS requires IL6 antagonist injections (e.g. Tocilizumab). Grade 3 CRS requires the addition of corticosteroid therapy, even though it compromises CAR-T function (unlike Tocilizumab). The grade of CRS does not appear to correlate with the overall response rate, but most responding patients experience CRS.

On-target, off-tumor toxicity: Unexpected toxicities due to the expression of the target antigen in healthy tissue have been described. For example, one fatal pulmonary edema was reported following infusion a HER2 CAR T-cell therapy in a patient with metastatic colon cancer; interestingly, another trial also evaluating HER2 CAR T-cells did not report lung toxicity, potentially because of different treatment modalities (lower dose, absence of post-infusion IL-2 administration, absence of lymphodepletion and different scFv) [89]. Similarly, a carboxy-anhydrase-IX (CAIX) CAR-T-cell evaluated in patients with metastatic renal cell carcinoma was associated with Grade 2–4 liver enzymes elevation; liver biopsies revealed CAIX expression on bile duct epithelium.

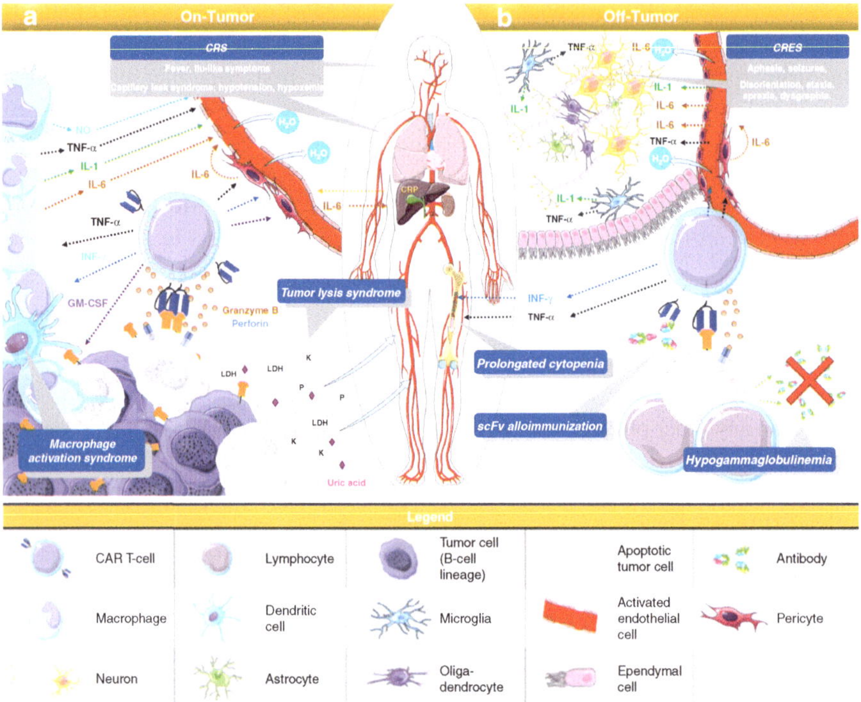

Fig. 15.4 On-target and off-target toxicities of autologous chimeric antigen receptor (CAR) T-cell therapy. (**a**) After specific antigen binding, CAR T-cell induce the activation of nearby macrophages, antigen-presenting cells and endothelial cells leading to the production of INFγ, TNF-α and GM-CSF, as well as massive release of other cytokines such as IL-1 and IL-6. This causes major systemic modifications which underlie clinical symptoms of CRS, including fever, chills, anorexia and asthenia. Severe CRS cause capillary leak syndrome, associated with hypotension or lung edema. Tumor lysis syndrome can also occur. (**b**) CRES manifestations are the consequence of increased blood-brain barrier permeability and capillary leak. Activated brain endothelial cells and microglia can produce IL-6 and VEGF, potentially causing brain edema. *CRES* CAR-T related encephalopathy syndrome, *CRS* cytokine release syndrome, *GM-CSF* granulocyte-macrophage colony-stimulating factor, *INFγ* interferon gamma, *LDH* lactate dehydrogenase, *scFv* single-chain variable fragments, *TNF-α* Tumor necrosis factor alpha

Off-target, off-tumor toxicity: CAR T-cell-related encephalopathy syndrome (CRES) often occurs together with CRS approximately 5 days after infusion in up to 71% of patients [90]. CRES results from the association of capillary leak, blood-brain barrier disruption and possibly microglia activation. CRS are scaled using the CARTOX-10. Grade 1 CRES is characterized by a range of symptoms, such as ataxia, apraxia, dysgraphia and disorientation in time and space. Grade 3 CRES consists of global aphasia (the most characteristic feature), depressed level of consciousness, seizures and sometime cerebral edema potentially leading to death. Tocilizumab is inefficient on CRES and high-dose steroids should be prescribed [91]. Other life-threatening AEs, such as prolonged cytopenias and severe anaphylaxis have also been reported.

15.3.10 Towards Phase 1 Efficacy Studies

Phase 1 trials are increasingly becoming efficacy-searching and potentially FDA breakthrough therapy designation studies. For example, the Keynote-001 study, initially planned as an initial dose-finding study of approximately 50 patients, ended up being a multi-cohort efficacy study that enrolled 1235 patients, following a seamless design, and led to the approval of pembrolizumab in melanoma only 3 years after study initiation [92]. A combination of adaptive, basket and umbrella trial design allowed testing various regimens in several histologies, while evaluating (and eventually registering) companion biomarkers of response (Fig. 15.3). Data of this study eventually served as basis for the approval of pembrolizumab in several diseases, including non-small cell lung cancer [21], MSI-high cancer, head and neck cancer and urothelial cancer, among others. The MASTERKEY-265 phase 1/3 trial evaluating talimogene laherparepvec (T-VEC) with pembrolizumab is another example of this "phase 1 registration trial" evolution [93]. Such seamless designs should be encouraged as they allow the continued redefinition of the trial by incorporating the latest biomarker, safety or efficacy updates, while limiting the administrative burden and number of open trials, thereby optimizing drug development.

15.4 IO Combination Trials

In view of the high benefit rates brought by IBC with regards to improved patient outcomes, combinations of immune therapies (IO-IO combinations), or of one immunotherapy and another anticancer agent have rapidly been developed, either to improve survival and/or to potentiate the action of one or the other anticancer therapy, and/or to overcome acquired resistance to ICI. Currently, more than 1500 early phase trials are evaluating IO combinations and this number continues to grow [1]. Studies described below are based on the results of a search performed on clinicaltrial.gov accessed in April 2019 (Figs. 15.5 and 15.6).

15.4.1 Methodological Considerations

In 2017, Nikanjam et al. reported that only 50% of studies that evaluated ICI in combination (63% and 36% for anti-PD(L)1 and anti-CTLA4 combinations, respectively) could deliver full dose of all agents [94]. Interestingly, drug development strategies have differed according to the type of combination. Most studies evaluating IO-IO combinations have followed a traditional dose-escalation process for at least one of the agents. Contrarily, almost all combinations with cytotoxic regimens have started at full dose of all therapies, which has proven to be feasible in most cases [94]. For targeted agents, strategies have varied, with approximately half of the studies performing a dose-escalation of the targeted therapy, and another half starting at full dose of all agents. However, severe and unexpected toxicities have been observed in most of these studies, often leading to trial discontinuation. Therefore, even if additive toxicities or drug-drug interactions are not expected, caution should be recommended when designing phase 1/2 trials of immunotherapies in combination, either by using traditional dose-escalation design (that would have the advantage of establishing the lowest safe and active dose) or by making provisions in the protocol to allow rapid dose de-escalation (in case both agents are started at full dose and unexpected toxicities are observed). Adaptive designs, including toxicity-based go/no-go decisions and biomarker-based endpoints, should also be favored. Specific guidelines have been established on this matter [95].

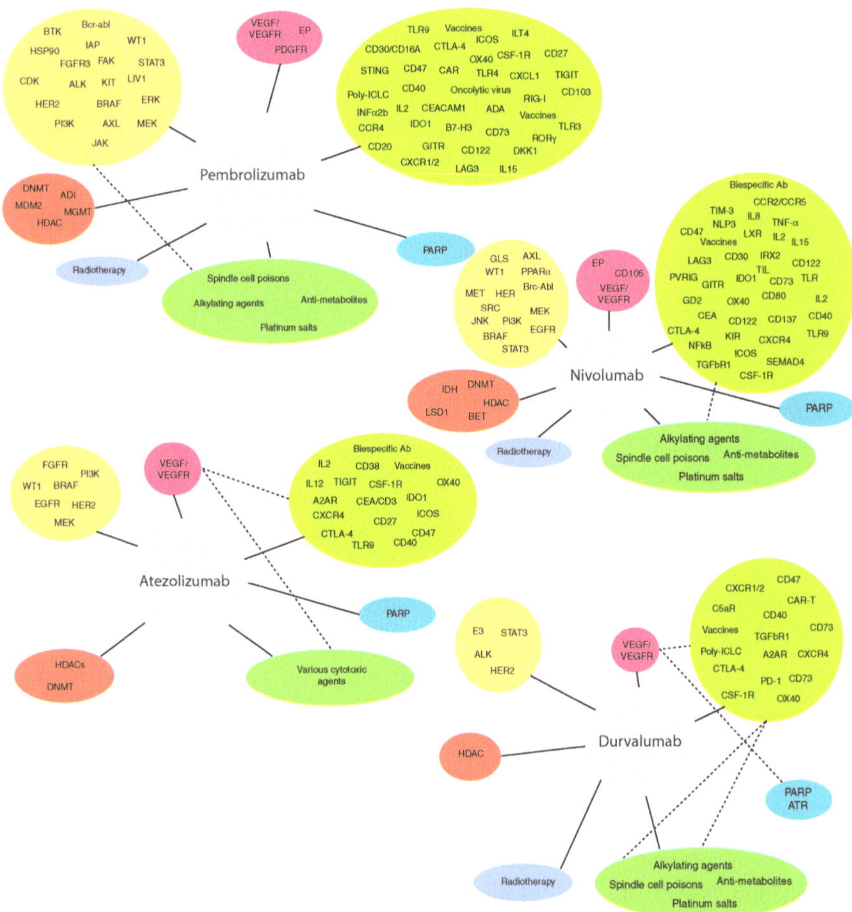

Fig. 15.5 Examples of ongoing phase 1 trials evaluating combinations with approved anti-PD-1 or anti-PD-L1 therapies. The main target classes that are currently being evaluated in association with some anti-PD-1 or anti-PD-L1 agents are depicted, with targeted therapies in yellow, epigenetic modifiers in orange, conventional cytotoxic chemotherapies in dark green, DNA repair inhibitors in blue, immune therapies in light green and antiantiogenic agents in pink. Dotted lines represent associations of three different therapeutic classes, on the anti-PD-1 or anti-PD-L1 therapy backbone. Only some trials are depicted here, but others may exist. Based on clinicaltrials.gov, accessed April 1st 2019, with phase 1 trials currently recruiting only

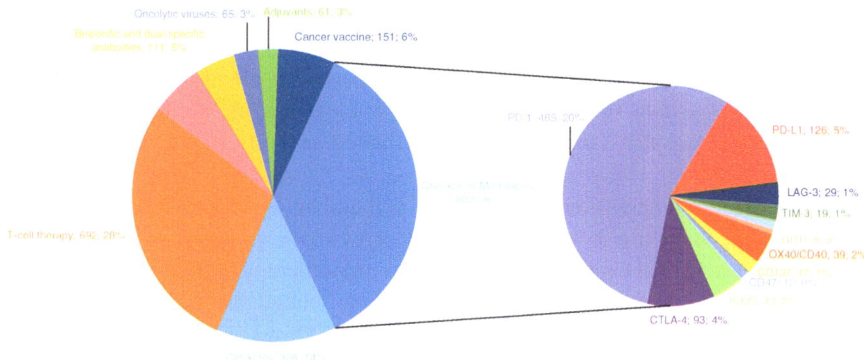

Fig. 15.6 Phase 1 trials of IO therapies. Search was performed for phase 1 trials recruiting only, with keywords "anticancer class" AND "cancer", where "anticancer class" corresponds to each of the category detailed in Fig. 15.5. (clinicaltrial.gov, accessed April 10, 2019)

15.4.2 IO–IO Combinations

15.4.2.1 Combinations with Co-inhibitory Molecules: T-Cell Antagonists

Cytotoxic T lymphocyte-associated antigen 4 (CTLA4) was the first ICI assessed in combination with anti-PD1 agents. Although the combination led to improved ORR (58%, 45% and 42% in patients with advanced-stage melanoma, renal cell cancer and NSCLC, respectively), G3-4 irAEs were reported in 59% of patients (*versus* 21% and 28% for single-agent nivolumab and ipilimumab, respectively) [96]. Noteworthy, irAE led to treatment discontinuation in 39% of patients receiving combination therapy, as opposed to 12% and 16% of patients receiving monotherapy nivolumab and ipilimumab, respectively. Currently, approximately 30 early phase clinical trials are evaluating anti-CTLA4 in combination with other IO agents, sometimes as a triple-combination with chemo and/or radiotherapy.

Lymphocyte activation gene 3 (LAG-3) is a co-inhibitory receptor that controls effector T-cell activity and regulatory T-cell immunosuppressive function. Preliminary activity of the anti-LAG-3 and anti-PD-(L)1 combination has shown promising results in immunotherapy-pretreated melanoma patients, notably in patients with LAG-3 expression ≥1% [97].

TIM-3 is a co-inhibitory receptor whose co-expression with PD-1 identifies the most exhausted CD8+ T-cell population. Dual TIM-3 and PD-(L)1 targeting is synergistic in inducing tumor shrinkage and IFN-γ. Results of early phase clinical studies evaluating TIM-3 inhibitors have been mitigated so far. The AMBER phase 1 clinical trial (NCT02817633) evaluating TSR-022 (anti-TIM-3) and TSR-042 (a PD-1 inhibitor) in patients who progressed after anti-PD-1 treatment showed that the combo was generally well-tolerated in patients with non-small cell lung cancer (NSCLC) [62]. Interestingly, the response rate (RR) and disease control rate (DCR) appeared to increase with dose, from 9% (n = 1/11) and 36% (n = 4/11) in the 100 mg group to 15% and 55% in the 300 mg group, respectively. The 300 mg dose was also suggested to be insufficient to maintain a maximal pharmacodynamic effect; results of the 900 mg dose have not been reported yet.

Other compounds, such as LY3321367, have been well-tolerated so far, mostly leading to dose-independent immune-related toxicities. Responses have been observed in monotherapy, e.g. one partial response in a patient with anti-CTLA4 and anti-PD1-resistant small cell lung cancer [62]. Bispecific TIM3/PD-1 targeting antibodies are also currently being evaluated in early phase clinical trials (NCT03708328).

TIGIT receptor expression on activated T-cell and natural killer (NK)-cell inhibits T-cell-dependent tumor killing and effector cytokine production. Recent data from the Phase 1a trial evaluating etigilimab in monotherapy at doses ranging from 0.3 to 20 mg/kg reported Grade 3 or higher immune-related rash in 17% of patients, together with other irAEs at frequencies >5%; the MTD was not reached. The phase 1 study assessing MK-7684 as monotherapy or in combination with pembrolizumab evaluated flat doses from 2.1 to 210 mg following a modified toxicity probability interval design with a target DLT rate during cycle 1 [62]. Among 68 enrolled patients, 34 patients received MK-7684 and 34 received MK-7684 + pembrolizumab. TrAEs occurred in 53% and 65% of patients receiving monotherapy and the combination, respectively, without any deaths or discontinuations due to treatment-related AEs. The most common irAEs were fatigue (15%) and pruritus (12%) with MK-7684 and pruritus (21%) and rash (15%) with MK-7684 plus pembrolizumab. RECIST partial responses were observed in 3% and 18% with monotherapy and combination therapy, respectively. Dose confirmation and the evaluation of efficacy for monotherapy and combination therapy are ongoing (NCT02964013 [62]). Other phase1/2 studies are evaluating anti-TIGIT agents in monotherapy and in combination with anti-PD(L)1 (NCT03563716; NCT02794571).

15.4.2.2 Combination with Co-stimulatory Molecules: T-Cell Agonists

CD137 is a costimulatory member of the TNF receptor superfamily whose activation on T-cells and NK-cells result in enhanced cytokine production, survival and proliferation. Preclinical data suggest that combining a CD137 agonist with anti-PD1 enhances T-cell trafficking to the tumor and reverses T-cell inhibition. Urelumab caused dose-dependent severe liver toxicity at doses >1 mg/kg, supporting the determination of the MTD at a pharmacodynamically active dose of 0.1 mg/kg q3weeks. Conversely, utomilumab could be dose-escalated (using a mixed 3 + 3 and continuous reassessment dose-escalation method) without DLT till 10 mg/kg q4weeks (monotherapy) or 5 mg/kg q3weeks (with pembrolizumab) [98]. RECIST partial responses were observed in 3% and 27% of patients in monotherapy and combination, respectively, with promising complete responses. Other trials evaluating CD137 agonists and anti-PD-1 agents are ongoing (NCT02253992, NCT03792724, NCT02534506).

OX40 is a potent costimulatory receptor expressed primarily on effector and activated T-cells; OX40 agonists improve antitumor immunity and tumor-free survival in non-clinical models. The phase 1 trial evaluating MEDI0562 (NCT02318394) was dose escalated from 0.03 to 10 mg/kg in 55 patients, with 10 mg/kg established as the MTD. The most common irAEs included fatigue (31%) and infusion-related reactions (15%). Grade 3 irAEs occurred in 16% of patients and none led to permanent discontinuation of MEDI0562. Of 50 efficacy-evaluable patients, 2 patients had RECIST partial responses at the first tumor assessment and 20 of the 22 patients with SD had responses lasting >3 months [62]. Other OX40 agonists are currently being evaluated in monotherapy or in combination with anti-PD-1 and/or anti-CTLA-4 agents (NCT01689870, NCT02410512, NCT02221960, NCT02528357, NCT02554812, NCT03241173).

Inducible T-cell co-stimulator (ICOS) is a co-stimulatory receptor belonging to the CD28/CTLA immunoglobulin super family whose expression is highly induced on effector T-cells upon T-cell receptor (TCR) engagement and activation. ICOS-positive effector T-cells have also been reported to be increased in tumors that respond to anti-CTLA-4 antibodies. Combination of ICOS agonists and other ICI are ongoing (NCT02723955, NCT02904226, NCT03693612).

Glucocorticoid-induced tumor necrosis factor receptor-related protein (GITR) is expressed on effector and regulatory T-cells, NK-cells, B-cells and dendritic cells; GITR signaling enhances activation of effector T-cells and abrogates regulatory T-cell-mediated antitumor immune suppression. Safety and efficacy evaluation of MEDI1873 was evaluated in the NCT02583165 phase 1 study. Dose escalation was performed following an accelerated-titration design (2-patient cohorts at 1.5 and 3 mg, followed by 3 + 3 in the following 6 cohorts, 7.5, 25, 75, 250, 500 and 750 mg); 75 and 250 mg doses were subsequently expanded in pharmacodynamic cohorts enrolling patients with NSCLC and HNSCC. Although the MTD was not reached, 3 DLTs occurred: Grade 3 worsening tumor pain (250 mg), Grade 3 nausea and vomiting (500 mg) and Grade 3 non-ST-elevation myocardial infarction (750 mg). Any-grade irAEs occurred in 82.5% of pts, most commonly headache (25%) and IRR (20%). Best overall response was SD in 43% of pts, including a 18% with SD lasting ≥24 weeks [62]. Other phase I trials evaluating GITR agonists with anti-PD1 agents are ongoing (NCT02583165; NCT02740270, NCT01239134, NCT03335540, NCT02553499, NCT02598960).

15.4.2.3 Combination with Agents Targeting the Tumor Microenviroment (TME)

High adenosine levels in the TME disable cytotoxic functions of NK and CD8+ T-cells, inhibits CD4+ T-cell response and promotes proliferation of regulatory T-cells and pro-tumor myeloid-derived suppressor cells. Multiple agents targeting the adenosine pathway including anti-CD39, anti-CD73 and anti-adenosine receptor—are evaluated in early phase trials. Preliminary results of the anti-CD73 BMS-986179 in combination with nivolumab are promising with efficacy and minimal toxicity [99].

Indoleamine 2,3-dioxygenase 1 (IDO1), which catalyzes tryptophan degradation, favors immune tolerance by inhibiting T-cell function following tryptophan depletion and increased kynurenine concentrations. IDO1 tumor expression correlates with increased regulatory T-cell infiltrates and shorter patient survival. The development of IDO inhibitors illustrates well the importance of thoroughly exploiting phase 1 data prior to developing combination studies. In the first-in-human phase 1 study, the MTD was not established and no objective responses were observed; plasma kynurenine was decreased at all dose levels although no changes in plasma proteins related to immunity or inflammation could be detected, potentially suggesting insufficient dosing in monotherapy. The 100 mg BID and 300 mg BID doses were subsequently evaluated in combination with nivolumab in the ECHO 204 phase I/II trial, which reported a 65% ORR in immune-naïve melanoma patients; similarly, data from the phase I/II trial KEYNOTE-037 combining epacadostat and pembrolizumab reported an ORR of 55% in patients with IO-naïve melanoma, with a rate of G3-4 irAEs in 24% of patients [100]. Unfortunately, these results were not confirmed by the large ECHO-301/KEYNOTE-252 study, where no difference in PFS or OS was observed. Many phase 1 trials are currently evaluating other anti-IDO-1 agents in combination with anti-PD1 agents and results are awaited (NCT03343613, NCT03695250, NCT02658890).

Next generation early phase IO combination trials will certainly assess multiple combinations of ICI and IO small molecules using novel designs, such as the NCT03459222 study, which will assess relatlimab (anti-LAG-3) and nivolumab with either an IDO1 Inhibitor or Ipilimumab [61].

15.4.3 Combinations with Molecularly Targeted Therapies

15.4.3.1 Combinations with Targeted DNA Damage Repair Inhibitors

Tumors with highest prevalence of somatic mutations, particularly melanoma, non-small cell lung cancer, bladder cancer, and microsatellite-instability (MSI)-high tumors have shown an improved response to immunotherapies. In line with these observations and with the physiopathology of neoantigen generation, genomic instability and mutational load have been identified as putative predictive biomarkers of response to immunotherapies [101]. Further, agents targeting DNA damage repair (DDRi), such as poly(ADP-ribose) polymerase (PARP) inhibitors, display intrinsic immunomodulatory properties in specific contexts, especially through the modulation of innate cGAS/STING signaling [102]. More than 20 phase 1/2 trials are currently evaluating PARPi in combination with ICI in various histologies including, ovarian, breast, NSCLC and urothelial cancer (NCT02734004; NCT02484404, NCT02953457; NCT02944396; NCT03061188; NCT03101280; NCT03810105; NCT03775486; NCT02660034; NCT03572478; NCT03308942; NCT03574779; NCT03824704; NCT03404960). This combination has proven to be safe with no additional toxicities when compared to either component drug.

Results from the MEDIOLA seamless phase 1 trial evaluating the combination of the PARPi olaparib with durvalumab has reported encouraging efficacy data, with a >80% disease control rate at 12 weeks in *BRCA1/2* mutant ovarian and breast cancer patients [103]. The TOPACIO phase 1/2 trial (NCT02657889), evaluating the combination of niraparib and pembrolizumab in patients with triple-negative breast cancer or non-platinum-refractory ovarian cancer [104], reported an objective response rate of 25% (15/60 evaluable patients) in the intention-to-treat population, and of 45% (5/11 evaluable patients) in the *BRCA1/2* mutant population.

Other DDRi are currently evaluated in combination with ICI, including Ataxia Telangiectasia and Rad3 kinase inhibitors (ATRi). Preliminary results of the phase 1/2 trial evaluating the ATRi AZD6738 with durvalumab (NCT02264678) in NSCLC and HNSCC patients has reported an encouraging 19% response rate (1 RECIST CR, 2 RECIST PRs, 1 RECIST uPR out of 21 evaluable patients). Interestingly, activity was independent of ATM loss or PD-L1 expression. Translational studies showed that, during AZD6738 treatment, peripheral monocytes, proliferating T-cells and immunostimulatory cytokine IL-12 were suppressed, followed by a rebound during the off-drug period.

15.4.3.2 Combinations with Epigenetic Modifiers

Chromatin remodeling and epigenetic processes significantly influence antitumor immunity, both at the cancer cell level (antigen presentation process, neo-antigen expression, endogenous retrovirus expression, cytokine production, etc.) and at the immune cell level (T-cell lineage determination, reversion of T-cell exhaustion phenotype, enhancement of memory T-cells, macrophage polarization, etc.), as reviewed in Aspeslagh et al. [105].

Several clinical trials are currently evaluating the immunomodulatory potential of epigenetic agents, including combinations of anti-PD(L)1 agents with BET, DNMT, EZH2 or HDAC inhibitors in both solid and hematological cancers. Like DDRi, such combinations seem to be feasible and no unexpected toxicities have been observed so far. Preliminary results of the combination of the HDAC inhibitor entinostat with pembrolizumab reported a response rate of 24% (14/17 patients) and 10% (3/31 patients) in the anti-PD(L)1-naive and anti-PD(L)1-resistant patient groups, respectively [106]. Translational studies comparing baseline and on-treatment biopsies revealed a decrease in MDSCs (−35.7%) and an increase in CD8+ T-cells (47.4%). In contrast, results of the randomized phase 2 study evaluating the DNMT inhibitor CC-486 with pembrolizumab versus pembrolizumab monotherapy did not show any significant benefit. Combinations with epigenetic modifiers raise specific challenges, such as scheduling, dose and patient selection, which should be evaluated in Phase 1 trials [105].

15.5 Conclusion and Perspectives

The advent of immunotherapies has led to a paradigm shift in drug development and has led to a significant transformation in phase 1 trial designs. Current challenges not only include the traditional trial endpoints of toxicity, safety, PK/PD characteristics and recommended phase 2 dose determinations, but also determination of efficacy, biomarker discovery and potentially drug registration. Novel trial designs—such as seamless designs or, in the case of combinations, MIDAS designs (Multicandidate Iterative design with Adaptive Selection) [107]—may be relevant in the expansion phase of phase 1 immunotherapy trials to allow transforming "phase 1 safety trials" to "phase 1 registration trials"; recent successes in drug development nicely illustrate this evolution [21, 73, 92, 93].

Despite these changes, the primary aim of phase 1 trials should remain the identification of the optimal dose that can be administered safely and which will lead to maximal efficacy. The identification of novel agents displaying bell-shaped curves highlights the importance of performing thorough phase 1 dose-escalation studies with comprehensive pharmacokinetic and pharmacodynamic analyses; further, the observation of unexpected dose-limiting toxicities (and potentially deleterious effects) in trials evaluating ICI in combination with targeted therapies during Phase 2 trials urgently calls for caution and rational drug development, especially during phase I studies.

These are very exciting times in early drug development in immuno-oncology and the wide implementation of immunotherapies to the oncology therapeutic armamentarium has been increasing at an unprecedented speed. The highest level of clinical, scientific and ethical rigor will be instrumental in successfully optimizing, prioritizing and expediting immunotherapy drug development to improve patient benefit.

Key Expert Opinion Points

- Immunotherapies have led to unprecedented transformation in the design and conduct of phase 1 trials, challenging all traditional phase 1 paradigms.
- Phase 1 trials evaluating immunotherapies should be designed as seamless trials, favoring novel adaptive designs that allow exploring safety, biomarkers and efficacy and in pre-defined populations and at multiple dose levels.
- Comprehensive translational analyses should be recommended at all stages of phase 1 trials in order to investigate biomarkers of toxicity, pharmacodynamic, pharmacokinetics and efficacy, together with their dose-, drug- or patient-dependency.
- The primary objective of phase 1 trials should remain the determination of the optimal dose and schedule, which should be done cautiously based on pharmacodynamic, pharmacokinetic and efficacy data.
- Phase 1 immunotherapy combination trials should be justified by robust rationale and preclinical data; redundancy should be limited.

References

1. Tang J, Yu JX, Hubbard-Lucey VM, Neftelinov ST, Hodge JP, Lin Y. Trial watch: the clinical trial landscape for PD1/PDL1 immune checkpoint inhibitors. Nat Rev Drug Discov. 2018;17(12):854–5.
2. Postel-Vinay S, Aspeslagh S, Lanoy E, Robert C, Soria JC, Marabelle A. Challenges of phase 1 clinical trials evaluating immune checkpoint-targeted antibodies. Ann Oncol. 2016;27(2):214–24.
3. Smith MR. Rituximab (monoclonal anti-CD20 antibody): mechanisms of action and resistance. Oncogene. 2003;22(47):7359–68.
4. Park S, Jiang Z, Mortenson ED, Deng L, Radkevich-Brown O, Yang X, et al. The therapeutic effect of anti-HER2/neu antibody depends on both innate and adaptive immunity. Cancer Cell. 2010;18(2):160–70.
5. Heiss MM, Murawa P, Koralewski P, Kutarska E, Kolesnik OO, Ivanchenko VV, et al. The trifunctional antibody catumaxomab for the treatment of malignant ascites due to epithelial cancer: results of a prospective randomized phase II/III trial. Int J Cancer. 2010;127(9):2209–21.
6. Gokbuget N, Dombret H, Bonifacio M, Reichle A, Graux C, Faul C, et al. Blinatumomab for minimal residual disease in adults with B-cell precursor acute lymphoblastic leukemia. Blood. 2018;131(14):1522–31.
7. Kantarjian H, Stein A, Gokbuget N, Fielding AK, Schuh AC, Ribera JM, et al. Blinatumomab versus chemotherapy for advanced acute lymphoblastic leukemia. N Engl J Med. 2017;376(9):836–47.
8. Kaufman HL, Kohlhapp FJ, Zloza A. Oncolytic viruses: a new class of immunotherapy drugs. Nat Rev Drug Discov. 2015;14(9):642–62.
9. Moore AE. Effect of inoculation of the viruses of influenza A and herpes simplex on the growth of transplantable tumors in mice. Cancer. 1949;2(3):516–24.
10. Lal R, Harris D, Postel-Vinay S, de Bono J. Reovirus: rationale and clinical trial update. Curr Opin Mol Ther. 2009;11(5):532–9.
11. Andtbacka RH, Kaufman HL, Collichio F, Amatruda T, Senzer N, Chesney J, et al. Talimogene laherparepvec improves durable response rate in patients with advanced melanoma. J Clin Oncol Off J Am Soc Clin Oncol. 2015;33(25):2780–8.
12. Lotze MT, Grimm EA, Mazumder A, Strausser JL, Rosenberg SA. Lysis of fresh and cultured autologous tumor by human lymphocytes cultured in T-cell growth factor. Cancer Res. 1981;41(11 Pt 1):4420–5.
13. Lu PH, Negrin RS. A novel population of expanded human CD3+CD56+ cells derived from T cells with potent in vivo antitumor activity in mice with severe combined immunodeficiency. J Immunol. 1994;153(4):1687–96.
14. Kershaw MH, Westwood JA, Darcy PK. Gene-engineered T cells for cancer therapy. Nat Rev Cancer. 2013;13(8):525–41.
15. Brentjens RJ, Davila ML, Riviere I, Park J, Wang X, Cowell LG, et al. CD19-targeted T cells rapidly induce molecular remissions in adults with chemotherapy-refractory acute lymphoblastic leukemia. Sci Transl Med. 2013;5(177):177ra38.
16. Neelapu SS, Locke FL, Bartlett NL, Lekakis LJ, Miklos DB, Jacobson CA, et al. Axicabtagene ciloleucel CAR T-cell therapy in refractory large B-cell lymphoma. N Engl J Med. 2017;377(26):2531–44.
17. Dranoff G, Jaffee E, Lazenby A, Golumbek P, Levitsky H, Brose K, et al. Vaccination with irradiated tumor cells engineered to secrete murine granulocyte-macrophage colony-stimulating factor stimulates potent, specific, and long-lasting anti-tumor immunity. Proc Natl Acad Sci U S A. 1993;90(8):3539–43.
18. Kantoff PW, Higano CS, Shore ND, Berger ER, Small EJ, Penson DF, et al. Sipuleucel-T immunotherapy for castration-resistant prostate cancer. N Engl J Med. 2010;363(5):411–22.

19. Topalian SL, Taube JM, Anders RA, Pardoll DM. Mechanism-driven biomarkers to guide immune checkpoint blockade in cancer therapy. Nat Rev Cancer. 2016;16(5):275–87.
20. Weber JS, O'Day S, Urba W, Powderly J, Nichol G, Yellin M, et al. Phase I/II study of ipilimumab for patients with metastatic melanoma. J Clin Oncol. 2008;26(36):5950–6.
21. Hodi FS, O'Day SJ, McDermott DF, Weber RW, Sosman JA, Haanen JB, et al. Improved survival with ipilimumab in patients with metastatic melanoma. N Engl J Med. 2010;363(8):711–23.
22. Ribas A, Kefford R, Marshall MA, Punt CJ, Haanen JB, Marmol M, et al. Phase III randomized clinical trial comparing tremelimumab with standard-of-care chemotherapy in patients with advanced melanoma. J Clin Oncol Off J Am Soc Clin Oncol. 2013;31(5):616–22.
23. Topalian SL, Hodi FS, Brahmer JR, Gettinger SN, Smith DC, McDermott DF, et al. Safety, activity, and immune correlates of anti-PD-1 antibody in cancer. N Engl J Med. 2012;366(26):2443–54.
24. Robert C, Soria JC, Eggermont AM. Drug of the year: programmed death-1 receptor/programmed death-1 ligand-1 receptor monoclonal antibodies. Eur J Cancer. 2013;49(14):2968–71.
25. Lamm DL, Blumenstein BA, Crawford ED, Montie JE, Scardino P, Grossman HB, et al. A randomized trial of intravesical doxorubicin and immunotherapy with bacille Calmette-Guerin for transitional-cell carcinoma of the bladder. N Engl J Med. 1991;325(17):1205–9.
26. Scholch S, Rauber C, Tietz A, Rahbari NN, Bork U, Schmidt T, et al. Radiotherapy combined with TLR7/8 activation induces strong immune responses against gastrointestinal tumors. Oncotarget. 2015;6(7):4663–76.
27. Corrales L, McWhirter SM, Dubensky TW Jr, Gajewski TF. The host STING pathway at the interface of cancer and immunity. J Clin Invest. 2016;126(7):2404–11.
28. Corrales L, Glickman LH, McWhirter SM, Kanne DB, Sivick KE, Katibah GE, et al. Direct activation of STING in the tumor microenvironment leads to potent and systemic tumor regression and immunity. Cell Rep. 2015;11(7):1018–30.
29. Negrier S, Escudier B, Lasset C, Douillard JY, Savary J, Chevreau C, et al. Recombinant human interleukin-2, recombinant human interferon alfa-2a, or both in metastatic renal-cell carcinoma. Groupe Francais d'Immunotherapie. N Engl J Med. 1998;338(18):1272–8.
30. Weber JS, Kahler KC, Hauschild A. Management of immune-related adverse events and kinetics of response with ipilimumab. J Clin Oncol. 2012;30(21):2691–7.
31. Postel-Vinay S, Gomez-Roca C, Molife LR, Anghan B, Levy A, Judson I, et al. Phase I trials of molecularly targeted agents: should we pay more attention to late toxicities? J Clin Oncol Off J Am Soc Clin Oncol. 2011;29(13):1728–35.
32. Postel-Vinay S, Collette L, Paoletti X, Rizzo E, Massard C, Olmos D, et al. Towards new methods for the determination of dose limiting toxicities and the assessment of the recommended dose for further studies of molecularly targeted agents - dose-Limiting Toxicity and Toxicity Assessment Recommendation Group for Early Trials of Targeted therapies, an European Organisation for Research and Treatment of Cancer-led study. Eur J Cancer. 2014;50(12):2040–9.
33. Brahmer JR, Tykodi SS, Chow LQ, Hwu WJ, Topalian SL, Hwu P, et al. Safety and activity of anti-PD-L1 antibody in patients with advanced cancer. N Engl J Med. 2012;366(26):2455–65.
34. Lutzky J, Antonia S, Blake-Haskins A, Li X, Robbins PB, Shalabi A, et al. A phase 1 study of MEDI4736, an anti–PD-L1 antibody, in patients with advanced solid tumors. J Clin Oncol. 2014;32(5s):3001.
35. Johnson DB, Friedman DL, Berry E, Decker I, Ye F, Zhao S, et al. Survivorship in immune therapy: assessing chronic immune toxicities, health outcomes, and functional status among long-term ipilimumab survivors at a single referral center. Cancer Immunol Res. 2015;3(5):464–9.
36. Agrawal S, Feng Y, Roy A, Kollia G, Lestini B. Nivolumab dose selection: challenges, opportunities, and lessons learned for cancer immunotherapy. J Immunother Cancer. 2016;4:72.

37. Qiao M, Jiang T, Ren S, Zhou C. Combination strategies on the basis of immune checkpoint inhibitors in non-small-cell lung cancer: where do we stand? Clin Lung Cancer. 2018;19(1):1–11.
38. Bargou R, Leo E, Zugmaier G, Klinger M, Goebeler M, Knop S, et al. Tumor regression in cancer patients by very low doses of a T cell-engaging antibody. Science. 2008;321(5891):974–7.
39. De Velasco G, Je Y, Bosse D, Awad MM, Ott PA, Moreira RB, et al. Comprehensive meta-analysis of key immune-related adverse events from CTLA-4 and PD-1/PD-L1 inhibitors in cancer patients. Cancer Immunol Res. 2017;5(4):312–8.
40. Wang PF, Chen Y, Song SY, Wang TJ, Ji WJ, Li SW, et al. Immune-related adverse events associated with anti-PD-1/PD-L1 treatment for malignancies: a meta-analysis. Front Pharmacol. 2017;8:730.
41. Bertrand A, Kostine M, Barnetche T, Truchetet ME, Schaeverbeke T. Immune related adverse events associated with anti-CTLA-4 antibodies: systematic review and meta-analysis. BMC Med. 2015;13:211.
42. Cuzzubbo S, Javeri F, Tissier M, Roumi A, Barlog C, Doridam J, et al. Neurological adverse events associated with immune checkpoint inhibitors: review of the literature. Eur J Cancer. 2017;73:1–8.
43. Thompson JA, Schneider BJ, Brahmer J, Andrews S, Armand P, Bhatia S, et al. Management of Immunotherapy-related toxicities, version 1.2019. J Natl Compr Cancer Netw. 2019;17(3):255–89.
44. Champiat S, Lambotte O, Barreau E, Belkhir R, Berdelou A, Carbonnel F, et al. Management of immune checkpoint blockade dysimmune toxicities: a collaborative position paper. Ann Oncol. 2016;27(4):559–74.
45. Brahmer JR, Lacchetti C, Schneider BJ, Atkins MB, Brassil KJ, Caterino JM, et al. Management of immune-related adverse events in patients treated with immune checkpoint inhibitor therapy: American Society of Clinical Oncology clinical practice guideline. J Clin Oncol Off J Am Soc Clin Oncol. 2018;36(17):1714–68.
46. Wang W, Wang EQ, Balthasar JP. Monoclonal antibody pharmacokinetics and pharmacodynamics. Clin Pharmacol Ther. 2008;84(5):548–58.
47. Long GV, Tykodi SS, Schneider JG, Garbe C, Gravis G, Rashford M, et al. Assessment of nivolumab exposure and clinical safety of 480 mg every 4 weeks flat-dosing schedule in patients with cancer. Ann Oncol. 2018;29(11):2208–13.
48. Roopenian DC, Akilesh S. FcRn: the neonatal Fc receptor comes of age. Nat Rev Immunol. 2007;7(9):715–25.
49. Ratain MJ, Goldstein DA. Time is money: optimizing the scheduling of Nivolumab. J Clin Oncol. 2018:Jco1800045.
50. Ascierto PA, Del Vecchio M, Robert C, Mackiewicz A, Chiarion-Sileni V, Arance A, et al. Ipilimumab 10 mg/kg versus ipilimumab 3 mg/kg in patients with unresectable or metastatic melanoma: a randomised, double-blind, multicentre, phase 3 trial. Lancet Oncol. 2017;18(5):611–22.
51. Camacho LH, Antonia S, Sosman J, Kirkwood JM, Gajewski TF, Redman B, et al. Phase I/II trial of tremelimumab in patients with metastatic melanoma. J Clin Oncol Off J Am Soc Clin Oncol. 2009;27(7):1075–81.
52. Robert C, Thomas L, Bondarenko I, O'Day S, Weber J, Garbe C, et al. Ipilimumab plus dacarbazine for previously untreated metastatic melanoma. N Engl J Med. 2011;364(26):2517–26.
53. Basak EA, Koolen SLW, Hurkmans DP, Schreurs MWJ, Bins S, Oomen-de Hoop E, et al. Correlation between nivolumab exposure and treatment outcomes in non-small-cell lung cancer. Eur J Cancer. 2019;109:12–20.
54. Spiess C, Zhai Q, Carter PJ. Alternative molecular formats and therapeutic applications for bispecific antibodies. Mol Immunol. 2015;67(2 Pt A):95–106.
55. Kontermann RE, Brinkmann U. Bispecific antibodies. Drug Discov Today. 2015;20(7):838–47.
56. Portell CA, Wenzell CM, Advani AS. Clinical and pharmacologic aspects of blinatumomab in the treatment of B-cell acute lymphoblastic leukemia. Clin Pharmacol. 2013;5(Suppl 1):5–11.

57. Lesterhuis WJ, Bosco A, Millward MJ, Small M, Nowak AK, Lake RA. Dynamic versus static biomarkers in cancer immune checkpoint blockade: unravelling complexity. Nat Rev Drug Discov. 2017;16:264–72.
58. Brahmer JR, Drake CG, Wollner I, Powderly JD, Picus J, Sharfman WH, et al. Phase I study of single-agent anti-programmed death-1 (MDX-1106) in refractory solid tumors: safety, clinical activity, pharmacodynamics, and immunologic correlates. J Clin Oncol. 2010;28(19):3167–75.
59. Niemeijer AN, Leung D, Huisman MC, Bahce I, Hoekstra OS, van Dongen G, et al. Whole body PD-1 and PD-L1 positron emission tomography in patients with non-small-cell lung cancer. Nat Commun. 2018;9(1):4664.
60. Curti BD, Kovacsovics-Bankowski M, Morris N, Walker E, Chisholm L, Floyd K, et al. OX40 is a potent immune-stimulating target in late-stage cancer patients. Cancer Res. 2013;73(24):7189–98.
61. Kerr WG, Chisholm JD. The next generation of immunotherapy for cancer: small molecules could make big waves. J Immunol. 2019;202(1):11–9.
62. Butterfield LH, Disis ML, Fox BA, Kaufman DR, Khleif SN, Wang E. SITC 2018 workshop report: immuno-oncology biomarkers: state of the art. J Immunother Cancer. 2018;6(1):138.
63. Ji Y, Wang SJ. Modified toxicity probability interval design: a safer and more reliable method than the 3 + 3 design for practical phase I trials. J Clin Oncol. 2013;31(14):1785–91.
64. Seymour L, Bogaerts J, Perrone A, Ford R, Schwartz LH, Mandrekar S, et al. iRECIST: guidelines for response criteria for use in trials testing immunotherapeutics. Lancet Oncol. 2017;18(3):e143–e52.
65. Borcoman E, Kanjanapan Y, Champiat S, Kato S, Servois V, Kurzrock R, et al. Novel patterns of response under immunotherapy. Ann Oncol. 2019;30:385–96.
66. Champiat S, Dercle L, Ammari S, Massard C, Hollebecque A, Postel-Vinay S, et al. Hyperprogressive disease is a new pattern of progression in cancer patients treated by Anti-PD-1/PD-L1. Clin Cancer Res. 2017;23(8):1920–8.
67. Lo Russo G, Moro M, Sommariva M, Cancila V, Boeri M, Centonze G, et al. Antibody-Fc/FcR interaction on macrophages as a mechanism for hyperprogressive disease in non-small cell lung cancer subsequent to PD-1/PD-L1 blockade. Clin Cancer Res. 2019;25(3):989–99.
68. Arkenau HT, Barriuso J, Olmos D, Ang JE, de Bono J, Judson I, et al. Prospective validation of a prognostic score to improve patient selection for oncology phase I trials. J Clin Oncol. 2009;27(16):2692–6.
69. Bigot F, Castanon E, Baldini C, Hollebecque A, Carmona A, Postel-Vinay S, et al. Prospective validation of a prognostic score for patients in immunotherapy phase I trials: the Gustave Roussy immune score (GRIm-Score). Eur J Cancer. 2017;84:212–8.
70. Hodi FS, Oble DA, Drappatz J, Velazquez EF, Ramaiya N, Ramakrishna N, et al. CTLA-4 blockade with ipilimumab induces significant clinical benefit in a female with melanoma metastases to the CNS. Nat Clin Pract Oncol. 2008;5(9):557–61.
71. Margolin K, Ernstoff MS, Hamid O, Lawrence D, McDermott D, Puzanov I, et al. Ipilimumab in patients with melanoma and brain metastases: an open-label, phase 2 trial. Lancet Oncol. 2012;13(5):459–65.
72. Arbour KC, Mezquita L, Long N, Rizvi H, Auclin E, Ni A, et al. Impact of baseline steroids on efficacy of programmed cell death-1 and programmed death-ligand 1 blockade in patients with non-small-cell lung cancer. J Clin Oncol Off J Am Soc Clin Oncol. 2018;36(28):2872–8.
73. Garon EB, Rizvi NA, Hui R, Leighl N, Balmanoukian AS, Eder JP, et al. Pembrolizumab for the treatment of non-small-cell lung cancer. N Engl J Med. 2015;372(21):2018–28.
74. Marabelle A, Routy B, Michels J, Kroemer G, Zitvogel L. Prime time for immune-checkpoint targeted therapy at ASCO 2015. Oncoimmunology. 2015;5(3):e1068494.
75. Brahmer J, Reckamp KL, Baas P, Crino L, Eberhardt WE, Poddubskaya E, et al. Nivolumab versus docetaxel in advanced squamous-cell non-small-cell lung cancer. N Engl J Med. 2015;373(2):123–35.
76. Armand P. Immune checkpoint blockade in hematologic malignancies. Blood. 2015;125(22):3393–400.

77. Jelinic P, Ricca J, Van Oudenhove E, Olvera N, Merghoub T, Levine DA, et al. Immune-active microenvironment in small cell carcinoma of the ovary, hypercalcemic type: rationale for immune checkpoint blockade. J Natl Cancer Inst. 2018;110(7):787–90.
78. Marabelle A, Tselikas L, de Baere T, Houot R. Intratumoral immunotherapy: using the tumor as the remedy. Ann Oncol. 2017;28(suppl 12):xii33–43.
79. Galluzzi L, Buque A, Kepp O, Zitvogel L, Kroemer G. Immunogenic cell death in cancer and infectious disease. Nat Rev Immunol. 2017;17(2):97–111.
80. Riley RS, June CH, Langer R, Mitchell MJ. Delivery technologies for cancer immunotherapy. Nat Rev Drug Discov. 2019;18(3):175–96.
81. Huck BRKL, Urbahns K. Small molecules drive big improvements in Immuno-oncology therapies. Angew Chem Int Ed Engl. 2018;57(16):4412–28.
82. Ramanjulu JM, Pesiridis GS, Yang J, Concha N, Singhaus R, Zhang SY, et al. Design of amidobenzimidazole STING receptor agonists with systemic activity. Nature. 2018;564(7736):439–43.
83. Tyring SK, Rosen T. Beyond a decade of 5% imiquimod topical therapy. J Drugs Dermatol. 2009;8(5):467–74.
84. Uemura MI, Haymaker CL, Murthy R, James M, Cornfeld M, Chunduru S, et al. Intratumoral (i.t.) IMO-2125 (IMO), a TLR9 agonist, in combination with ipilimumab (ipi) in PD-(L)1 refractory melanoma (RM). J Clin Oncol. 2017;35(suppl 7):136.
85. Fesnak AD, June CH, Levine BL. Engineered T cells: the promise and challenges of cancer immunotherapy. Nat Rev Cancer. 2016;16(9):566–81.
86. Pettitt D, Arshad Z, Smith J, Stanic T, Hollander G, Brindley D. CAR-T cells: a systematic review and mixed methods analysis of the clinical trial landscape. Mol Ther. 2018;26(2):342–53.
87. Lee DW, Kochenderfer JN, Stetler-Stevenson M, Cui YK, Delbrook C, Feldman SA, et al. T cells expressing CD19 chimeric antigen receptors for acute lymphoblastic leukaemia in children and young adults: a phase 1 dose-escalation trial. Lancet. 2015;385(9967):517–28.
88. Maude SL, Frey N, Shaw PA, Aplenc R, Barrett DM, Bunin NJ, et al. Chimeric antigen receptor T cells for sustained remissions in leukemia. N Engl J Med. 2014;371(16):1507–17.
89. Ahmed N, Brawley VS, Hegde M, Robertson C, Ghazi A, Gerken C, et al. Human epidermal growth factor receptor 2 (HER2)-specific chimeric antigen receptor-modified T cells for the immunotherapy of HER2-positive sarcoma. J Clin Oncol Off J Am Soc Clin Oncol. 2015;33(15):1688–96.
90. Maude SL, Laetsch TW, Buechner J, Rives S, Boyer M, Bittencourt H, et al. Tisagenlecleucel in children and young adults with B-cell lymphoblastic leukemia. N Engl J Med. 2018;378(5):439–48.
91. Santomasso BD, Park JH, Salloum D, Riviere I, Flynn J, Mead E, et al. Clinical and biological correlates of neurotoxicity associated with CAR T-cell therapy in patients with B-cell acute lymphoblastic leukemia. Cancer Discov. 2018;8(8):958–71.
92. Robert C, Ribas A, Wolchok JD, Hodi FS, Hamid O, Kefford R, et al. Anti-programmed-death-receptor-1 treatment with pembrolizumab in ipilimumab-refractory advanced melanoma: a randomised dose-comparison cohort of a phase 1 trial. Lancet. 2014;384(9948):1109–17.
93. Long GV, Dummer R, Ribas A, Puzanov I, Michielin O, VanderWalde A, et al. A phase I/III, multicenter, open-label trial of talimogene laherparepvec (T-VEC) in combination with pembrolizumab for the treatment of unresected, stage IIIb-IV melanoma (MASTERKEY-265). J Immunother Cancer. 2015;3(2):P181.
94. Nikanjam M, Patel H, Kurzrock R. Dosing immunotherapy combinations: analysis of 3,526 patients for toxicity and response patterns. Onco Targets Ther. 2017;6(8):e1338997.
95. Smoragiewicz M, Bogaerts J, Calvo E, Marabelle A, Perrone A, Seymour L, et al. Design and conduct of early clinical studies of immunotherapy agent combinations: recommendations from the task force on methodology for the development of innovative Cancer therapies. Ann Oncol. 2018;29(11):2175–82.

96. Wolchok JD, Chiarion-Sileni V, Gonzalez R, Rutkowski P, Grob JJ, Cowey CL, et al. Overall survival with combined nivolumab and ipilimumab in advanced melanoma. N Engl J Med. 2017;377(14):1345–56.
97. Ascierto PA, Bono P, Bhatia S, Melero I, Nyakas MS, Svane I-M, et al. LBA18Efficacy of BMS-986016, a monoclonal antibody that targets lymphocyte activation gene-3 (LAG-3), in combination with nivolumab in pts with melanoma who progressed during prior anti–PD-1/PD-L1 therapy (mel prior IO) in all-comer and biomarker-enriched populations. Ann Oncol. 2017;28(suppl 5)
98. Segal NH, Logan TF, Hodi FS, McDermott D, Melero I, Hamid O, et al. Results from an integrated safety analysis of Urelumab, an agonist anti-CD137 monoclonal antibody. Clin Cancer Res. 2017;23(8):1929–36.
99. Siu LL, Burris H, Le DT, Hollebecque A, Steeghs N, Delord J-P, et al. Abstract CT180: preliminary phase 1 profile of BMS-986179, an anti-CD73 antibody, in combination with nivolumab in patients with advanced solid tumors. Cancer Res. 2018;78(13 Suppl):CT180.
100. Mitchell TC, Hamid O, Smith DC, Bauer TM, Wasser JS, Olszanski AJ, et al. Epacadostat plus pembrolizumab in patients with advanced solid tumors: phase i results from a multicenter, open-label phase I/II trial (ECHO-202/KEYNOTE-037). J clin Oncol. 2018:Jco2018789602.
101. Chabanon RM, Pedrero M, Lefebvre C, Marabelle A, Soria JC, Postel-Vinay S. Mutational landscape and sensitivity to immune checkpoint blockers. Clin Cancer Res. 2016;22(17):4309–21.
102. Chabanon RM, Muirhead G, Krastev DB, Adam J, Morel D, Garrido M, et al. PARP inhibition enhances tumor cell-intrinsic immunity in ERCC1-deficient non-small cell lung cancer. J Clin Invest. 2019;129(3):1211–28.
103. Penson RT, Alvarez RH, Kaufman B, Gresty C, Angell HK, Meyer K, et al. 448TiPMEDIOLA: a phase I/II trial of olaparib (PARP inhibitor) in combination with durvalumab (anti-PD-L1 antibody) in pts with advanced solid tumours – new ovarian cancer cohorts. Ann Oncol. 2018;29(suppl 8)
104. Konstantinopoulos PA, Matulonis UA. PARP inhibitors in ovarian cancer: a trailblazing and transformative journey. Clin Cancer Res. 2018;24(17):4062–5.
105. Aspeslagh S, Morel D, Soria JC, Postel-Vinay S. Epigenetic modifiers as new immunomodulatory therapies in solid tumours. Ann Oncol. 2018;29(4):812–24.
106. Hellmann M, Jänne P, Opyrchal M, Hafez N, Raez L, Gabrilovich D, et al. OA05.01 efficacy/safety of entinostat (ENT) and pembrolizumab (PEMBRO) in NSCLC patients previously treated with anti-PD-(L)1 therapy. J Thorac Oncol. 2018;13(10):S330.
107. Yuan Y, Guo B, Munsell M, Lu K, Jazaeri A. MIDAS: a practical Bayesian design for platform trials with molecularly targeted agents. Stat Med. 2016;35(22):3892–906.

Chapter 16
Radiotherapy Considerations and Strategic Approaches in Phase I Trials

Lauren E. Colbert, Ying Yuan, Jaap D. Zindler, Clifton D. Fuller, and Charles R. Thomas

Abstract Cellular damage by ionizing radiation relies on time to consider DNA damage, repair, reoxygenation, repopulation and redistribution. This means that both tumor kill and toxicity must be considered differently in phase I trials than those from drugs, and the combination of targeted agents and immunotherapy agents with radiation must also be carefully considered. Additionally, timing and logistics of radiation therapy may cause delays or interruptions in phase I study designs in combination with drugs that must also be carefully considered when designing trials. Dose limiting toxicity trials and maximum tolerated dose trials including RT may require longer follow up to fully evaluate toxicity. Adaptive phase I trial designs that consider longer term toxicity in their study design are advantageous for this purpose.

Keywords Radiotherapy · Phase I trials · Radiatiation · Radiation oncology Radiation biology

---

L. E. Colbert · C. D. Fuller
Department of Radiation Oncology, University of Texas MD Anderson Cancer Center, Houston, TX, USA
e-mail: LColbert@mdanderson.org; CDFuller@mdanderson.org

Y. Yuan
Department of Biostatistics, University of Texas MD Anderson Cancer Center, Houston, TX, USA
e-mail: yyuan@mdanderson.org

J. D. Zindler
Department of Radiation Oncology, Erasmus MC, Rotterdam, The Netherlands
e-mail: j.zindler@erasmusmc.nl

C. R. Thomas (✉)
Department of Radiation Medicine, Oregon Health and Science University Knight Cancer Institute, Oregon, USA
e-mail: thomasch@ohsu.edu

T. A. Yap et al. (eds.), *Phase I Oncology Drug Development*,
https://doi.org/10.1007/978-3-030-47682-3_16

Key Points

- Radiation relies on cellular repair, reoxygenation, repopulation and redistribution for both tumor kill and repair from toxicity. These should be taken into account when combining with new drug agents.
- The delivery of radiation often involves complex planning, and may take multiple weeks to prepare. This should be considered in design of a phase I trial involving radiation.
- Radiation dose and fractionation are not summative. Shorter courses may actually cause more toxicity than longer courses, if the single fraction dose is higher.
- Radiation toxicity may be extremely elevated by synergistic drug combinations, and new combinations should be tested with care.
- MTD and DLT trials including radiation must consider delayed onset toxicity, often up to 3–6 months post radiation.

16.1 General Introduction to Radiation Therapy

16.1.1 Basic Radiation Biology

In estimating clinical success or failure of radiation therapy, radiation oncologists often refer to the "Four R's" of radiation biology, namely *Repair, Reoxygenation, Repopulation* and *Redistribution* (within the cell cycle). These four biologic principles govern how much DNA damage is induced and, in turn, how much tumor kill will occur.

Repair refers to the DNA repair that results in between given fractions of radiation. This repair occurs generally via non-homologous end joining and homologous recombination pathways. This repair can be capitalized on by combination with specific targeted therapies that affect either of these pathways, such as poly(ADP-ribose) polymerase (PARP) inhibitors.

Reoxygenation refers to the principle that DNA damage is much more effective in oxygenated cells, and thus the "hypoxic fraction" of a tumor may not be damaged by a single dose of radiation therapy. In addition to direct DNA damage, radiation induces oxygen radicals that cause secondary DNA damage. Under hypoxic conditions, these are not present and cellular repair is much quicker, resulting in less cell kill. Allowing time for reoxygenation to occur will allow for greater cell killing. Combination of radiation with therapies that increase oxygenation, such as vascular endothelial growth factors (VEGF) inhibitors (Willett CG, Boucher Y, di Tomaso E, et al. Direct evidence that the VEGF-specific antibody bevacizumab has antivascular effects in human rectal cancer. Nat Med) or paclitaxel chemotherapy [1], may increase tumor kill.

Repopulation refers to the fact that both tumor cells and normal cells multiply in between fractions of radiation therapy. This is disadvantageous for radiation therapy, and is in part the reason that treatment time should be kept as short as possible with minimal interruptions in therapy, particularly for tumor types that exhibit rapid repopulation, such as head and neck or cervical cancers [2].

Redistribution refers to the redistribution of cells within the cell cycle. Sensitivity to DNA damage as a result of ionizing radiation is variable based on its position within the cell cycle, with cells being most prone to double stranded DNA damage in G2/M phases of the cell cycle, as the cell does not have adequate time to repair DNA damage before dividing. Cells are least sensitive in late S phase. This is partially due to the fact that repair via homologous recombination is most prominent during late S phase, when sister chromatids are available and most of the DNA has been replicated; repair via non-homologous end joining is predominant and more error prone during G1, when no sister chromatids are available. Targeted therapies that result in cell cycle arrest or redistribution, such as those that target cyclin-dependent kinases [3–5] can improve antitumor responses to radiation.

16.1.2 Dose and Fractionation

Radiation therapy accomplishes tumor control by causing double strand breaks in cancer cells' DNA, leading to an inability to divide. Unfortunately, these breaks can also be created in normal cells. In order to overcome this and capitalize on differences in reproduction between normal and cancer cells, radiation therapy is given in multiple doses, or "fractions," over a course of time. This allows repeated damage to cancer cell DNA, while allowing normal tissue time to repair. An important point for the non-radiation oncologist is that total "dose" of radiation is not cumulative; i.e., administering 1.8 Gy for 25 fractions to a total dose of 45 Gy is not equivalent to administering 9 Gy for 5 fractions to a total dose of 45 Gy. These treatment regimens have grossly different tumor control and normal tissue toxicities due a principal referred to as the alpha/beta ratio. Put simply, this ratio quantifies the amount of damage and repair that occurs for a tumor tissue versus a normal tissue, which is different for large doses versus small doses. Multiple equations exist to convert from different dose sizes to reach a biological equivalent dose (BED) that is comparable between different dose and fractionation regimens. Specific doses (in terms of BED) to normal tissue and their associated risk of toxicity have been estimated based on previous modeling; for instance, treating the spinal cord to 50 Gy is associated with a < 1% risk of myelopathy, while treating the spinal cord to 60 Gy is associated with a 6% risk of myelopathy, and to 69 Gy is associated with a nearly 50% risk of myelopathy (2010 PMID 20171502 – "Use of normal tissue complication probability models in the clinic." [6]. For this reason, the spinal cord is rarely treated above doses of 50 Gy. This total dose limit to specific tissues limits the tumoricidal dose that can be delivered, and is often the reason that reirradiation is challenging. Toxicity rates can be much higher with reirradiation, and thus deciding whether reirradiation is possible requires reviewing previous treatment plans, reviewing normal tissue constraints, and weighing the clinical risks and benefits carefully. This should be considered in eligibility criteria when designing trials involving radiation therapy.

16.1.3 Treatment Delivery

Another key concept for the non-radiation oncologist designing trials involving radiation is that radiation therapy is a tool that works only where radiation is delivered, meaning that toxicity, other than fatigue, is generally only observed in areas where the radiation dose is delivered. This component of spatial cooperation is evident in trials using combined modalities ([7], IJROBP). For instance, in a patient receiving pelvic radiation therapy, alopecia of the scalp or headache is likely attributable to other causes. Additionally, for trials involving systemic therapies with specific associated toxicities, this should be considered; for example, an immunotherapy that is associated with high rates of colitis or diarrhea should be cautiously administered with full pelvic or abdominal radiation therapy. One of the greatest advances in external beam radiation therapy (EBRT) has been the ability to "shape" the dose delivery to target tumor tissues while avoiding normal tissues. This can lead to a favorable increase in the therapeutic ratio, e.g. the ratio of tumor control probability/normal tissue complication probability. 3D conformal radiation therapy (3D-CRT) is "standard" radiation therapy, and can be described as similar to square flashlight beams (Fig. 16.1); although tumor is covered, normal tissues receive a large volume of radiation. Intensity modulated radiation therapy (IMRT) allows the dose to be "painted" over the target, resulting in a much more conformal radiation treatment to the tumor. IMRT has become even more advanced to allow narrower margins on the treatment volume, by incorporating better patient immobilization, management of respiratory movement, and high-quality diagnostic imaging known as image-guided radiotherapy (IGRT) including advanced MRI and PET/CT. The combination of IGRT and IMRT results in increased accuracy and precise delivery of radiotherapy. Stereotactic body radiation therapy (SBRT) involves delivering high doses of radiation therapy (generally greater than 5–6 Gy per fraction) using tight margins and advanced IMRT treatment planning techniques. Because these techniques are so tightly and carefully planned, they require skill and thought on the part of the radiation oncologist, and a solid understanding of the tumor location, borders and clinical picture, and careful treatment plan design by radiation dosimetrists and physicists.

16.1.4 Logistics of Radiation Delivery

There are multiple steps involved in developing and delivering radiation therapy that must be accounted for logistically in preparation for a clinical trial. Prior to radiation delivery, patients must undergo a planning CT scan, known as a radiation simulation, which the radiation oncologist will use to design the treatment plan. This planning scan must be done in the treatment position on a specially calibrated CT machine, so a standard diagnostic CT scan cannot be substituted. Diagnostic CT, MRI or PET/CT scans may be required to supplement tumor delineation and will be fused with the planning scan, if necessary. After this

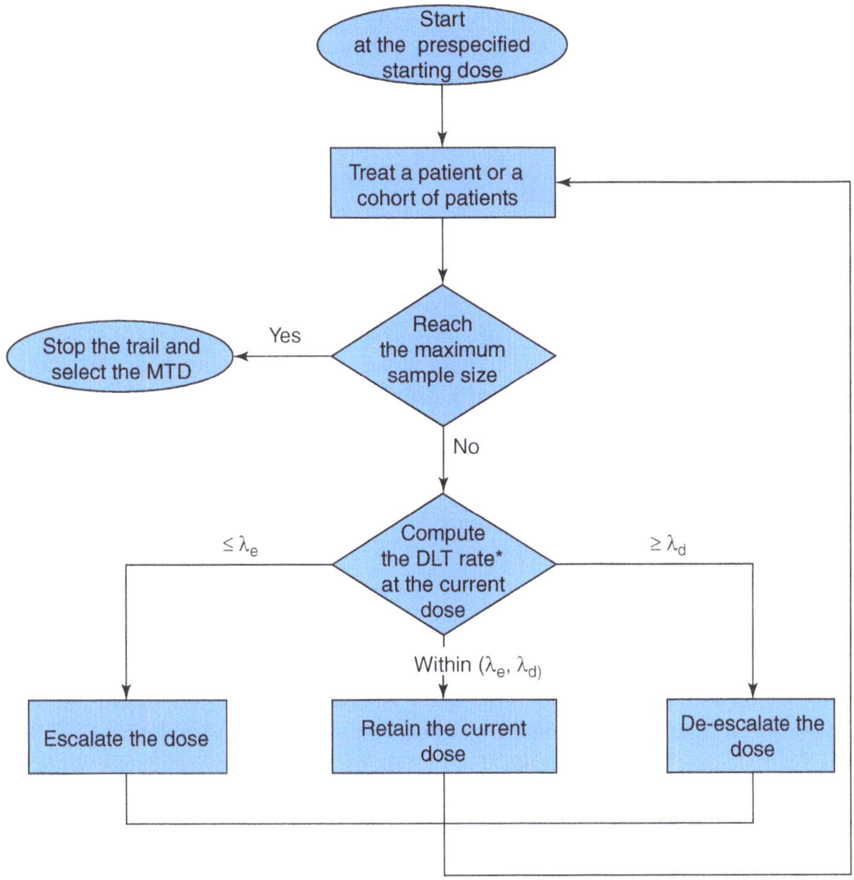

$$\text{* DLT rate} = \frac{\text{Total number of patients who experienced DLT at the current dose}}{\text{Total number of patients treated at the current dose}}$$

Fig. 16.1 The flowchart of the BOIN design, where λ_e and λ_d are two prespecified optimal dose escalation and de-escalation boundaries, as shown in Table 16.1

simulation scan, the radiation oncologist will delineate on each individual slice of the scan the tumor volumes (gross tumor volume or GTV) and "at risk" volumes (clinical target volume or CTV), in addition to a margin for setup and positioning error (planning target volume or PTV). The radiation oncologist will then make a decision regarding a prescription to each of these volumes, and often there will be multiple layers of individual doses to multiple CTV's or PTV's. This may take several days. Once these decisions are made, a radiation dosimetrist will compute a treatment plan to achieve these goals. The radiation oncologist, dosimetrist and radiation physicist will go through multiple iterations of this plan to create an optimized plan, which may take another several days. The plan must then go through quality checks with the radiation physicist to ensure the machine appropriately delivers the specified plan. The length of time for this whole process can vary between departments, but could be between one week and four weeks, with longer time required for more complex treatment planning such as SBRT or reirradiation.

16.2 Novel Trial Designs

The objective of phase I oncology trials is to find the maximum tolerated dose (MTD), which is defined as the dose with the dose-limiting toxicity (DLT) probability closest to the target DLT rate, e.g., 30%. Depending on the trial setting, we may be interested in finding (1) the MTD of RT alone or in combination with a fixed dose of chemotherapy, or (2) the MTD of a drug in combination with a fixed dose of RT. In case 1, the RT-related DLT is the main focus that drives dose finding. In case 2, the drug-related DLT (rather than RT-related DLT) is of main focus. Because of the different nature of RT-related and drug-related DLTs, these two types of trials require different design considerations and strategies. We have illustrated this through different case studies below:

Case 1: Glioblastoma Trial
A phase I trial was designed to establish the MTD of TG02, combined with concomitant temozolamide and radiotherapy for adult patients with recurrent anaplastic astrocytoma and glioblastoma. TG02 is a pyrimidine-based multi-kinase inhibitor that has been shown to have inhibitory effects on cyclin-dependent kinases (CDKs) and Janus Kinase 2 (JAK2). Four dose levels of TG02 are investigated, with the target DLT rate of 0.3. The maximum sample size comprised 24 patients, treated in cohort sizes of 3 patients. DLT was graded using CTCAE 4.0 over a time frame of 4 weeks.

Case 2: SBRT Boost Trial
A phase I trial was developed to establish the MTD of stereotactic body radiotherapy (SBRT) boost with concurrent chemoradiotherapy for patients with advanced pancreatic cancer. Five doses of SBRT, i.e., 6, 7, 8, 9 or 10 Gy X 3Fr, were studied. Patients are treated in cohort sizes of 3 patients. The dose escalation was based on the DLT occurring within a time frame of 9 months post radiotherapy, with a target DLT rate of 0.3. The DLT was defined as grade 3 or 4 gastro-intestinal or other non-hematological toxicity related to radiotherapy to the upper abdomen, graded as per CTCAE 4.0.

In classic phase I RT trials, the RT dose was prescribed based on tumor volume; for example, brain metastases will get single fractions of 20 Gy, 22 Gy, and 24 Gy in a trial. The problem with this strategy is that tumors may have different volumes. This will have an effect on the RT dose impacting the surrounding healthy brain tissue. It may occur that with a single fraction of 24 Gy, the volume of healthy brain tissue that receives 12 Gy or more (e.g. V12 Gy) is 6 cm^3. At an earlier phase in the trial, a larger brain metastasis received 20 Gy. Because of its large size, the V12 Gy of the healthy brain tissue was 14 cm^3 in this trial. While receiving a lower tumor dose, the risk of complications, e.g. radionecrosis was higher in the low dose arm because of a higher V12 Gy. This may hamper the reliability of the results of phase I trials. A relatively new approach to overcome this issue is through the use of isotoxic dose prescription. With this strategy, the RT dose is not prescribed based on the target volume, but on the normal tissue tolerance level. In the setting of a phase I trial, the dose to the target volume is escalated, but several normal tissue tolerance levels are tested. If this strategy indeed provides more reliable results, it will ultimately still require clinical validation [8–10]. In the following case 3, an example is provided of a phase I RT trial using isotoxic dose prescription.

Case 3: Stereotactic Radiosurgery Trial with Isotoxic Dose Prescription
A phase I trial was designed to find the MTD of healthy brain tissue, e.g. normal tissue tolerance level. Three normal tissue tolerance levels were studied and the dose in the target volume was escalated to the highest technical dose achievable (V12 Gy_{brain} of 7 cm^3, V12 Gy_{brain} of 10 cm^3, and V12 Gy_{brain} of 13 cm^3), while respecting the normal tissue tolerance level.

16.2.1 Finding the MTD of a Drug in Combination with Radiotherapy

When the objective is to find the MTD of a drug in combination with a fixed dose RT, the drug-related DLT is often of primary interest. As the drug-related DLT is often acute, the determination of the MTD and dose escalation/de-escalation is typically based on the DLTs observed in the first cycle of treatment (e.g., the first 21 days). Under this assumption, various phase I trial designs have been proposed to find the MTD. These designs are generally classified into algorithm-based designs, model-based designs, and model-assisted designs [11–13]. Algorithm-based designs use a set of simple, pre-specified rules (or algorithm) to determine the dose escalation and de-escalation, without assuming any model on the dose-toxicity curve, for example, the conventional 3 + 3 design. The 3 + 3 design is simple and easy to implement, but has long been criticized for its poor operating characteristics e.g., no specific target DLT rate, poor accuracy to identify and estimate the MTD, and a greater tendency to underdose patients [14].

In contrast to algorithm-based designs, model-based designs utilize a statistical model, e.g., the logistic model, to describe the dose-toxicity relationship and guide the dose escalation and de-escalation process. As information accrues during the trial, the model-based design updates the estimate of the model and uses it to guide the dose allocation for subsequent patients. An example of a model-based design is the continuous reassessment method (CRM; [15]). Studies show that the CRM has a substantially better performance than the 3 + 3 design; however, the use of the CRM remains limited due to several reasons. Because of statistical and computational complexity of the CRM, it remains a challenge to communicate to clinical investigators how the design works, leading them to perceive dose allocations as coming from a "black box". In addition, as a model-based approach, although generally robust, the CRM is still subject to the influence of model misspecification [16–18].

Mode-assisted designs merge as an attractive, cutting-edge approach that combines the simplicity of algorithm-based designs and the performance of model-based designs. Similar to the model-based design, the model-assisted design utilizes a statistical model (e.g., the binomial model) to derive the design. Like the algorithm-based design, the model-assisted design's rule of dose escalation and de-escalation can be pre-tabulated before the onset of the trial [11]. Examples of model-assisted designs include the modified toxicity probability interval (mTPI) design [19], Bayesian optimal interval (BOIN) design [20–22], and Keyboard design [23]. Large-scale numerical study shows that the model-assisted design, in particular the BOIN design, yields substantially better operating characteristics than the 3 + 3 and mTPI designs [12, 13], while is similarly easy to implement. Thus, in what follows, we focus on the BOIN design.

With the BOIN design, decisions of dose escalation and de-escalation only requires a simple comparison of the observed DLT rate at the current drug dose with a pair of fixed, prespecified dose escalation and de-escalation boundaries. For example, let $\hat{p}$ denote the observed DLT rate at the current dose, defined as $\hat{p} = n_{DLT} / n$, where n_{DLT} is the number of patients who have experienced a DLT at the current dose, and n is the total number of patients treated at the current dose. Let λ_e and λ_d denote two prespecified cutoffs, representing dose escalation and de-escalation boundaries, respectively. The BOIN design is described as follows:

1. Patients in the first cohort are treated at the lowest dose or the physician-specified dose.
2. Assuming that the current dose level for treating the latest cohort of patients is j^{cur}, to assign a dose to the next cohort of patients:
   - escalate the dose to level $j^{cur} + 1$ if $\hat{p}_j \leq \lambda_e$;
   - de-escalate the dose to level j^{cur} - 1 if $\hat{p}_j \geq \lambda_d$;
   - otherwise, retain the current dose.
3. Repeat step 2 until the maximum sample size N is reached. At that point, select the MTD using a statistical tool known as the isotonic estimate [20].

Table 16.1 provides the optimal dose escalation and de-escalation boundaries (λ_e, λ_d) for commonly used target DLT rates (Fig. 16.1). For example, if the target DLT rate of a trial is $\phi = 0.3$, the corresponding escalation and de-escalation boundaries are $\lambda_e = 0.236$ and $\lambda_d = 0.359$, respectively. Such dose escalation and de-escalation decision rules can be equivalently expressed as Table 16.2, which may be more convenient to use in practice. Interestingly, in this case, the 3 + 3 rule is nested within the BOIN design, i.e. escalate/de-escalate/retain the current dose if 0/3 or 2/3 or 1/3 patients have DLT. The optimal dose escalation and de-escalation boundaries are derived to minimize the chance of making incorrect

Table 16.1 The optimal escalation/de-escalation boundaries (λ_e, λ_d) under the BOIN design for different target toxicity rates (ϕ) with its default setting

	Target toxicity rate ϕ					
Boundaries	0.15	0.20	0.25	0.30	0.35	0.40
λ_e (Escalation)	0.118	0.157	0.197	0.236	0.276	0.316
λ_d (De-escalation)	0.179	0.238	0.298	0.359	0.419	0.480

Table 16.2 Dose escalation/de-escalation rule for the glioblastoma trial using the BOIN design

	The number of patients treated at the current dose														
Actions	1	2	**3**	4	**5**	6	**7**	8	**9**	10	**11**	12	**13**	14	**15**
Escalate if # of DLT <=	0	0	**0**	0	**1**	1	**1**	1	**2**	2	**2**	2	**3**	3	**3**
De-escalate if # of DLT >=	1	1	**2**	2	**2**	3	**3**	3	**4**	4	**4**	5	**5**	6	**6**
Eliminate if # of DLT >=	NA	NA	**3**	3	**4**	4	**5**	5	**5**	6	**6**	7	**7**	8	**8**

dose escalation and de-escalation decisions (i.e., only escalating/de-escalating the dose when the current dose is actually toxic/safe), see Liu and Yuan [20] for technical details.

For safety, during the trial conduct, the BOIN design imposes a dose elimination (or overdose control) rule as follows: if $\Pr(p_j > \phi | n_j, y_j) > 0.95$ and $n_j \geq 3$, dose level j and higher are eliminated from the trial, and the trial is terminated if the lowest dose level is eliminated. This rule says that if the observed data indicate that there is more than 95% chance that the true DLT rate of the current dose (i.e., p_j) is higher than the target DLT rate ϕ, that dose is deemed overly toxic and should be eliminated from the trial.

The BOIN design has been used in variety of oncology trials, including trials for pediatric tumors, adult tumors, solid tumors, and liquid tumors, see Yuan et al. [11] for a list of trials.

16.2.2 Finding MTD of RT Alone or in Combination with a Drug

In phase I trials aiming to find the MTD of RT, alone or in combination with a drug, the RT-related DLT is often of the main interest. Compared to drug-related DLT described previously, the challenge is that RT-related DLT is often late-onset and may take several months or longer to be ascertained. This causes a major logistical difficulty for conducting such a trial. For example, if the DLT takes up to 9 months to evaluate and the accrual rate is 1 patient/month, on average, six new patients will be accrued while waiting to evaluate the previous three patients' outcomes. The challenge is determining how new patients will receive timely treatments when the outcomes of previous patients are still pending.

The time-to-event BOIN (TITE-BOIN) design provides a simple solution to address late-onset toxicity. TITE-BOIN is built upon the BOIN design described above. In the presence of late-onset toxicity, the standard BOIN cannot be used directly because the DLT data from some patients will still be pending, and as such, the value of the n_{DLT} will be unknown; therefore, $\hat{p}$ cannot be calculated, and thus, the dose escalation/de-escalation rule described in Fig. 16.1 cannot be applied. TITE-BOIN overcomes this difficulty by imputing the DLT outcome for patients whose DLT data are pending (hereafter denoted as "pending patients"). After the imputation, n_{DLT} becomes known and $\hat{p}$ can be calculated and compared with λ_e and λ_d to determine dose escalation/de-escalation. Imputation is a well-established statistical technique for handling missing data (18–20). One innovation of TITE-BOIN is to utilize data from all patients, including DLT data from patients who have completed DLT assessment and also the follow-up time data from the pending patients. The latter is quantified by the standardized total follow-up time (STFT), defined as the sum of the follow-up times for all currently pending patients at the current dose, divided by the length of DLT assessment window.

The time-to-event CRM (TITE-CRM; [24]), a model-based method, also uses the follow-up time to improve the design efficiency. Compared to TITE-CRM, one prominent advantage of the TITE-BOIN is that it maintains the simplicity of the BOIN—the dose escalation/de-escalation rule of TITE-BOIN can be tabulated prior to trial conduct. Table 16.3 shows the TITE-BOIN decision rule for the SBRT boost trial described in **case 2** above. To conduct the trial, no complicated model fitting or computation is needed. Instead, the number of patients and those who experienced a DLT, as well as the number of pending patients and their STFT at the current dose are counted, before using the table to make a dose escalation/de-escalation decision. For example, if 3 patients have been treated at the current dose, and one patient has a DLT, one has no DLT, and one is pending. If the follow-up time of the pending patient exceeds (or is less than) 7.92 months, or equivalently STFT = 7.92/9 = 0.88, we will retain (or de-escalate) the current dose for treating the next cohort of patients. In contrast, the TITE-CRM is less transparent and works in a "black-box" fashion, requiring the selection of the dose-toxicity model prior to trial conduct, as well as real-time model fitting and estimation during the trial. Table 16.3 shows the decision rule up to 9 patients treated at a dose. The TITE-BOIN allows any prespecified cohort size and total sample size, and the corresponding decision table can be easily generated using the software described later.

The use of the pending patients' follow-up time distinguishes TITE-BOIN from the Rolling 6 design and renders it substantially higher accuracy to identify the MTD. Rolling 6 design is a modification of the 3 + 3 design that allows for the continuous accrual of up to six patients when some of the patients' DLT data are pending (11). As an algorithm-based design, the Rolling 6 design inherits the drawbacks of the 3 + 3 design, such as low accuracy for MTD identification, treating a large

Table 16.3 Dose escalation and de-escalation boundaries for TITE-BOIN with a target DLT rate of 0.3 and cohort size of 3 up to 9 patients at a dose

No. treated	No. DLTs	No. data pending	STFT			No. treated	No. DLTs	No. data pending	STFT		
			Escalate	Stay	De-escalate				Escalate	Stay	De-escalate
3	0	≤1	Y			6	≥4	≤2			Y&Elim
3	0	≥2	Suspend accrual			9	0	≤4	Y		
3	1	0		Y		9	0	≥5	Suspend accrual		
3	1	1		>0.88	≤0.88	9	1	≤4	Y		
3	1	≥2	Suspend accrual			9	1	≥5	Suspend accrual		
3	2	≤1			Y	9	2	0	Y		
3	3	0			Y&Elim	9	2	1	≥0.59	<0.59	
6	0	≤3	Y			9	2	2	≥1.65	<1.65	
6	0	≥4	Suspend accrual			9	2	3	≥2.71	<2.71	
6	1	≤1	Y			9	2	4	≥3.77	<3.77	
6	1	2	≥0.6	<0.6		9	2	≥5	Suspend accrual		
6	1	3	≥1.96	<1.96		9	3	0		Y	
6	1	≥4	Suspend accrual			9	3	1	>0.58	≤0.58	
6	2	0		Y		9	3	2	>1.65	≤1.65	
6	2	1		>0.73	≤0.73	9	3	3	>2.72	≤2.72	
6	2	2		>1.8	≤1.8	9	3	4	>3.79	≤3.79	
6	2	3		>2.87	≤2.87	9	3	≥5	Suspend accrual		
6	2	≥4	Suspend accrual			9	4	≤5			Y
6	3	≤3			Y	9	≥5	≤4			Y&Elim

Note: "No. treated" is the total number of patients treated at the current dose level, "No. DLTs" is the number of patients who experienced DLT at the current dose level, "No. data pending" denotes the number of patients whose DLT data are pending at the current dose level, "STFT" is the standardized total follow-up time (in months) for the patients with data pending, defined as the total follow-up time for the patients with data pending divided by the length of the DLT assessment window. "Y" represents "Yes", and "Y&Elim" represents "Yes & Eliminate". When a dose is eliminated, all higher doses should also be eliminated

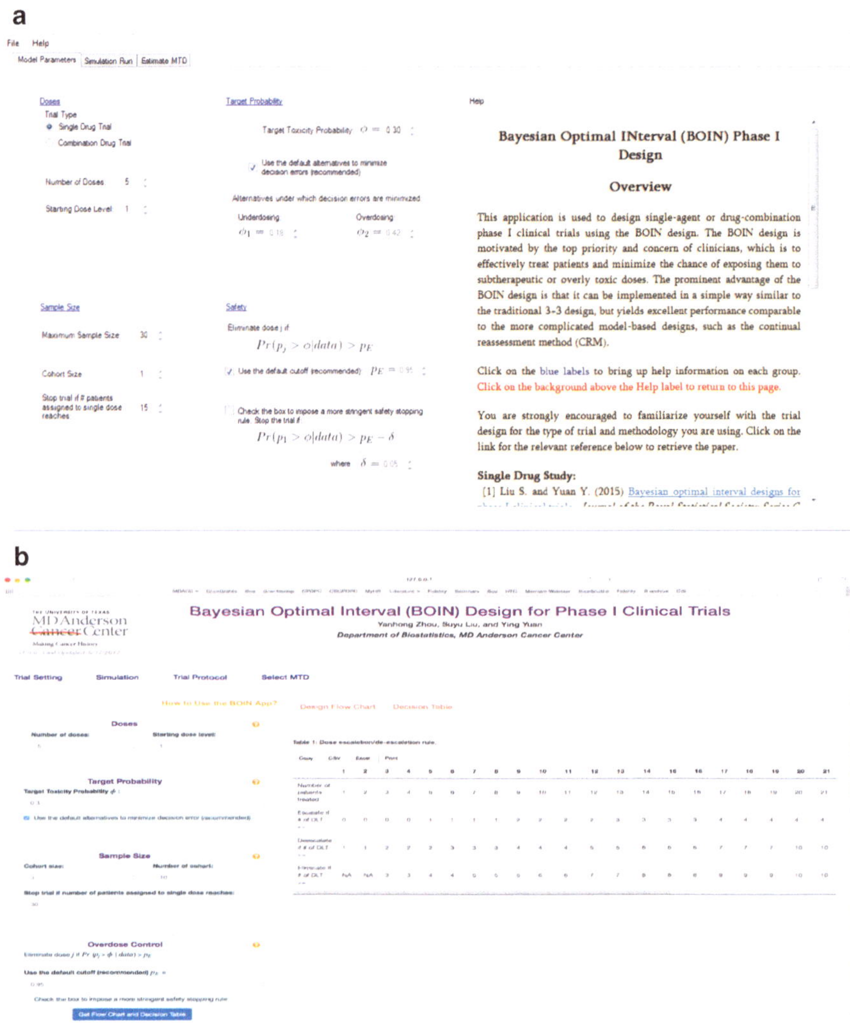

Fig. 16.2 Windows desktop program (**a**) and web app (**b**) for the BOIN design

proportion of patients at low (potentially subtherapeutic) doses, and harbors an inability to target a specific DLT rate for the MTD. In addition, the Rolling 6 design is inefficient because it ignores the follow-up time of the pending patients, which contains rich information for decision making. For example, a pending patient who is 3 days away from completing a DLT assessment is less likely to experience a DLT than a pending patient who has been followed for only 3 days, as the latter has a greater chance of experiencing a DLT during the remaining follow-up time.

16.2.3 Software

The BOIN and TITE-BOIN design can be easily implemented using Windows desktop program freely available from https://biostatistics.mdanderson.org/software-download/SingleSoftware.aspx?Software_Id=99, and web apps freely available at http://www.trialdesign.org. Each software package comes with intuitive graphical user interface, detailed documents, and step-by-step tutorial on how to use it to design phase I trials. It allows users to generate the decision table for dose escalation and de-escalation, perform simulation studies to generate the operating characteristics of the design, and create the protocol template for trial protocol preparation. Figure 16.2 shows the user interface of the BOIN Windows desktop program and the corresponding web app.

Key Expert Opinion Points

- An expert radiation oncologist should always be involved in the design of any phase I trial including radiation therapy. The unique risks of radiation with new drug agents should not be underestimated.
- The dose and fractionation of radiation used in combination trials can have vastly different effects. These should be carefully chosen in consultation with an expert radiation oncologist. Normal tissue tolerances may be vastly different in the presence of new combination agents.
- Phase I trial designs involving radiation should include longer term toxicity evaluation, even up to years post radiation, as radiation toxicities can continue to accrue over time.
- Similarly, response endpoints may need a longer timepoint for evaluation. Often, initial imaging may demonstrate treatment related inflammation that might be mistaken for or impossible to distinguish from disease progression.
- Radiation treatment design and delivery is important and can be much more variable than chemotherapy drug administration. In fact, radiation delivery is much more similar to the technical aspects of surgery. Phase I trials including radiation should have centralized, rigourous QA by disease site experts.

References

1. Milas L, Hunter NR, Mason KA, et al. Role of reoxygenation in induction of enhancement of tumor response by paclitaxel. Cancer Res. 1995;55:3564–8.
2. Shuryak I, Hall EJ, Brenner DJ. Dose dependence of accelerated repopulation in head and neck cancer: supporting evidence and clinical implications. Radiother Oncol. 2018 Apr;127(1):20–26. https://doi.org/10.1016/j.radonc.2018.02.015. Epub 2018 Mar 10.
3. Cristofanilli M, Turner NC, Bondarenko I, Ro J, Im SA, Masuda N, et al. Fulvestrant plus palbociclib versus fulvestrant plus placebo for treatment of hormone-receptor-positive, HER2-negative metastatic breast cancer that progressed on previous endocrine therapy (PALOMA-3):

final analysis of the multicentre, double-blind, phase 3 randomised controlled trial. Lancet Oncol. 2016;17(4):425–39.
4. Finn RS, Aleshin A, Slamon DJ. Targeting the cyclin-dependent kinases (CDK) 4/6 in estrogen receptor-positive breast cancers. Breast Cancer Res. 2016;18(1):17.
5. Hortobagyi GN, Stemmer SM, Burris HA, Yap YS, Sonke GS, Paluch-Shimon S, et al. Ribociclib as first-line therapy for hr-positive, advanced breast cancer. N Engl J Med. 2016;375(18):1738–48.
6. Marks LB. Int J Radiat Oncol Biol Phys. 2010 Mar 1;76(3 Suppl):S10–S19.
7. Steel and Peckham. https://doi.org/10.1016/0360-3016(79)90044-0.
8. Zindler JD, Schiffelers J, Lambin P, Hoffmann AL. Improved effectiveness of stereotactic radiosurgery in large brain metastases by individualized isotoxic dose prescription: an in silico study. Strahlenther Onkol 2018 Jun;194(6):560–569. https://doi.org/10.1007/s00066-018-1262-x. Epub 2018 Jan 18.
9. Zindler JD, Thomas CR Jr, Hahn SM, Hoffmann AL, Troost EG, Lambin P. Increasing the therapeutic ratio of stereotactic ablative radiotherapy by individualized isotoxic dose prescription. J Natl Cancer Inst. 2015 Oct 16;108(2). pii: djv305. https://doi.org/10.1093/jnci/djv305. Print 2016 Feb. Review.
10. Hartgerink D, van der Heijden B, De Ruysscher D, Postma A, Ackermans L, Hoeben A, Anten M, Lambin P, Terhaag K, Jochems A, Dekker A, Schoenmaekers J, Hendriks L, Zindler J. Stereotactic radiosurgery in the management of patients with brain metastases of non-small cell lung cancer: indications, decision tools and future directions. Front Oncol. 2018 May 9;8:154. https://doi.org/10.3389/fonc.2018.00154. eCollection 2018. Review.
11. Yuan Y, Lee JJ, Hilsenbeck SG. Model-assisted designs for early-phase clinical trials: simplicity meets superiority. JCO Precis Oncol. 2019; https://doi.org/10.1200/PO.19.00032.
12. Zhou H, Murray T, Pan H, Yuan Y. Comparative review of toxicity probability interval designs for phase I clinical trials. Stat Med. 2018a;37(14):2208–22.
13. Zhou H, Yuan Y, Nie L. Accuracy, safety and reliability of novel phase I trial designs. Clin Cancer Res. 2018b;24(18):4357–64.
14. Le Tourneau C, Lee JJ, Siu LL. Dose escalation methods in phase I cancer clinical trials. JNCI J Natl Cancer Inst. 2009;101:708–20.
15. O'Quigley J, Pepe M, Fisher L. Continual reassessment method: a practical design for phase I clinical trials in cancer. Biometrics. 1990;46(1):33–48.
16. Yin G, Yuan Y. Bayesian dose finding in oncology for drug combinations by copula regression. J R Stat Soc Ser C (Appl Stat). 2009a;58(2):211–24.
17. Yin G, Yuan Y. Bayesian model averaging continual reassessment method in phase I clinical trials. J Am Stat Assoc. 2009b;104(487):954–68.
18. Yin G, Yuan Y. A latent contingency table approach to dose finding for combinations of two agents. Biometrics. 2009c;65(3):866–75.
19. Ji Y, Liu P, Li Y, Nebiyou Bekele B. A modified toxicity probability interval method for dose-finding trials. Clin Trials. 2009;7(6):653–63.
20. Liu S, Yuan Y. Bayesian optimal interval designs for phase I clinical trials. J R Stat Soc Ser C (Appl Stat). 2015;64(3):507–23.
21. Yuan Y, Hess K, Hilsenbeck S, Gilbert M. Bayesian optimal interval design: a simple and well-performing design for phase I oncology trials. Clin Cancer Res. 2016a;22:4291–301.
22. Yuan Y, Nguyen HQ, Thall PF. Bayesian designs for phase I/II clinical trials. Boca Raton, FL: CRC Press; 2016b.
23. Yan F, Mandrekar SJ, Yuan Y. Keyboard: a novel Bayesian toxicity probability interval design for phase I clinical trials. Clin Cancer Res. 2017;23(15):3994–4003. https://doi.org/10.1158/1078-0432.CCR-17-0220.
24. Cheung YK, Chappell R. Sequential designs for phase I clinical trials with late-onset toxicities. Biometrics. 2000;56(4):1177–82. https://doi.org/10.1111/j.0006-341x.2000.01177.x.

Chapter 17
The Paradigm of Early Phase Studies in Hematological Malignancies

Vishwanath Sathyanarayanan and Swaminathan P. Iyer

Abstract Hematological Malignancies are at the forefront of rapid advances in molecular technology which has enabled the understanding of the biology and brought us to the cutting edge of diagnosis and therapy. Today, it is possible to routinely sequence the entire genome of patients with blood cancers, providing us with a panorama of the genomic changes that underlie these malignancies. These advances have undoubtedly revolutionized how we diagnose and treat patients with these diseases and other cancers as well.

While we understand the pathogenesis of these malignancies in the context of newer therapies, the general approach to diagnosis and treatment are very different in various leukemias, lymphomas, and myeloma. Moreover, the course of the natural history of these various entities is varied; however, the overall goal of treatment is the prolongation of survival and ultimate cure. In this review, we provide a detailed look at the various drugs that have changed the course of treatment of the major types of hematologic malignancies. We discuss a few "gems" in clinical studies that have provided both initial proofs-of-concept and informative testing ground for a variety of targeted/immune-based therapeutics. The key points covered in this chapter include:

1. Early phase clinical trials and evolution of molecular-based assays
2. Phase 1 studies and understanding the biology of the disease
3. Goals of treatment
4. Challenges in designing clinical trial protocols in hematological malignancies
5. Role of biomarkers and bioimaging; approval of new drugs
6. Future studies on the horizon

Keywords Hematologic malignancies · Phase I · Kinase inhibitors · Monoclonal antibodies · Accelerated approval

---

V. Sathyanarayanan
Medical Oncologist, Apollo Hospitals, Bangalore, India

S. P. Iyer (✉)
Department of Lymphoma/Myeloma, The University of Texas, MD Anderson Cancer Center, Houston, USA
e-mail: spiyer@mdanderson.org

T. A. Yap et al. (eds.), *Phase I Oncology Drug Development*,
https://doi.org/10.1007/978-3-030-47682-3_17

Key Points

- Despite several challenges, several clinical trials have led to successful FDA approvals in hematological malignancies; there is still a need for more trials which combine the three-pronged approach.
- Several genomic and signaling pathways have been dissected which have highlighted several targets.
- Molecular-based assays: PCR, Sanger's sequencing and whole exome sequencing have led to better understanding of the biology and the immune microenvironment of the tumors with the discovery of potential targets.
- Several small molecule inhibitors and monoclonal antibodies have been developed against these targets successfully.

17.1 Hematology in the Forefront of Drug Development

According to the Cancer Facts & Figures 2018, there will be an estimated 1,735,350 new cancer cases diagnosed and 609,640 cancer deaths in the United States, out of which approximately 200,000 will be attributable to hematological malignancies [1].

With the increasing disease burden, treatment options for hematological malignancies have also evolved significantly over the last two decades. Personalized medicine refers to tailoring treatments to each based on an analysis of one's molecular and genetic makeup [2]. The advent of molecular technology like next-generation sequencing (NGS), the microenvironment of the tumor is being dissected, and clinical trials of novel drugs targeting the microenvironment, have led to accelerated approval of several drugs which has improved the outcome of these cancers. Moreover, hematologic malignancies have striking models for successful radiation therapy, chemotherapy, immunotherapy, immunomodulators, adoptive t-cell, oncolytic virus, interferons, cytokines, cancer vaccines, and chimeric antigen receptor T cell therapies. In this chapter, we focus on the early phase clinical trials and evolution of molecular-based assays, phase 1 studies and understanding the biology of the disease, the challenges in designing clinical trial protocols in hematological malignancies, the role of biomarkers and bioimaging; approval of new drugs and the future studies on the horizon.

Historically, early-phase clinical trials have been the last resort for patients whose cancers had progressed on standard of care therapies. These studies looked at achieving the optimal dose with least toxicities and with the goal of quickly moving across various cancer types including a few hematological cancers particularly lymphomas. Moreover, these studies were empirical with no design to match patients with best therapies; not surprisingly, only a few patients would respond to these experimental approaches (ranged from 5% to 7%) [3]. Understanding the biology of the disease better has been one of the three essential factors in drug discovery. The other two reasons are the discovery of newer Small Molecular inhibitors

(SMI) and Monoclonal Antibodies (MAbs) and the advent of precise molecular techniques. The utilization of polymerase chain reaction (PCR) based genomic analysis, Sanger's sequencing and subsequently next-generation sequencing (NGS) have allowed choosing the right drug for the right patient (personalized medicine), which ultimately translates into improved outcomes. With this three-pronged approach early phase clinical trials have significantly evolved in the last 10 years. With the current clinical trial designs, at least a third of the patients achieve disease control in treatment-refractory patients. In this evolving era of precision medicine, the response rates can be as high as 80–100% [4]. Several studies to decipher the complex genomic alterations in Acute Myeloid Leukemia (AML) including analysis of The Cancer Genome Atlas (TCGA), have helped better prognostication and understanding the pathogenesis of the disease [5]. Mutational and structural analysis by whole exome sequencing in diffuse large B cell lymphomas (DLBCL) is evidence to the genetic heterogeneity of the disease and also its dynamic nature with the acquisition of new driver mutations during disease progression [6]. Gene expression analysis has also been prognostic in follicular lymphoma [7]. Serine/threonine PIM protein kinases regulate the tumorigenesis in several hematological malignancies. PIM Inhibitor SMI-4a Induces Cell Apoptosis and Cell Cycle Arrest in B-Cell Acute Lymphocytic Leukemia Cells through inhibition of the JAK2/STAT3 Pathway [8].

Bruton tyrosine kinase (BTK) amplification is noted in several low- and high-grade lymphomas (Fig. 17.1). The prototype drug-ibrutinib and subsequently acalabrutinib are now approved by the Food and Drug Administration (FDA) following encouraging results in clinical trials. The FDA approval of Ibrutinib in relapsed mantle cell lymphoma and chronic lymphocytic leukemia is based on studies by Wang et al. and Byrd et al. and acalabrutinib received accelerated approval based on a phase 2 single-arm study in relapsed mantle cell lymphoma [9–11].

17.2 Phase I Trials as Gateways Between Science and Clinical Studies

Phase I studies are the gateway between pre-clinical research and translational medicine, and the outcome of these trials have a significant impact on the next steps of any prospective drug. The primary objectives of a phase I study are to provide information on the safety and tolerability along with the pharmacokinetics (PK) and pharmacodynamics (PD) of a molecule that has gone through successful preclinical and toxicology testing. Subsequently, further studies are designed to measure potential interaction effects of different substances on the metabolism of the new drug, and to evaluate the effect of food, and genetic differences and also study the effect of biomarkers.

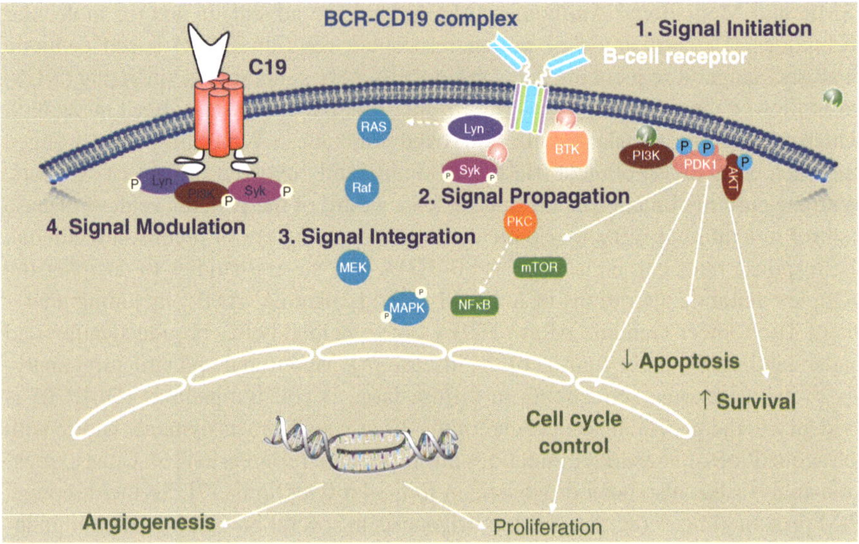

Fig. 17.1 B cell receptor (BCR) Signaling Pathways. The B cell receptor signaling mechanism involves the BCR co-receptor molecule CD19, an integral transmembrane glycoprotein along with other signaling proteins such as Lyn, BTK, PI3K among others. Upon BCR ligation (1. Signal Initiation), tyrosines within the cytoplasmic tail of CD19 are phosphorylated by Lyn and BTK (2. Signal Propagation)-to create binding sites for the SH2 domains of the p85 adaptor subunit of PI-3K. Association of PI-3K with CD19 localizes to its lipid substrates in the plasma membrane and increases the activity of the p110 catalytic subunit of PI-3K (3. Signal Integration and 4. Modulation)

The drug development process typically involves discovery, preclinical development, and the Phase I clinical trial. This continuum between preclinical development and clinical trial is sharply defined by the filing of an Investigational New Drug. The transition from discovery to preclinical development rests on the ultimate understanding of the cancer biology and how the target in question can be optimized through in vitro and in vivo studies to cause active cell killing through the purported survival pathway inhibition.

17.3 Some Examples in Hematological Malignancies on How Putting the Biology at the Basis for Investigational New Drug (IND) Studies Helped Drug Development

- *Cell Survival Pathways:* Chromosomal translocations/Cell cycle and Survival: Cancer cells display abnormalities in the regulation of cell cycle and survival. Although solid and hematological cancer cells share these abnormalities, they differ in their origin. In contrast with most solid cancers, mature B-cell malignancies harbor recurrent chromosomal translocations (with or without gene fusion) that, in some cases, can be used to diagnose that specific malignancy. Directly or indirectly, these translocations lead to the dysregulated expression of genes involved in cell survival and/or proliferation. For instance, mantle cell lymphoma (MCL), multiple myeloma (MM), Burkitt's lymphoma (BL) and follicular lymphoma (FL) cells harbor translocations between chromosomes that encode the IgH locus and different genes such as (i) CCND1 in MCL, (ii) CCND1; FGFR in MM, (iii) MYC in BL, and (iv) BCL2 in FL. Other mature B-cell malignancies i.e., diffuse large B-cell lymphoma (DLBCL), hairy cell leukemia (HCL), Waldenström Macroglobulinemia (WM), splenic marginal zone lymphoma (SMZL), mucosa-associated lymphoid tissue lymphoma (MALT) and chronic lymphocytic leukemia (CLL), do not have recurrent translocations involving IgH locus but show other recurrent mutations in several genes involved in the BCR, MAPK, NOTCH, NFkB and mTOR pathways, which govern survival and proliferation. The translocations and/or mutations in driver genes is the first event in the process of malignant transformation, followed by secondary events such as RB1 deletion, RAS and TP53 mutation/deletion and/or additional chromosomal loss or gain [12, 13].

- *Apoptotic pathways:* Many hematological malignancies express high levels of anti-apoptotic proteins such as Bcl-2 or Mcl-1, yet are primed to undergo apoptosis. This is correlated with the overexpression of the pro-apoptotic Bcl-2 family of proteins which counteract the anti-apoptotic counterparts in the mitochondria. This opens strategies for therapeutic targeting; many of these malignancies are sensitive to BH3 mimetic molecules that target the anti- and pro-apoptotic complexes at the mitochondria. Survival deregulation is also related to aberrations in pathways upstream of mitochondria such as BCR or NFkappaB pathways (Fig. 17.1), and these dysregulated pathways can also be therapeutically targeted with specific inhibitors (e.g., BTK, proteasome inhibitors) [14].
- *Directly targeting the cell surface tumor antigens:* By identifying the lineage markers in the hematopoietic cells, subpopulation-specific surface antigens like CD20 in malignant B cells which have helped us discover targets like rituximab. Similarly, Bi-specific T cell engagers (BiTE) work on the principle of linking cytotoxic T lymphocytes (CTLs) and their tumoricidal activity with the targeting platform of a mAb. Blinatumomab is a bispecific antibody recognizing CD3 and the B cell-specific marker CD19. It has shown promising results in patients with relapsed/refractory acute lymphoblastic leukemia in the TOWER trial which led to its FDA approval [15].

17.4 Molecular Techniques Used in Early Clinical Trials in Hematological Malignancies

- *Conventional Cytogenetics (Karyotyping)*—Cytogenetics is the study of chromosomes. In contrast to the epithelial carcinoma, genetic aberrations in hematological malignancies frequently involve balanced or reciprocal chromosomal translocations. It remains the cornerstone for the diagnosis of Chronic Myelogenous Leukemia since it was described for the first time by Dr. Janet Rowley [16]. It is also used to prognosticate the disease, particularly in AML and MM. Cytogenetic analysis of chronic lymphocytic leukemia (CLL) and multiple myeloma (MM) patients is often difficult because of the low proliferating rate of the malignant cells. This problem was overcome by using the Fluorescent In-Situ Hybridization (FISH) technique that identifies chromosomal abnormalities using single-stranded DNA labeled with fluorochrome) which are hybridized to a patient's sample and the hybridization is visualized using a fluorescence microscope. This technique can be performed both on dividing as well as on non-dividing interphase cells [17].

- *Polymerase Chain Reaction (PCR)*—PCR is the most commonly used molecular assay in the diagnosis of hematological malignancies. Basics of most PCR techniques involve amplification of a desired segment of DNA by using primers, and enzymes like reverse transcriptase and DNA polymerases. In clinical practice, Real-time PCR (RQ-PCR) is commonly used for detecting fusion genes such as BCR-ABL and PML-RARA for assessment of treatment response. Besides, PCR makes it easy to detection of mutations, for determining lymphoid clonality, for post-transplant chimerism analysis and minimal residual disease (MRD) detection.
- *Next Generation Sequencing (NGS)*—NGS is a high throughput parallel sequencing technique that allows thousands of genomes to be studied in a short time. Not only can the whole genome be sequenced by NGS, but targeted sequencing of exome, the mRNA-Transcriptome and the Epigenome. The Cancer Genome Atlas (TCGA) project has incorporated this detailed genomic information from patient samples with AML and DLBCL into the existing prognostic scoring systems and helped optimize therapeutic plans. With the growing list of mutated genes has enabled choosing a specific treatment plan including transplant in TP53 or targeted agents like IDH1 and IDH2. In cytogenetically normal AML presence of FLT-3-ITD mutation confers poor outcomes and would need the incorporation of the FLT-3-ITD inhibitor [5].
- *Flow cytometry*—Flow cytometry is a well-established immunophenotyping tool for the diagnosis, classification, prognostic stratification, and monitoring of hematological malignancies.

17.5 Basic Considerations for Treatment

- *Defining the disease:* The correct clinical research use of terminology associated with hematological cancers requires familiarity and understanding. The World Health Organization (WHO) has been updating the classification system that not only uses cell morphology from the peripheral blood or bone marrow or the lymph nodes, but also includes assessments of cellular genetics and immunophenotype, cell of origin, and clinical patterns [18, 19]. It is also essential to know the clinical urgency of treating these neoplasms—whereas the need to treat is imminent for acute promyelocytic leukemia, Burkitt's lymphoma within even 48 h of diagnosis, the considerations may be different for CLL or multiple myeloma.

- *Goals of Treatment: Cure vs. Prevention vs. Supportive care:* The general goals of treatment in Hematological malignancies is not only to improve the symptoms but also potentially cure the underlying diseases. However, the cure rates even with allogeneic stem cell transplantation are at best between 30–50%. Therein lies the need to have novel therapies that can achieve this goal. It is therefore vital to understand the challenges faced by these patients, particularly the degree of prognostic uncertainty associated with these diagnoses, and their different illness trajectories. In a tertiary center, participation in clinical studies is highly encouraged, and often the unwritten goal of a study is to serve as a bridge to stem cell Transplant. Furthermore, to appropriately drive development strategy in hematological oncology, an understanding of the treatment landscape is important to assess the potential benefit of an investigational treatment's effect on the underlying disease both concerning efficacy and safety. While determining the developmental strategy for a compound, the choice of endpoints is very important and can often start with Phase I study with expansion cohorts.
- *Therapeutic Immune responsiveness in hematologic malignancies:* A key clinical feature of the blood malignancies is their immune responsiveness. Moreover, they are easily sampled and hence accurate characterization of cellular surface markers, and differentiation of a malignant cell from an immune cell has been possible. The delineation of the tumor microenvironment by directly sampling relevant tissues before and after immunotherapy has been useful. Paralleling the early successes of chemotherapy for the treatment of blood malignancies were the spontaneous tumor regressions in lymphomas and durable remissions of leukemias following allogeneic hematopoietic stem cell transplantation (allo-HSCT). Indeed, the efficacy of allo-HSCT derives mainly from the graft-versus-leukemia effect (GvL) and a donor-derived immune eradication of malignant cells. Development of immunodeficient host mice has been the key to better engraft PDX models. Next-generation sequencing has helped us understand the genomic landscape of human cancers. Based on this concept, we may be able to replicate tumor heterogeneity in the xenograft model as well [20]. With the advent of immunotherapy, PD 1 and PD L1 blockers are currently in several phases of clinical trials in hematological malignancies, especially in lymphomas. Nivolumab is already FDA approved for relapsed/ refractory HL. Predictive biomarkers beyond PDL1 need to be developed to select patients who may benefit from immunotherapy. Another major treatment breakthrough in 2017 was the approval of the first 2 chimeric antigen receptor (CAR) T-cell (or gene) therapies for cancer. The first CAR T-cell therapy, tisagenlecleucel (Kymriah), was approved in August 2017 for the treatment of relapsed/ refractory acute lymphoblastic leukemia (ALL). In a planned analysis, 75 patients received an infusion of tisagenlecleucel and the overall remission rate within 3 months was 81%, The rates of event-free survival (EFS) and overall survival (OS) were 73% (95% confidence interval [CI], 60 to 82) and 90% (95% CI, 81 to 95), respectively, at 6 months and 50% (95% CI, 35

to 64) and 76% (95% CI, 63 to 86) at 12 months [21]. Neelapu et al. presented results of the second CAR-T therapy axicabtagene ciloleucel (Yescarta), with the ZUMA 1 study which has transformed the outcomes in R/R high-grade B cell lymphomas including double hit lymphomas. The FDA approved Yescarta in 2017 for refractory aggressive B-cell non-Hodgkin lymphoma, based on a single-arm clinical trial that showed an ORR of 72% and a complete response rate of 51% in patients with aggressive refractory disease. [22]

- *Other considerations in management:* Since many of these diseases have their origin in the bone marrow, a certain level of cytopenias are accepted per protocol stipulations. It is therefore essential to understand the significance and implications of blood count shifts as well as of transfusions and dosing timing.

  An additional side effect that is a clinical eventuality is the Tumor Lysis Syndrome. The increased sensitivity to the given agents and the rapidity to cell death can create a spectrum of biochemical changes in uric acid, lactate dehydrogenase (LDH) and potassium or a fulminant acute renal injury requiring dialysis. This was a case in point with Phase I studies with Lenalidomide and Venetoclax. Both the protocols were revamped with slower dose escalation and careful clinical observations [23].

  Another consideration is age-historically, older patients and those with comorbidities have been excluded from clinical trials [24]. Among the FDA approved treatments for cancer, only 9% of patients enrolled in registration trials were older than 75 years of age, whereas one-third of patients with cancer fall within that age group [25]. The CLL study with Chlorambucil(C) vs. C + Obinutuzumab vs. C + Rituximab allowed entry of older patients with specific co-morbidities into this clinical study. In this randomized, phase III trial in patients with untreated comorbid CLL, the overall response rate was significantly higher (78% vs. 65%, $P < 0.0001$) and median progression-free survival was significantly prolonged (26.7 vs. 15.2 months, $P < 0.0001$) for obinutuzumab plus chlorambucil vs. rituximab plus chlorambucil [26]. Furthermore, treatment goals for older patients are not always the same as for younger patients. Although willing to receive chemotherapy [27], elderly patients are generally less willing to accept toxicity for additional survival time.

17.6 Clinical Trial Design Considerations

- *Protocol development and optimization of design:* A learning curve in early phase studies is the applicability to the given patient population. Some of this is offset by a broad-based understanding of the early work done as part of the pre-clinical IND (toxicology, animal studies, targeted starting dose established, appropriate formulation and manufacturing stability and scalability). The high stakes involved with advanced disease and sick patients especially in Leukemia and lymphoma should allow for protocol amendments. Often, there is a constant interaction between the principal investigator (PI) and the Medical teams and flexible approaches to protocol development can help with appropriate protocol amendments without affecting the overall costs of the project.

- Early Phase clinical studies often invoke significant efforts and cost the collection of large amounts of information. Given the different clinical events that ensue with the treatment, the different endpoints in assessment and the unique complications seen, the protocols are individualized for optimal data collection through the electronic case report forms (eCRFs). Therefore, a thorough understanding and dissemination of the biology, assessment endpoints and side effect reporting are necessary for sponsors, researchers, and contract research organizations (CROs). This can reduce the data collection as well as the costs for the sponsor and CRO.
- *Endpoints in treatment:* The varied nature of blood-based cancers requires that treatment trials rely on different end-point measurements to determine treatment-related changes and disease progression, which can add more complexity to trial design, conduct, and assessment. The gold standard is still the Overall survival (OS) when evaluating cancer treatment effectiveness. However, instead of OS, the most commonly used surrogate endpoint is progression-free survival (PFS) for trials involving advanced cancers. Other surrogate endpoints include disease-free or event-free survival (EFS), response rate (RR) or objective response rate (ORR), time to treatment failure (TTF) and time to progression (TTP) [28]. Major molecular response endpoints are also common and require great specificity in determining the measurements and the techniques, based on the disease. In CML, for example, the PCR assay can evaluate depth of molecular responses and was the secondary end-point for two large Phase III studies involving Imatinib and Nilotinib and Dasatinib.
- *Importance of adaptive design in early phase clinical trials:* It is possible to use PK/PD to guide dose escalation decisions and develop adaptive designs that enable adjustments to the study design and/or specific patient population. Whereas conventional study design methods (such as 3 + 3 designs) are still used, interest in adaptive design study hold promise for improving drug development. Traditional designs often start with a dose well below animal toxicity with no effect and may not allow reaching higher doses quickly. The more progressive adaptive design algorithms permit a change in dose level after each patient is treated based on the accumulated responses of previously enrolled subjects. Pooled PK studies are useful in determining the clinical predictors of drug pharmacokinetics and to compare the pharmacokinetics of drugs in the same class [29, 30]. These algorithms can increase the speed of the dose escalation and reduce patient exposure to doses that are not effective. The National Cancer Institute (NCI) Web Reporting System and Toxicity over Time (ToxT) package are tools which augment graphical representation of adverse effects (AE) which may be useful in the era of novel/targeted therapies. Standardization of irAEs and case definitions including grades of these may be useful in the era of immunotherapy and CAR-T cell therapies [31].
- *Bioimaging:* Hematological oncology trials have pioneered the use of technology including Imaging to provide specificity and measure survival. For example,

the 2011 biologics license application (BLA) submitted to the FDA for Brentuximab vedotin- an Antibody Drug Conjugate (ADC) was the first to use the agency's response criteria for lymphoma drugs, outlined in 2007 which included FDG-PET (18F-fluorodeoxyglucose positron emission tomography) scans in the response assessments. The FDA considered PFS acceptable as an endpoint to confirm clinical benefit because an OS endpoint would not likely occur within a reasonable time frame. The BLA used data from two single-arm studies, both designed to show superiority using PFS as a primary endpoint and OS as a secondary endpoint. The FDA used these data to grant approval of BV in combination with CHP in untreated CD30+ peripheral T cell lymphoma (ECHELON-2). It is also approved for relapsed/refractory HL and as a maintenance post-ASCT in HL [32–34].
- *Biomarkers:* The FDA has developed a guidance document to help investigators who are planning to use minimal residual disease (MRD) as a biomarker in clinical trials conducted under an investigational new drug application or to support FDA approval of products intended to treat various hematologic malignancies. The guidance highlights considerations for MRD assessment that are specific to certain hematologic malignancies explains how MRD might be used in clinical trials, and lists requirements for regulatory submissions that utilize MRD. MRD could potentially be used as a biomarker in clinical trials—specifically as a diagnostic, prognostic, predictive, efficacy-response, or monitoring biomarker, according to the draft guidance. Additionally, MRD could be used as a surrogate endpoint or "to select patients at high risk or to enrich the trial population."

17.7 Lessons from Recent Approvals

A substantial number of New molecular entities (NMEs) move through Phase I into Phase II; however, progression from Phase I through approval each year has been very low. Development of rituximab began in the late 1980s. In 1994, rituximab received its first approval for the treatment of NHL by the United States Food and Drug Administration (FDA), and it has revolutionized the treatment of hematological malignancies [35]. It took another ten years to see the second wave of approvals. Between 2005 through 2013, FDA's Center for Drug Evaluation and Research (CDER) averaged approximately 25 novel new drug approvals per year (Tables 17.1 and 17.2). These include drugs for all diseases and all indications. In 2014, approximately 64% of drugs moved from Phase I to Phase II and 10.4% moved from Phase I through approval and 41 novel new drugs were approved—six in total for oncology. These drugs were approved under the FDA accelerated approval program, which allows early approval of a drug for serious or life-threatening illnesses that offer benefit over current treatment. Once accelerated approval is granted, these drugs must undergo additional testing. These approvals in oncology were based on

Table 17.1 Monoclonal antibodies, CAR-T cell therapies and PD-1 inhibitors approved for the treatment of hematological malignancies

Drug	Target	Type	Approvals
Rituximab	CD20	mAb	B-NHL
Ofatumumab	CD20	mAb	CLL
Obinutuzumab	CD20	mAb	CLL, FL
Ibritumomab tiuxetan (radioimmunotherapy)	CD20	mAb	FL
Rituximab and hyaluronidase human	CD-20	mAb	DLBCL, CLL
Elotuzumab	CS1	mAb	R/R MM
Daratumumab	CD38	mAb	R/R MM
Alemtuzumab	CD52	mAb	CLL
Denileukin diftitox	CD25	mAb	CTCL
Nivolumab/Pembrolizumab	PD1	mAb	HL and PMBCL
Mogamulizumab-kpkc	CCR-4	mAb	Relapsed MF
Siltuximab	IL-6	mAb	Multicentric Castleman's disease
Blinatumomab	CD19	CAR-T	B-ALL
Axicabtagene ciloleucel	CD19	CAR-T	DLBCL
Tagraxofusp-erzs	CD-123	CAR-T	BPDCN

B-NHL B-cell Non-Hodgkin lymphoma, *CLL* chronic lymphocytic leukemia, *FL* follicular lymphoma, *HL* Hodgkin lymphoma, *PTCL* peripheral T cell lymphoma, *CTCL* cutaneous T cell lymphoma, *B-ALL* acute lymphoblastic leukemia, *DLBCL* diffuse large B cell lymphoma, *BPDCN* blastic plasmacytoid dendritic cell neoplasm, *R/R MM* Relapsed/refractory multiple myeloma, *MF* mycosis fungoides, *mAb* Monoclonal antibody, *CAR-T* chimeric Antigen Receptor-T cell

a "surrogate endpoint" (e.g., a laboratory measure) or other clinical measure considered to predict the clinical benefit of a drug [36]. By 2016, 37 indications of 31 drugs for hematological malignancy were granted accelerated approval. Of these, 31 indications were relapsed or refractory hematological malignancy. Although post-marketing clinical trials for verifying clinical efficacy were completed regarding the other 6 indications, accelerated approval regarding only 13 of the 31 indications for relapsed or refractory hematological malignancy was converted to regular approval [37]. Moreover, 5 of the 13 indications were granted regular approval based on clinical data in different population from (earlier treatment line than) the indications granted accelerated approval as follows: ibritumomab tiuxetan for follicular lymphoma, alemtuzumab for chronic lymphocytic leukemia, imatinib for pediatric chronic myeloid leukemia, ofatumumab for chronic lymphocytic leukemia and brentuximab vedotin for Hodgkin lymphoma and PTCL. The other 8 of 13 indications were granted regular approval for very similar population to the indications granted accelerated approval as follows: relapsed or refractory cutaneous T-cell lymphoma (denileukin), relapsed or refractory chronic myeloid leukemia (dasatinib, nilotinib and omacetaxine), relapsed or refractory multiple myeloma (bortezomib, carfilzomib and pomalidomide) and relapsed or refractory chronic lymphocytic leukemia (ibrutinib) [37]. In 2017, the FDA approved 46 new drugs, a

Table 17.2 Newer small molecules/targeted therapies approved for the treatment of hematological malignancies

Drug	Target	Approval
Venetoclax	BCL-2	Relapsed CLL and elderly AML (in combination with cytarabine)
Ibrutinib	BTK	CLL relapsed MCL, WM, GVHD
Acalabrutinib	BTK	Relapsed MCL
Duvelisib	PI3K	Relapsed CLL, FL
Glasdegib	Sonic Hedgehog	Elderly AML in combination with cytarabine
Ivosidenib	IDH-1	Relapsed AML
Enasidenib	IDH-2	Relapsed AML
Midostaurin	FLT3-ITD	AML
Bortezomib	Proteasome inhibitor	MM
Carfilzomib	Proteasome inhibitor	Relapsed MM
Ixazomib	Oral proteasome inhibitor	Relapsed MM
Lenalidomide/ Pomalidomide	immunomodulator	Relapsed MM
Panobinostat	HDAC	Relapsed MM
Romidepsin/Belinostat	HDAC	Relapsed PTCL
Ponatinib	BCR-ABL	CML (T315I)
Omacetaxine mepesuccinate	Protein synthesis	CML
Bosutinib	BCR-ABL, SRC-ABL	CML

AML Acute myeloid leukemia, *BCL-2* B-cell lymphoma-2, *BTK* Bruton tyrosine kinase, *CML* Chronic myeloid leukemia, *CLL* Chronic lymphocytic leukemia, *FL* Follicular lymphoma, *GVHD* Graft Vs. host disease, *MM* multiple myeloma, *BCR-ABL* Breakpoint cluster region-Abelson murine leukemia gene, *HDAC* Histone deacetylase, *FLT3-ITD* FMS like tyrosine kinase 3-internal tandem duplication

21-year high. Approvals in Oncology were 16 of the 46 (35%) new drugs approved and for the first time 2 of the novel immune cell-based (or gene) therapies. More than 50% of the new therapies were oral agents. Of the 46 new drugs approved, 3 of these drugs were first-in-class in Blood cancers-inotuzumab ozogamicin (Besponsa), enasidenib (Idhifa) and midostaurin (Rydapt).

Other significant approvals in oncology involve 6 drugs for hematologic malignancies, including midostaurin (Rydapt) for patients with FLT3-positive acute myeloid leukemia (AML), acalabrutinib (Calquence) for mantle-cell lymphoma, the second FDA-approved BTK inhibitor and enasidenib (Idhifa), which targets IDH2-positive AML.

Drug delivery is critical to obtaining better responses. This can be achieved by conjugating cytotoxic drugs to a validated mAb. This improves the therapeutic window of the chemotherapeutic drug and reduces chemotherapy-related side effects. Based on this concept, Brentuximab vedotin has shown excellent results in peripheral T cell lymphoma and Hodgkin lymphoma [32, 34].

Some of these drug approvals are based on Phase II, and Phase III studies for patients with relapsed or refractory lymphoid malignancies have been mostly in multiple myeloma and chronic lymphocytic leukemia. However even Phase I studies with appropriate expansion cohorts have led to FDA approvals. A case in point is Ibrutinib which showed impressive results in phase 1 trials. In relapsed/refractory B cell lymphoid malignancies, the objective response rate in 50 evaluable patients was 60%, including the complete response of 16%. Median progression-free survival in all patients was 13.6 months [37]. Challenges remain with drugs like Imetelstat which has been studied in phase 1 and 1/2 clinical trials in patients with hematologic malignancies; however, it has failed in most trials [[38–40].

17.8 Conclusions

Hematologic malignancies account for one of the top 10 regarding incidence of cancers as well as the cause of death due to cancers. While the annual incidence rates of some of these cancers are trending up, there has also been a significant decline in mortality mainly because of the advances in the diagnosis and management. Cellular therapies may slowly but steadily replace allogenic stem cell transplantation. CAR-T cell therapies have shown excellent durable remissions in relapsed/refractory DLBCL.

Dramatic outcomes have been reported using next-generation precision medicine techniques based on molecular profiling and genomic analysis to match a patient's underlying biology (driving mutations, protein expression, gene amplifications, gene deletions, and epigenetic changes) to the most appropriate therapy. Nevertheless, there are limitations in Genome-based therapy decisions because of our incomplete understanding of the relationship between cancer phenotype and genotype, the microenvironment and the complex interplay resulting in the dynamic evolutionary survival processes. Future pioneering studies that also incorporate drug based functional assays that may provide proof of concept in the relevant ex-vivo genomic models that can predict the clinical response.

Key Expert Opinion Points

1. Hematological Malignancies are at the forefront of rapid advances in therapeutics and molecular technologies with a large impact on survival and even cure.
2. Cutting edge genomic sequencing technologies have now become routine and enabled us to have deeper predictive insights into the biology of various leukemias, lymphomas, and myeloma. This has implications into the future diagnostic classification systems that must rapidly incorporate newly discovered molecular subtypes.

3. Therapeutic progress in small molecules, monoclonal and bi-specific antibodies, chimeric antigen therapies have positively impacted many aggressive entities. Early phase clinical trials have been able to demonstrate proof of principle mechanism of action in changing the otherwise natural course of biology and provide long term response data. This has led to FDA approval of novel therapies
4. The challenges in designing clinical trial protocols are being overcome by multiple cohort studies using appropriate biomarkers and bioimaging.

References

1. Siegel RL, Miller KD, Jemal A. Cancer Statistics, 2017. CA Cancer J Clin. 2017;67(1):7–30.
2. Collins FS, Varmus H. A new initiative on precision medicine. N Engl J Med. 2015;372:793–5.
3. Von Hoff DD, Turner J. Response rates, duration of response, and dose response effects in phase I studies of antineoplastics. Investig New Drugs. 1991 February;9(1):115–22.
4. Kato S, Subbiah V, Kurzrock R. Counterpoint: successes in the pursuit of precision medicine: biomarkers take credit. J Natl Compr Canc Netw. 2017 July;15(7):863–6.
5. The Cancer Genome Atlas Research Network Genomic and epigenomic landscapes of adult de novo acute myeloid leukemia. N Engl J Med. 2013;368:2059–74.
6. Morin RD, Mungall K, Pleasance E, Mungall AJ, Goya R, Huff RD, Scott DW, Ding J, Roth A, Chiu R, et al. Mutational and structural analysis of diffuse large B-cell lymphoma using whole-genome sequencing. Blood. 2013;122:1256–65.
7. Dave SS, Wright G, Tan B, Rosenwald A, Gascoyne RD, Chan WC, Fisher RI, Braziel RM, Rimsza LM, Grogan TM, et al. Prediction of survival in follicular lymphoma based on molecular features of tumor-infiltrating immune cells. N Engl J Med. 2004 Nov 18;351(21):2159–69.
8. Kuang et al. PIM inhibitor SMI-4a induces cell apoptosis and cell cycle arrest in B-cell acute lymphocytic leukemia cells via the JAK2/STAT3 pathway. ASH 2018.
9. Wang ML, Rule S, Martin P, Goy A, Auer R, Kahl BS, et al. Targeting BTK with ibrutinib in relapsed or refractory mantle-cell lymphoma. N Engl J Med. 2013;369:507–16.
10. Byrd JC, Furman RR, Coutre SE, Flinn IW, Burger JA, Blum KA, et al. Targeting BTK with ibrutinib in relapsed chronic lymphocytic leukemia. N Engl J Med. 2013;369:32–42.
11. Wang M, Rule S, Zinzani PL, Goy A, Casasnovas O, et al. Acalabrutinib in relapsed or refractory mantle cell lymphoma (ACE-LY-004): a single-arm, multicentre, phase 2 trial. Lancet. 2018 Feb 17;391(10121):659–67.
12. Bernicot I, Douet-Guilbert N, Le Bris M-J, Herry A, Morel F, De Braekeleer M. Molecular cytogenetics of IGH rearrangements in non-Hodgkin B-cell lymphoma. Cytogenet Genome Res. 2007;118:345–52.
13. Nogai H, Dörken B, Lenz G. Pathogenesis of non-Hodgkin's Lymphoma. J Clin Oncol. 2011;29(14):1803–11.
14. Roberts AW, Huang D. Targeting BCL2 with BH3 mimetics: basic science and clinical application of venetoclax in chronic lymphocytic leukemia and related B cell malignancies. Clin Pharmacol Ther. 2016;101(1):89–98.
15. Kantarjian H, Stein A, Gökbuget N, et al. Blinatumomab versus chemotherapy for advanced acute lymphoblastic leukemia. N Engl J Med. 2017;376:836–47.
16. Rowley JD. The critical role of chromosome translocations in human leukemias. Annu Rev Genet. 1998;32:495–519.
17. Sreekantaiah C. FISH panels for hematologic malignancies. Cytogenet Genome Res. 2007;118(2–4):284–96.
18. Swerdlow SH, Campo E, Pileri SA, et al. The 2016 revision of the World Health Organization classification of lymphoid neoplasms. Blood. 2016;127:2375–90.
19. Leonard JP, Martin P, Roboz GJ. Practical implications of the 2016 revision of the World Health Organization classification of lymphoid and myeloid neoplasms and acute leukemia. J Clin Oncol. 2017;35(23):2708–15.

20. Aparicio S, Hidalgo M, Kung AL. Examining the utility of patient-derived xenograft mouse models. Nat Rev Cancer. 2015;15:311–6.
21. Maude SL, Laetsch TW, Buechner J, Rives S, Boyer M, et al. Tisagenlecleucel in children and young adults with B-cell lymphoblastic leukemia. N Engl J Med. 2018 Feb 1;378(5):439–48.
22. Neelapu SS, Locke FL, Bartlett NL, Lekakis LJ, Miklos DB, et al. Axicabtagene ciloleucel CAR T-cell therapy in refractory large B-cell lymphoma. N Engl J Med. 2017 Dec 28;377(26):2531–44.
23. Cheson BD, Heitner Enschede S, Cerri E, et al. Tumor lysis syndrome in chronic lymphocytic leukemia with novel targeted agents. Oncologist. 2017;22(11):1283–91.
24. Hutchins LF, Unger JM, Crowley JJ, et al. Underrepresentation of patients 65 years of age or older in cancer-treatment trials. N Engl J Med. 1999;341:2061–7.
25. Murthy VH, Krumholz HM, Gross CP. Participation in cancer clinical trials: race-, sex-, and age-based disparities. JAMA. 2004;291:2720–6.
26. Goede V, Fisher K, Busch R, et al. Obinutuzmab plus chlorambucil in patients with CLL and coexisting conditions. N Engl J Med. 2014;370:1101–10.
27. Extermann M, Albrand G, Chen H, et al. Are older French patients as willing as older American patients to undertake chemotherapy? J Clin Oncol. 2003;21(17):3214–9.
28. Booth CM, Eisenhauer EA. Progression-free survival: meaningful or simply measurable? JCO Apr. 2012;1:1030–103.
29. Jones AK, Freise KJ, Agarwal SK, Humerickhouse RA, Wong SL, et al. Clinical predictors of venetoclax pharmacokinetics in chronic lymphocytic leukemia and non-Hodgkin's Lymphoma patients: a pooled population pharmacokinetic analysis. AAPS J. 2016 Sep;18(5):1192–202.
30. Connarn JN, Hwang R, Gao Y, Palmisano M, Chen N. Population pharmacokinetics of lenalidomide in healthy volunteers and patients with hematologic malignancies. Clin Pharmacol Drug Dev. 2018 Jun;7(5):465–73.
31. Thanarajasingam G, Minasian LM, Baron F et al. (37 more authors). Beyond maximum grade: modernising the assessment and reporting of adverse events in haematological malignancies. Lancet Haematol. 2018; 5(11): e563–e598. ISSN 2352–3026.
32. Horwitz et al. The ECHELON-2 trial: results of a randomized, double-blind, active-controlled phase 3 study of Brentuximab vedotin and CHP (A+CHP) versus CHOP in the frontline treatment of patients with CD30+ peripheral T-cell lymphomas. ASH 2018.
33. Moskowitz CH, Nademanee A, Masszi T, et al. AETHERA Study Group. Brentuximab vedotin as consolidation therapy after autologous stem-cell transplantation in patients with Hodgkin's lymphoma at risk of relapse or progression (AETHERA): a randomised, double-blind, placebo-controlled, phase 3 trial. Lancet 2015;385(9980):1853–62.
34. Younes A, Gopal AK, Smith SE, et al. Results of a pivotal phase II study of Brentuximab vedotin for patients with relapsed or refractory Hodgkin's lymphoma. J Clin Oncol. 2012;30(18):2183–9.
35. Harrison AM, Thalji NM, Greenberg AJ, Tapia CJ, Windebank AJ. Rituximab for non-Hodgkin's lymphoma: a story of rapid success in translation. Clin Transl Sci. 2013;7(1):82–6.
36. Nagai S, Ozawa K. Analysis of drugs for hematological malignancy that were granted accelerated approval and feasibility of randomized phase 3 clinical trials for relapsed and refractory hematological malignancy. Blood. 2016 Dec;128(22):2387.
37. Advani RH, Buggy JJ, Sharman JP, et al. Bruton tyrosine kinase inhibitor ibrutinib (PCI-32765) has significant activity in patients with relapsed/refractory B-cell malignancies. J Clin Oncol. 2013;31(1):88–94.
38. Huff CA, Wang Q, Badros AZ, et al. The telomerase inhibitor, imetelstat, rapidly reduces myeloma cancer stem cells (CSCs) in a phase II trial [abstract]. Blood. 2012;120(21). Abstract 4898.24.
39. Baerlocher GM, OppligerLeibundgut E, Ottmann OG, et al. Telomerase inhibitor imetelstat in patients with essential thrombocythemia. N Engl J Med. 2015;373(10):920.
40. Tefferi A, Lasho TL, Begna KH, et al. A pilot study of the telomerase inhibitor imetelstat for myelofibrosis. N Engl J Med. 2015;373(10):908–19.

Chapter 18
Pharmacokinetic Considerations for Organ Dysfunction Clinical Trials in Early Drug Development

Analia Azaro, Mehmet Esat Demirhan, Joann Lim, and Jordi Rodon

Abstract It is not infrequent that patients with different cancers are affected by bodily organ dysfunction. Factors such as comorbidities, prior anticancer therapies and tumor-related issues are frequent causes of organ impairment. Since patients with bodily organ dysfunction are not frequently enrolled in conventional clinical trials due to standard study eligibility criteria, such patients are placed at a disadvantage in receiving appropriate anticancer treatment. Renal and hepatic impairment may also have potential detrimental effects on the pharmacokinetic profile of drugs, with subsequent implications for both safety and efficacy.

Renal function can be classified into 5 categories (normal, mild, moderate, severe and end-stage renal dysfunction), but the main classifications used (FDA, EMA and NCI-ODWG, KIDGO) currently have different cutoffs for each group, and also differ in their methods for calculating the eGFR. Renal impairment can be a consequence of damage through a range of mechanisms (glomerular filtration, tubular secretion, tubular absorption, and renal metabolism), likely differently affecting not only the excretion of drugs, but also other parameters such as absorption, distribution, protein binding, metabolism and excretion (ADME) of drugs even in those with low renal clearance.

A. Azaro (✉)
Molecular Therapeutics Research Unit (UITM), Medical Oncology Department,
Vall d'Hebron University Hospital, Barcelona, Spain

Early Clinical Drug Development Group,
Vall d'Hebron Institute of Oncology (VHIO), Barcelona, Spain
e-mail: aazaro@vhio.net

M. E. Demirhan · J. Lim
Investigational Cancer Therapeutics Department, The University of Texas MD Anderson Cancer Center, Houston, TX, USA
e-mail: MEDemirhan@mdanderson.org; jlim@mdanderson.org

J. Rodon
Investigational Cancer Therapeutics Department, The University of Texas MD Anderson Cancer Center, Houston, TX, USA

T. A. Yap et al. (eds.), *Phase I Oncology Drug Development*,
https://doi.org/10.1007/978-3-030-47682-3_18

Conversely, hepatic impairment is frequently classified as mild, moderate and severe. In oncology, the two most commonly used classifications are the Child-Pugh and NCI-ODWG scores. Both scores use objective variables that are easily measurable laboratory parameters (e.g. total bilirubin, prothrombin time, albumin and ALT/AST). Nevertheless, the Child-Pugh score also includes clinical variables including encephalopathy and ascites, which may not always accurately represent the severity of liver function in patients with different cancers. The severity of hepatic impairment varies between highly hepatic extracted drugs (EH > 7), blood flow-limited, intermediate (EH < 7–EH > 3) and low extracted drugs (EH < 3). Furthermore, hepatic impairment is also associated with variable and non-uniform reductions in CYP450 enzymes activity and changes in unbound drug, which also affect the disposition and exposure of drugs.

Understanding the degree of severity of organ dysfunction and the underlying responsible mechanisms, as well as the impact on pharmacokinetics are key challenges in patients with renal and hepatic impairment, which should be assessed in early phase clinical trials if appropriate.

Keywords Renal impairment · Hepatic impairment · Pharmacokinetics Pharmacodynamics · Anticancer drugs

Key Points

1. Organ dysfunction is frequently seen in patients with different cancers. Renal and hepatic impairment are the most relevant organ dysfunction, and they directly affect the pharmacokinetics of drugs and ultimately potentially their safety and efficacy.
2. Renal impairment, including deterioration of glomerular filtration, tubular secretion, tubular absorption, and renal metabolism, is likely to affect absorption, distribution, protein binding, metabolism and excretion (ADME) but especially renal clearance of many drugs.
3. Hepatic impairment is likely to affect hepatic clearance of drugs due to variable, non-linear changes in CYP450 enzymes and changes in protein binding. Depending on the degree of hepatic dysfunction, drugs with high hepatic extraction drugs, and eventually, with low extraction would have affected pharmacokinetic profiles.
4. The design of clinical trials in patients with renal impairment and hepatic impairment warrants a deep knowledge of the disease, evaluation of the organ dysfunction, pharmacokinetics and pharmacology of the agent.

18.1 Organ Dysfunction in Cancer Patients

Comorbidities are commonly observed in patients with different cancers, which ultimately influence the response to anticancer therapies and patient outcomes. Accordingly, renal and hepatic dysfunction are relatively frequent comorbidities that can have an impact on the pharmacokinetics (PK) of anticancer drugs. However, the

PK of many antitumor agents has not been sufficiently studied in patients with different cancers with organ dysfunction, which precludes them from receiving optimal anticancer therapies. In addition, these patients do not generally meet eligibility criteria in clinical trials. There are thus limited data available on the safety, PK profile, and optimal dosing of many different anticancer agents in patients with organ impairment.

18.2 Renal Impairment

End-stage kidney disease (ESKD) is defined as a medical condition in which renal function is below 15%. According to the pace of onset, kidney failure can be classified as acute kidney injury (AKI) or as chronic kidney disease (CKD). AKI is an abrupt (<48 h) reduction in renal function that is currently defined as an absolute increase in serum creatinine ≥0.3 mg/dl (≥ 26.4 μmol/l), a percentage increase in serum creatinine ≥50% (1.5-fold from baseline), or a reduction in urine output (documented oliguria of less than 0.5 ml/kg/h for more than six hours). On the other hand, CKD is defined as a decrease in renal function manifested as a glomerular filtration rate (GFR) of less than 60 ml/min/1.73 m^2 for at least three months accompanied or not by markers of kidney damage (e.g. albuminuria, urinary sediment alterations, electrolyte disturbances or other anomalies associated with tubular disorders, histological or imaging defects, history of kidney transplantation). When the GFR is below 15 ml/min/1.73 m^2, it is considered as ESKD [1–3].

The global prevalence of CKD has been consistently estimated in 11–13%, with the majority of cases having an estimated GFR around 30–59 ml/min [4]. The prevalence of CKD is directly related to age, although no significant differences were found in prevalence between age- and non-age-adjusted groups in a large meta-analysis [5]. Furthermore, CKD prevalence is also determined by gender having women a better prognosis. For example, it has been observed that renal disease progresses at a slower rate in women with polycystic kidney disease, IgA nephropathy, membranous glomerulopathy, and CKD of unknown etiology [6].

Increases in serum creatinine (SCr) as small as 10% (0.2 mg/dl–17.6 μmol/l) have been associated with a prolonged intensive care unit stay and increased mortality. The frequent comorbidities present in cancer patients directly influence their care, the selection of the initial treatment and the effectiveness of treatment [7, 8]. In sum, AKI jeopardizes the continuation of effective cancer treatment and limits cancer patient inclusion in clinical trials [9].

18.2.1 Causes of Renal Impairment in Cancer Patients

Patients with different cancers are at risk of CKD due to concomitant risk factors and morbidities, as well as because of specific kidney insults derived from their respective tumors or anticancer therapies (Tables 18.1 and 18.2). These aggressions include prior episodes of AKI, nephrotoxic anticancer agents, reduction in a kidney

Table 18.1 Risk factors of CKD in the global population [10]

Risk factors of CKD	Smoking
	Hypertension
	Diabetes mellitus type 1 and 2
	Obesity
	Aristolochic acid nephropathy and Balkan endemic nephropathy
	Polycystic kidney disease
	Glomerulonephritis (autoimmune diseases, diabetes, systemic infections)
	Pyelonephritis or interstitial nephritis
	HIV infection, hepatitis B infection, and hepatitis C infection
	Renal tubular disorders (renal tubular acidosis, nephrogenic diabetes insipidus, Fanconi syndrome), renal potassium wasting, renal magnesium wasting, cystinuria
	Vascular diseases (atherosclerosis, hypertension, ischemia, vasculitis, thrombotic microangiopathy)
	Prevalence of high-risk alleles in MYH9 and APOL1 genes
	Tubulointerstitial diseases, urinary tract infections, stones, obstructions, drug toxicity
	Environmental pollution, pesticides, analgesic abuse, herbal medications, unregulated food additives

mass following a nephrectomy, chronic obstructive nephropathy, or kidney irradiation. Remarkably, not all patients exposed to nephrotoxic chemotherapeutic agents develop kidney injury, which is suggestive that the risk of nephrotoxicity is a multifactorial phenomenon. In addition to innate drug toxicity, certain host characteristics and renal handling of the drug increase kidney injury. In general, one or more of these factors combine to increase the risk for kidney injury and renal vulnerabilities to drug-induced kidney disease in cancer patients [41, 42].

There are certain preceding risk factors in cancer patients, as is the case with elderly subjects with reduced total body water at baseline, increased levels of angiotensin-II/endothelin decreased GFR, and higher rates of renal oxidative stress. Another intrinsic non-modifiable risk factor is to have an underlying genetic tendency. Gene polymorphisms in the renal cytochrome P450 enzyme system, which favor reduced metabolism and renal excretion increase the risk of nephrotoxicity. Likewise, mutations in genes that regulate drug carrier proteins can impair drug excretion and induce nephrotoxicity by increasing intracellular drug concentrations [36].

Many cancers affect the kidneys either directly or indirectly, increasing the risk for kidney injury. Direct tumor effects include myeloma-related kidney injury, infiltration of the renal parenchyma as seen with leukemias and lymphomas, urinary tract obstruction, and secondary glomerulopathies. Lymphomatous invasion of the kidneys may occasionally present as AKI. Furthermore, metastatic extrarenal solid tumors rarely cause AKI, with lung cancer being the most common solid tumor to metastasize to the kidney, followed by gastric and breast cancer [43]. In such cases, AKI could be improved to some degree with anticancer treatment.

Table 18.2 Anticancer drugs associated with kidney injury

Anticancer drug	Kidney injury		References
IL-2, denileukin diftitox	Capillary leak syndrome	Acute kidney injury could be reversible or progress to chronic renal disease	Avarbock et al. [11], Sahni et al. [12]
Antiangiogenic drugs (bevacizumab), tyrosine kinase inhibitors, gemcitabine, cisplatin, mitomycin C	Thrombotic microangiopathy		Eremina et al. [13], Usui et al. [14], Sahni et al. [12], Rosner et al. [15], Glezerman and Edgar [16]
Antiangiogenic drugs (bevacizumab) pamidronate	Glomeruli Minimal change disease		Markowitz et al. [17], Stokes et al. [18], Usui et al. [14]
Antiangiogenic drugs (bevacizumab) pamidronate, zoledronate (rare), gefitinib	Glomeruli Focal segmental glomerulosclerosis		Markowitz et al. [17], Kumasaka et al. [19], Sahni et al. [12], Stokes et al. [18], Usui et al. [14]
Platinum-based drugs, zoledronate, ifosfamide, mithramycin, pentostatin, imatinib, diaziquone, pemetrexed, mTOR inhibitors, vemurafenib, dabrafenib, crizotinib	Tubulointerstitium Acute tubular necrosis		Glezerman et al. [20], Markowitz et al. [21], Sahni et al. [12], Izzedine et al. [22], Wanchoo [23], Izzedine [24]
Cisplatin, ifosfamide, azacitidine, diaziquone, imatinib, pemetrexed	Tubulopathies		Ciarimboli et al. [25], Zamlauski-Tucker et al. [26], Ciarimboli et al. [27], Glezerman et al. [20], Sahni et al. [12]
Platinum-based drugs azacytidine	Salt wasting		Sahni et al. [12]
Platinum-based drugs cetuximab, panitumumab	Magnesium wasting		Dietrich et al. [28], Schrag et al. [29], Muallem and Moe [30], Van Cutsem et al. [31]
Cisplatin, ifosfamide, pemetrexed	Nephrogenic diabetes insipidus		Zamlauski-Tucker et al. [26], Ciarimboli et al. [27], Glezerman et al. [20], Fung et al. [32]
Cyclophosphamide, vincristine	Syndrome of inappropriate antidiuresis		Bressler and Huston [33], Cutting [34]
Immunotherapeutic drugs (ipilimumab,nivolumab, Pembrolizumab) sorafenib, sunitinib	Acute interstitial nephritis		Azar [35], Perazella [36], Izzedine et al. [37], Rosner et al. [15], Cortazar et al. [38], Shirali et al. [39]
Methotrexate	Crystalline nephropathy		Widemann and Adamson [40]

Indirect cancer-related effects include volume depletion from nausea and vomiting, diarrhea, over-diuresis, metabolic disturbances, malignant ascites or pleural effusions, sepsis, and cardiac involvement, inducing a prerenal state that sensitizes the kidney to nephrotoxins [44]. In addition, comorbidities that affect baseline renal function are commonly present in cancer patients, including poor cardiac function, diabetes, hypertension, recent radiocontrast exposure or other nephrotoxic medications, poor oral intake, intravascular volume depletion, and genitourinary obstruction due to tumor infiltration.

Finally, there are many anticancer drugs that are associated with different types of kidney injuries (Table 18.2). The mechanism of nephrotoxicity with cisplatin involves signal pathways that lead to tubular cell death and inflammation by increasing intracellular drug concentration. Once cisplatin enters the tubular cell, several intracellular injury pathways are activated, causing renal tubular cell apoptosis and necrosis which, in turn, lead to clinical AKI and/or tubulopathy. Sodium wasting is another consequence of cisplatin treatment, and it can be associated with hypovolemia, orthostasis, and prerenal AKI. Moreover, cisplatin can impair the reabsorption of magnesium in the distal nephron, causing refractory hypomagnesemia. Finally, water absorption in the collecting duct can be disturbed, resulting in a form of nephrogenic diabetes insipidus [45–48].

For epidermal growth factor receptor (EGFR) inhibitors, the primary renal abnormality is magnesium wasting [28]. The incidence of severe hypomagnesemia in patients treated with cetuximab, for example, has been estimated in 10–15%, whilst patients treated with panitumumab experience hypomagnesemia in ~36% of cases, with an incidence of severe hypomagnesemia of 3% [29, 31].

The use of androgen deprivation therapy (ADT), on the other hand, is associated the lack of vasodilatation effects of testosterone on renal vessels, affecting tubular function [49].

In conclusion, cancer patients may develop various kidney lesions that impair their immediate survival and limit the adequate treatment of the underlying malignant process. Overall, kidney-related problems often hinder the administration of anticancer drugs in oncology practice, and pose challenges regarding cancer patient inclusion in clinical trials with new investigational drugs.

18.2.2 Impact of Renal Impairment on the Pharmacokinetics and Pharmacodynamics of Cancer Drugs

As seen, renal insufficiency/impairment has been shown to be highly prevalent in cancer patients, and, in addition to an increased cancer-related and unrelated mortality, renal insufficiency can also affect PK of anticancer therapy use, affecting one or several of the PK phases: absorption, distribution, metabolism and excretion (ADME). The differential effect of drugs in patients with renal insufficiency (efficacy or toxicity) is generally based on changes in these PK parameters and how they are affected. The clinical pharmacokinetics (ADME) effects and potential mechanisms of increased drug concentrations will be a consequence of accumulated uremic toxins [50, 51]

- Absorption and bioavailability: although the bioavailability of some drugs has been reported to be reduced, there are no consistent findings proving absorption impairment in patients with kidney disease. It is complex to assess because drugs that undergo a significant pre-systemic elimination (e.g. gut wall, liver) will have a moderate-to-low oral bioavailability, and patients with kidney disease would have a reduced pre-systemic elimination. However, drugs with reduced oral bioavailability and high pre-systemic elimination have shown to have a significant increase in area under the curve in patients with severe renal dysfunction.
- Volume of distribution: it can also significantly increase in patients with severe CKD due to fluid overload, decreased protein binding, and others.
- Metabolism and elimination: The two main organs responsible for the elimination of drugs and their metabolites from the body are the liver and the kidneys, and these two processes are directly affected by the anticancer drugs and the comorbidities and concomitant medications of the patient.

Consequently, it may be necessary to adjust the dosage those anticancer drugs to avoid drug accumulation and toxicities [52, 53]. For that, dedicated clinical trials for this patient population, and methods to assess the renal function and classify patients to standardize clinical research in this patient population are of major importance in a comprehensive drug development plan.

18.2.3 Assessment of Renal Function

Prior to discussing the assessment of renal function, it is necessary to review the normal GFR. This rate is equal to the sum of the filtration rates in all of the functioning nephrons. In other words, GFR estimates the number of functioning nephrons. The filtering units of the kidney, i.e. the glomeruli, filter about 180 l per day (125 ml/min) of plasma. However, the normal value of GFR depends on age, sex, and body size. It is approximately 120 and 130 ml/min/1.73 m^2 for women and men, respectively (with considerable variation among normal individuals). Not surprisingly, GFR is widely accepted as the best overall measurement method of renal function. Clinically, if the excretion rate of freely filtered substance and its concentration in plasma are known, GFR can be estimated by using the following formula:

$$GFR = \frac{Excretion\ rate}{C}$$

where the excretion rate (in mg/min) is the product of urine volume per unit of time and urine solute concentration, and C is the plasma solute concentration at the midpoint of the urine collection interval.

Both the FDA and EMA provide guidance on the methods to be used in clinical trials in patients with renal impairment. Although renal excretion of a drug may involve tubular secretion as well as glomerular filtration, the EMA and FDA guidelines have considered sufficient to use GFR as a global measure of renal function in PK studies. According to these guidelines, *measured* or *estimated* GFR refer to whereas GFR was determined by using an exogenous or an endogenous substance, respectively. The gold standard for assessing renal function is considered to be *measured* GFR using an exogenous substance such as inulin, ^{51}Cr-EDTA, ^{99}mDTPA, iothalamate sodium, or ^{125}I-iohexol as filtration marker [54]. Inulin was the classical gold standard method, but it is being replaced by radioisotope filtration markers owing to inulin methodological limitations [55] which showed low variability high accuracy [56–58] (Table 18.3). All these exogenous substances meet the criteria of an ideal filtration marker and are exclusively eliminated through the renal route. The use of non-radioisotopic exogenous substances or *estimating* GFR by using endogenous markers is based mainly on convenience.

Clinical situations in which it may important to have a more precise knowledge of GFR and use precise methods of GFR evaluation include: (i) prior to dose adjustment of medications, especially toxic medications with narrow therapeutic indices (e.g., chemotherapy); (ii) prior to kidney donation; and (iii) prior to determining the need for transplant. But measuring GFR is complex, time-consuming, and inconvenient to perform in clinical practice and for these reasons, GFR is usually estimated using serum markers (Table 18.4).

Serum creatinine is the most common endogenous filtration marker accepted for the estimation of the renal function. Creatinine is distributed in body water, not bound to plasma proteins, and it is freely filtered by the glomeruli. Still, creatinine serum creatinine can vary depending on its production and urinary excretion (Table 18.5), and it is also mildly secreted by proximal tubular cells, plus it undergoes extrarenal elimination. Therefore, the measurement of creatinine clearance (CL_{CR}) has become a useful estimator of GFR [59], but, although convenient, CL_{CR} it is not the best indicator of the efficiency of all the renal excretion pathways.

Many equations to estimate renal function have been developed and validated. These equations include variables like age, sex, race, and body size, as well as

Table 18.3 Relative accuracy and convenience of different exogenous and endogenous markers for GFR quantification [59, 60]

Markers	Accuracy	Convenience	Advantage	Disadvantage
Inulin clearance	++++	+	Good marker	Complex
Serum Cystatin C	++++	+	No affected by	methodology
Radioactive	++++	++	age, sex, race	Expensive
contrast agents	+++	++	Good marker	Radiation
(^{99}mTcDTPA)	++	+++	Good marker	exposure
Non-radioactive	++	++++	Easy to measure	Allergic reactions
contrast agents				24 h urine
Creatinine				collection
clearance				Variability
Serum creatinine				

Table 18.4 Exogenous and endogenous kidney pathway markers [60]

Pathway and marker		
Renal plasma/blood flow	Glomerular filtration	Tubular function
5-Hydroxyindoleacetic acid	Creatinine	5-Hydroxyindoleacetic acid
^{125}I- or	Creatinine and cimetidine	*p*-Aminohippurate
^{131}I-ortho-iodohippurate	Cystatin C	N1-Methylnicotinamide
p-Aminohippurate	Inulin	(1-NMN)
	^{125}I-Iothalamate	Probenecid
	Sinistrin	Pindolol
	^{99}mTc-DTPA	Fluconazol
	^{169}Y-DTPA	

Table 18.5 Variation of serum creatinine levels among subjects over time due to factors affecting serum creatinine levels [61, 62]

Factor	Known effect on serum creatinine
Age (neonates, elderly)	Decreased
Female sex	Decreased
Race or ethnic group	
Black	Increased
Hispanic	Decreased
Asian	Decreased
Body habitus	
Muscular	Increased
Amputation	Decreased
Obesity	No change
Drugs (e.g. trimethoprim, cimetidine)	Increased
Chronic illness	
Malnutrition, inflammation (e.g. cancer, cachexia, severe cardiovascular diseases, prolonged infections, hospitalized patients)	Decreased
Neuromuscular diseases (dystrophies, paralysis, Cushing syndrome)	Decreased
Diet	
Vegetarian diet	Decreased
Cooked meat	Increased

serum creatinine. All these formulas derive from regression techniques and they vary in accuracy. When the performance of equations using standardized creatinine has been assessed by comparing the results with measured GFR in a study population, it seems that the Modification of Diet in Renal Disease (MDRD) equation is less biased and has a greater accuracy than the Cockcroft-Gault (C-G) equation. Regarding the Chronic Kidney Disease Epidemiology Collaboration (CKD-EPI) equation, it seems to have a greater accuracy than other equations when used to classify CKD stages [63], but it performs better in healthy patients. In patients with GFR of less than 80 ml/min/ 1.73 m^2 [64], it seems that a direct measurement of GFR is better. The accuracy of these formulas can also be influenced by the use of actual or ideal body but, at the end of the day, the concordance between the MDRD, Chronic Kidney Disease Epidemiology Collaboration (CKD-EPI) and C-G equations it is around 82–88%. Because of that any of these equations are accepted by Regulatory Agencies' guidelines for PK studies in patients with impaired renal function (Pharmacokinetics in Patients with Impaired Renal Function—Study Design, Data Analysis, and Impact on Dosing and Labeling FDA guidance) [65] (EMA Guideline on the evaluation of the pharmacokinetics of medicinal products in patients with decreased renal function).

Since there are no endogenous anion markers, p-aminohippuric acid (PAH) and probenecid (500–1000 mg) are used in clinical studies to estimate tubular secretion [66].

18.2.4 Classification of Renal Impairment

Renal function groups have been defined using different criteria and diverse ranges, generating multiple classifications of renal impairment, i.e., KDIGO, FDA, EMA, and the NCI working group (Table 18.6). Consequently, there are subtle differences in the categorization of groups among clinical trials depending on which one is used.

The FDA classification of renal dysfunction studies have categorized patients as having mild, moderate, or severe renal dysfunction with CL_{CR} ranges of 40–59, 20–39, and 0–19 ml/min, respectively. In clinical trials and practice, CL_{CR} equal to or greater than 60 ml/min (or a $S_{CR} < 1.5$ mg/dl) is generally considered as an acceptable renal function. This is also the usual eligibility criterion for the enrolment of patients into oncology phase I studies. This threshold, though includes patients with mild renal dysfunction according to the FDA criteria. Still, it is recommended that all clinical trials apply the FDA/EMA categorization to homogenize and reduce the number of classifications used for renal dysfunction. This is also supported by a retrospective analysis of NCI/CALGB trials [67], where it was found that patients with an estimated CL_{CR} of 40–49 ml/min (included in the mild renal dysfunction category based on the NCI/CALGB, but in the moderate category according to the FDA) were primarily responsible for the differences in the frequency of toxicity (Table 18.6).

Albuminuria, the earliest marker of glomerular disease, can classified into several categories (but with poor correlation with the risk of CKD). Clinical trials, though, do rarely stratify renal impairment according to the values of albuminuria but proteinuria and/or albuminuria can be used as exclusion criteria in early clinical trials of drugs with potential nephrotoxicity (e.g. antiangiogenics).

Neither GFR nor albuminuria alone can completely capture the prognosis of a patient with CKD. Consequently, integration of both parameters has been proposed for a classification of renal dysfunction, the KDIGO2012's risk classification of CKD according to international guidelines using albuminuria and GFR, but in clinical trials the sole use of GFR alone is more established.

Table 18.6 Comparison of thresholds used in the classification of renal impairment

Stage	GFR group	KDIGO	Estimated CrCl/GFR–FDA/EMA	Estimated CL_{CR}–NCI (ml/min/1.73 m^2)
1	Normal	≥90 ml/min	≥90 ml/min	≥60 ml/min
2	Mild decrease	60–89 ml/min	60–89 ml/min	40–59 ml/min
3	Moderate decrease	59–30 ml/min	59–30 ml/min	20–39 ml/min
4	Severe decrease	15–29 ml/min	15–29 ml/min	<20 ml/min
5	ESKD	Kidney failure	<15 ml/min not on dialysis	Any
			Requiring dialysis	

Abbreviations: CL_{CR} creatinine clearance based on the Cockcroft-Gault equation, *GFR* glomerular filtration rate based on the MDRD equation

18.3 Hepatic Impairment

In the early development of cytotoxic chemotherapy agents with a narrow therapeutic index, only cancer patients were enrolled on such trials based on ethical concerns over short and long-term toxicities of these agents. But in the development of molecularly targeted therapeutics, healthy volunteer studies have been used to assess single-dose exposure PK parameters. When assessing the effect of liver dysfunction, such studies may be performed using patients with varying degrees of hepatic impairment with or without cancer. For assessing long-term tolerability, only the latter group of patients could be evaluated. Therefore, the Cancer Therapy Evaluation Program (CTEP) at the NCI prioritized hepatic dysfunction phase I clinical trials (HDCT) to determine safe administration parameters of antineoplastic agents for subjects with varying degrees of liver dysfunction. Since then, studies from the HDCTs, sponsored by the CTEP, along with other clinical trials, have provided relevant clinical data on the optimal dosing of antineoplastic agents in subjects with different degrees of liver abnormalities, offering administration guidance in the labels for patients with abnormal organ function [68, 69]

18.3.1 Causes of Liver Failure in the Cancer Patient

Liver failure in cancer patients can occur as a result of pre-existing conditions, viral or drug-induced hepatitis and/or cirrhosis (including anticancer treatments), or liver infiltration by primary or metastatic tumors. Based on recent studies, the main causes are chronic hepatitis B/C infection, alcohol-induced liver disease, non-alcoholic fatty liver disease, and non-alcoholic steatohepatitis [70–72], and due to the frequency of chronic liver diseases (CLDs), they represent a major world public health problem.

Many chemotherapeutic agents can cause liver damage, ranging from transient changes in liver biochemical tests (Table 18.7) to more severe and chronic damage. Most adverse reactions are idiosyncratic due to differences in susceptibility to drug-induced liver injury or inability to recover from the injury among patients. However,

Table 18.7 Hepatoxicity and liver pattern damage of some anticancer agents

Liver pattern damage	Anticancer agent	Frequency	Clinical relevance	References
Increased AST, ALT and AP, with or without increased bilirubin	*Paclitaxel* *Nabpaclitaxel*	High doses, up to 37% CYP2C8 type II polymorphism in 18% of African Americans	Reversible	Villano et al. [73]
	Cisplatin	Common	Reversible	Hill et al. [74]
	Imatinib	Up to 10%	Severe 2–4%	Mando [75], Mindikoglu [76]
Cholestasis or intrahepatic cholestasis	*Cytarabine*	Common	Reversible	Slavin et al. [77]
	Gemcitabine	Rare	Life-threatening	Robinson et al. [78]
Veno-occlusive disease	*Etoposide*	At high doses or in transplantation 10–25%	Life-threatening	Tran et al. [79]
	Dacarbazina	Rare, with fever and eosinophilia	Fulminant liver failure	Asbury et al. [80], Friedman et al. [81]
Bilirubin increase (hemolysis)	Capecitabine	Common (23–25%)	Severe	Scheithauer [82], Van Cutsem et al. [83]
Fibrosis, cirrhosis or liver necrosis s	*Methotrexate*	At cumulative dose, up to 30%	Potentially irreversible	Chu and Allegra [84]
	Etoposide	Rare	Severe	Tran et al. [79]
Steatosis	*Irinotecan*	Up to 50%	Steatohepatitis can increase morbidity	Morris-Stiff et al. [85]
Sinusoidal obstruction or dilatation síndrome	*Oxaliplatin*	20–80%	Increase morbidity after liver resection	Doroshow et al. [86, 87], Rubbia-Brandt et al. [88], Vauthey et al. [89], Morris-Stiff et al. [85]

Abbreviations: *ALT* alanine aminotransferase, *AP* alkaline phosphatase, *AST* aspartate aminotransferase some drugs are particularly hepatotoxic [90]. Moreover, pre-existing liver disease or previous liver irradiation might increase susceptibility to drug-induced liver damage.

Liver dysfunction in cancer patients can be also secondary to malignancy (i.e. primary liver tumor or liver metastases), but these are uncommon causes of acute liver failure. Tumors in or around the liver and the biliary tree can affect liver function by multifactorial mechanisms that include direct loss of healthy functional liver volume or intra/extra-hepatic biliary obstruction. Similarly, portal vein occlusion secondary to thrombosis—by hypercoagulation syndromes or direct tumor infiltration—may compromise vascular supply to healthy liver parenchyma and thus drug metabolism.

Furthermore, cancer might indirectly affect drug metabolism in the liver. Tumors can generate a host inflammatory response that involves cytokines, such as IL-6 and TNF-α, which manifest clinically through the observation of increased acute-phase reactants in serum, cachexia, and fever. They can also contribute to cholestasis or inflammation in the liver [91]. This inflammatory response is associated with decreased CYP3A4 activity in the liver [92], with a secondary effect in the expression of drug transporters and, thus, drug clearance [93]. Albumin levels can also be affected, which might modify the amount of free or unbound drug in plasma and the volume of distribution. Although the magnitude of these effects is thought to be minor in most subjects, their impact on elderly patients could be higher, particularly in those who are frail due to multiple comorbidities and whose liver function is compromised by the tumor.

Potential interactions between the liver and chemotherapy agents fall into two categories: direct chemotherapy-induced hepatotoxicity and potentiation of pre-existing liver disease (especially, viral hepatitis). Altered hepatic drug metabolism due to an underlying liver disease can result in higher or more persistent drug levels in the body, thereby causing an increased systemic toxicity (mainly, myelosuppression), and/or worsening of liver function due to chemotherapy-induced hepatotoxicity.

But liver injury during cancer treatment may not always be related with anticancer agents but potential reactions to antibiotics, analgesics, antiemetics, and other medications. The susceptibility of patients to liver injury may be affected by pre-existing medical conditions such as the ones mentioned before, and also by nutritional deficiencies or parenteral nutrition. Therefore, the attribution of liver injury may be difficult. Complicating things even more, most hepatotoxic drug reactions are idiosyncratic and have non-dose-dependent effects, either through immunologic mechanisms or due to differences in metabolic responses among individuals.

18.3.2 Impact of Hepatic Impairment on the Pharmacokinetics and Pharmacodynamics of Cancer Drugs

The liver plays a central role in key PK parameters such as absorption/bioavailability/metabolism of first pass, distribution, metabolism and elimination of most drugs and many drug metabolites. Certain parameters that can potentially influence drug PK (e.g. liver blood flow, binding to plasma proteins, or biliary excretion) depend on the normal functioning of this organ. Hepatic disease results in numerous pathophysiologic structural changes that may affect hepatic drug clearance, as is the case with cirrhotic livers, where a 50% reduction in such function has been observed [94, 95]. Some of the PK parameters affected by liver dysfunction include:

- Although some metabolic transformation can occur in the intestinal epithelial cells, hepatic clearance is the cornerstone of drug PKs. The hepatic clearance of highly extracted drugs is blood-flow-limited and relatively insensitive to changes in drug binding to blood components or to enzyme/transporter activity (i.e. CL_{int}). Liver diseases (cirrhosis, primary tumors or metastases) are associated with alterations in liver blood flow and porto-systemic shunting due to portal vein occlusion or infiltration. The resulting vascular compromise of the liver parenchyma could have a significant impact on the hepatic drug clearance and particularly in the case of highly extracted drugs.
- A significant decrease in reversible drug binding to plasma proteins is often found in CLDs due to reduced albumin and α1-acid glycoprotein synthesis. Moreover, the accumulation of endogenous compounds, such as bilirubin, inhibit plasma protein binding of certain drugs. Similarly, ascites produces qualitative changes in albumin and α1-acid glycoprotein levels.
- The metabolism of drugs is decreased in liver dysfunction due to a certain degree of oxidization impairment and sinusoidal capillarization. Chronic liver disease is associated with variable and non-uniform reductions in the activity of CYP450 enzymes, and this can be further influenced by blood flow alterations and hypoxia and intrahepatic shunting [96–99].
- Differences in cytochrome-dependent clearance have also been associated with differences in genotype. For instance, there is a trend towards higher clearance capacity in subjects CYP3A5*1 homozygous. Consequently, it has been demonstrated that the clearance of drugs metabolized by CYP3A4/5, such as midazolam, nifedipine and everolimus, is altered depending on the genotype.
- Liver disease may also modify the expression and function of hepatic transporters such as BCRP NTCP, OATP1B1, OCT1, or P-gp [100, 101].

18.3.3 Measurement of Liver Function: Exogenous and Endogenous Markers

Conventional biochemical tests are used to evaluate liver function by assessing endogenous substances whose production is affected by the liver, such as bilirubin, albumin, and prothrombin time. Hepatic synthesis can be evaluated by albumin levels because it is exclusively produced by the liver (as well as the prothrombin time, a marker of the extrinsic pathway of the coagulation cascade) Likewise, plasma levels of bilirubin reflect hepatic clearance.

Dynamic liver function tests have been developed to quantitatively assess hepatic dysfunction. Several exogenous substances are used as marker substrates for liver clearance, including indocyanine green (ICG), antipyrine [102], caffeine, galactose [103], and monoethylglycinexylidide (MEGX) [104]. Some of them, like ICG, galactose and sorbitol, are bloodflow limited substances (therefore, they have a high extraction ratio), and when hepatic uptake mechanisms are significantly altered, the clearance of these substances is substantially altered [105, 106]. The most frequent exogenous marker used in this setting is ICG, a substance selectively taken up by the hepatocytes and later excreted unmodified into the bile via an ATP-dependent transport system. Thus, the ICG excretion rate in bile reflects the hepatic ATP levels and energy status. The plasma disappearance rate of ICG (PDR_{ICG}) is the most commonly used parameter for clinical and experimental assessment of liver function, with a normal range of 18–25%/min. Notably, the PDR_{ICG} does not represent the liver blood flow, but rather the ICG uptake by hepatocytes and its excretion into the bile, which is blood flow/energy status dependent. Since ICG excretion is an ATP-dependent process, a decrease in ATP levels during hepatic dysfunction can be detected.

For assessment of the metabolic function of the liver, one could use substances whose liver elimination is minimally influenced by total hepatic blood flow or portal-systemic shunting, such as low-extraction drugs, include antipyrine, caffeine, and midazolam. Depending on their metabolic pathway, they reflect the activity of different liver functions (antipyrine by multiple CYP450 isoforms such as CYP1A2, CYP2B6, CYP2C8, CYP2C9, CYP2C18, and CYP3A4 [107]; caffeine mostly by CYP1A2 [108]; midazolam almost exclusively by CYP3As [109]; MEGX by CYP3A and CYP1A2 [110, 111]).

18.3.4 Classification of Hepatic Impairment

Liver function can be assessed by various combinatorial indices, the most relevant of which are the Child-Pugh (CP) score, the Model of End-Stage Liver Disease (MELD) and the NCI index. They differ in the parameters used for assessment of the liver function (some objective parameters such as prothrombin time/INR, total bilirubin, AST or albumin, some subjective parameters such as ascites, hepatic encephalopathy), the availability of those parameters in the clinical setting and their validation status. The CP and MELD scores are the most used classification systems to assess prognosis in patients with CLDs, the former being the most widely used to evaluate liver function. However, it must be noted that the CP score was developed as a prognostic marker in patients undergoing transection of hepatic varices, rather than as a predictor of drug elimination (Table 18.8) [112, 113].

However, this classification has several practical limitations in cancer patients, which include: (i) potential overestimation of the influence of proteins synthesized by the liver since albumin and coagulation factors strongly correlate with each other; (ii) use of arbitrary cutoff values; (iii) homogeneous weight given to all

Table 18.8 Modified Child-Pugh (CP) score (nutritional status was replaced by prothrombin time) and categories of liver dysfunction

Points			
Parameters	1	2	3
Encephalopathy	None	Minimal	Advanced (coma)
Ascites	Absent	Controlled	Refractory
Bilirubin (μmol/l)	<34	34–51	>51
Albumin (g/l)	>35	28–35	<28
Prothrombin (s)[a]	<4	4–6	>6
Categories of modified Child-Pugh score			
Group	Description		Child-Pugh score
A	Mild liver dysfunction		5–6
B	Moderate liver dysfunction		7–9
C	Severe liver dysfunction		10–15

[a]Prothrombin time values of 4 s and 6 s approximately correspond to 50% and 40% of normal, respectively

variables; (iv) non-inclusion of creatinine, a relevant prognostic factor present in other scores and considered relevant by some authors [114, 115]; (v) some of its parameters are subjective (ascites and encephalopathy) and most of the parameters can be affected by the disease or its therapy or other factors (encephalopathy and brain metastasis; albumin levels and nutritional status, ascites and peritoneal disease [116]).

Approaches based only on standard liver biochemistry tests have been suggested such as the NCI Organ Dysfunction Working Group (NCI-ODWG) classification, and have been evaluated in hepatic impairment cancer trials (Table 18.9) [69]. This classification is based on two objective and readily measurable laboratory parameters, i.e. total bilirubin and AST/ALT levels.

Another approach, preferred by hepatologists is the Model of End-Stage Liver Disease (MELD). The MELD score, uses only three biochemical parameters (serum bilirubin, serum creatinine, and INR [116, 117]), and its value has been demonstrated in different settings: variceal bleeding [118], infections in cirrhotic patients [119], liver failure [120, 121], alcoholic hepatitis [122], and other chronic diseases [123].

Neither the FDA nor the EMA guidelines on hepatic dysfunction have included the MELD score among the recommended classifications to be used in phase I pharmacokinetic studies in cancer patients with hepatic dysfunction, mainly because this score is a predictor of mortality. The current FDA guidelines for hepatic dysfunction for studies that aim to stratify hepatic impairment recommend the use of the CP classification. Nonetheless, few published phase I trials in cancer patients have used this score (e.g. buparlisib ([124] #30), erlotinib ([125] #31), tipifarnib ([126] #32)). In Oncology, NCI-ODWG criteria constitutes the most commonly used classification system in phase I studies of anticancer agents.

Table 18.9 Comparison of the liver function categories by Child Pugh classification or by NCI Organ Dysfunction Working Group classification

Categorization of hepatic impairment			
	Child Pugh classification (by FDA and EMA)	NCI Organ Dysfunction Working Group	
		Total bilirubin	ALT or AST
Normal			
Mild	A (5–6 ponts)	B1: ≤ ULN B2: > 1–1.5x ULN	B1: > ULN B2: Any
Moderate	B (7–9 points)	> 1.5–3x ULN	Any
Severe	C (10–15 points)	>3x ULN	Any

Abbreviations: *ALT* alanine aminotransferase, *AST* aspartate aminotransferase, *EMA* European Medicines Agency, *FDA* Food and Drug Administration, *NCI* National Cancer Institute, *ULN* upper limit of normal

18.4 Study Designs in Organ Dysfunction Population

Some preclinical models of CKD have been developed have been developed, including Genetically Engineered Models, Vascular injury models (such as Spontaneously hypertensive rats), Glomerular and interstitial injury models (such as animals that develop Lupus nephritis), or models with induced damage (either immune-induced models such as Thy-1 nephritis or non-immune such as nephrectomy, radiation nephropathy, lateral ureteral obstruction or chemically induced). Despite this, none is considered a good *in vivo* RI models to assess the impact on pharmacokinetic parameters and in most cases, a phase 1 trial in patients with renal function impaired is required [127].

The FDA and EMA have published guidelines for conducting of studies in patients with RI or HI. These are generic recommendations, and are not specific for anticancer agents. They also focus on determining primarily the PK parameters in these patient population, rather than the safety or tolerability of the agents. These guidelines recognize the uncertainties surrounding the assessment of hepatic and renal Because of that, the NCI-Organ dysfunction Working Group has provided specific instructions and protocol templates for organ impaired function studies in oncology. Studies in organ impairment are not mandatory in all circumstances, but may be justified in some circumstances, and this as well as what groups of organ impairment need to be studied are based on the drug pharmacological characteristics, and the expected effects of organ dysfunction on its PK. Organ impairment investigations are usually required in a new drug application (NDA) submission for drugs with a narrow therapeutic range or if the mechanism of metabolism and excretion of a drug is unknown. The Regulatory agencies have also issued recommendations on when such studies are needed (Table 18.10):

Table 18.10 FDA and EMA recommendations on the convenience of studies in renal or liver dysfunction

Renal			Liver		
When renal impairment studies may be considered?	FDA	EMA	When hepatic impairment studies may be not considered?	FDA	EMA
The drug is likely to be used in patients with impaired renal function	x	x	The drug is likely to be used in patients with impaired hepatic function	x	x
Renal impairment is likely to mechanistically alter the PK of the drug and/or its active metabolites.	x	x	Hepatic metabolism and/or excretion accounts substantially (>20%) to the metabolism and/or elimination of a drug or its active/toxic metabolites	x	
Dose excreted unchanged in urine is >30%	x		Hepatic metabolism and/or excretion accounts substantially (>20%) but there is a narrow therapeutic index	x	
If the drug is primarily metabolized or secreted in bile, because renal impairment can inhibit some pathways of hepatic and gut drug metabolism and transport.	x	x	If the route of metabolism is unknown and it cannot be shown that hepatic elimination is minor	x	
Therapeutic proteins and biologics with molecular weight <69 kDa	x (<50 kDa)		HI is likely to significantly alter the PKs of the drug and/or its active metabolites		x
ESRD patients undergoing dialysis, PK should be studied under both dialysis and non-dialysis conditions to determine the extent to which dialysis contributes to the elimination of the drug and active metabolites	x	x	A posology adjustment may be needed for such patients taking into account the PK/PD relationship		x
When renal impairment studies may be not considered?			When hepatic impairment studies may be not considered?		
Gaseous or volatile drugs	x	x	Lack of data may be justified if the drug is not intended to be used in patients with HI		x
Single-dose administration if prolonged elimination of the drug/active metabolite is not a safety problem	x	x	If relevant information exists		x
Monoclonal antibodies	x	x	The drug is excreted entirely via renal routes of elimination with no involvement of the liver.	x	

Other			The drug is metabolized in the liver to a small extent (<20 percent), and the therapeutic range of the drug is wide.	x	
1. Administered agents without relevant systemic absorption			The drug is gaseous or volatile, and the drug and its active metabolites are primarily eliminated via the lungs.	x	
2. Hepatically eliminated drugs which safety data were available indicating that dose adjustments are not necessary even at a markedly increased exposure of the drug		x	Single-dose administration, unless clinical concerns suggest otherwise.	x	
3. Hepatically eliminated drugs where increases in exposure due to renal impairment can be monitored in clinical practice					
4. Drug cannot be safely administered to healthy subjects and a study in patients is not feasible or justifiable.					

aSee CHMP/EWP/89249/2004 Guidelines on the clinical investigation of the pharmacokinetics of therapeutic proteins CHMP/EWP/89249 [128, 129]

Many of the anticancer agents, however, do not have specific studies or recommendations for these patient populations. The main reasons for this include:

- Some of the earlier drugs were developed before the guidelines were developed, such as carboplatin, the anthracyclines and etoposide [130–133].
- A strict implementation of these guidelines, especially in oncology, where they are especially difficult to incorporate, make these studies impractical.
- Some of the studies are performed after drug approval, and are initiated by clinicians independently of regulatory agencies.
- Interpretation and application of the results are occasionally difficult. For example, in the case of eribulin, researchers observed a 50% increase in eribulin exposures in patients with moderate renal dysfunction despite the fact that it has a limited urinary elimination and there is no correlation between renal function and PK parameters. Based on this, the FDA recommended a prudent dose reduction in patients with moderate or severe renal impairment [134].

The convenience of, as well as when and how to study the effect of the organ dysfunction of a specific drug may vary. A dedicated stand-alone organ dysfunction study may be warranted in some cases, while in others, this information could be collected within the context of large late phase clinical trials (e.g. using a population PK with sparse sampling in a patient population with varying degrees of organ dysfunction) (Tables 18.11 and 18.12).

A dedicated organ dysfunction study performed in the early stages of development may provide some guidance on how to better define the patient population to

Table 18.11 Types of organ impairment studies and their characteristics based on FDA and EMA guidelines (Pharmacokinetics in Patients with Impaired Renal Function—Study Design, Data Analysis, and Impact on Dosing and Labeling FDA guidance) (EMA Guideline on the evaluation of the pharmacokinetics of medicinal products in patients with decreased renal function)

Organ impairment study designs	Characteristics
Full study	Includes subjects covering the full renal/ hepatic function range Equal number of patients in each group May include a "normal function" control group
Reduced study or staged study	Two groups studied initially (mild dysfunction and normal) If the organ impairment is anticipated not to be clinically relevant If initial study does shows an effect on impairment, then evaluate intermediate impairment group
Population pharmacokinetics	Based on conducted Phase I/II/III trials Studies should have included patients with different degrees of organ impairment Need to adjust for differences in frequencies of patients with and without organ dysfunction
Hemodialysis/peritoneal dyalisis	Only in renal impairment The drug is normally administered between dialysis sessions Unlikely to be important for most anticancer drugs It may be integrated in a full-range study

Table 18.12 Selected examples of studies of anticancer agents in renal and liver dysfunction

Renal Impairmet				
Drug Study design	Population (RI classification used)	GFR equation used	Outcome Statistically significant/ clinical impact	References
Oxaliplatin Full study	Normal: CrCL >60 mL/min Mild: CrCL 40–59 mL/min Moderate: CrCL 20 39 mL/min Severe: CrCL <20 mL/min (ODWGI)	CLCR by 24 h-urine collection	Yes/No	Takimoto [135]
Imatinib Mesilate Full study	Normal: CrCL >60 mL/min Mild: CrCL 40–59 mL/min Moderate: CrCL 20 39 mL/min Severe: CrCL <20 mL/min (ODWGI)	CLCR by 24 h-urine collection	Yes/No	Gibbons et al. [136]
Abiraterone Reduced study	ESRD (requiring hemodialysis)	MDRD	No/No	Marbury et al. [137]
Eribulin (Mild group not included)	Normal: GFR ≥ 80 mL/min; Moderate: GFR 30–50 mL/min; Severe: GFR 15–29 mL/min	Cockcroft–Gault	No/Yes	Tan et al. [134]
Hepatic impairment				
Drug	Population (HI classification used)	Liver function dynamic test	Outcome	References
Oxaliplatin	Normal: TB, AST, AP ≤ ULN Mild TB ≤ ULN, AST > ULN–2.5 × ULN, AP ULN–5× ULN Moderate: TB > ULN–3 mg/dL, AST >2.5 × ULN, AP >5x ULN Severe: TB > 3 mg/dL, AST any, AP any Liver transplant: TB, AST, AP any (Ad-hoc score)	No	Dose 130 mg/m^2 every 21 days without CL alteration and tolerated by all groups	Doroshow et al. [86, 87], Synold et al. [138]

Table 18.12 (continued)

Renal Impairmet				
Drug Study design	Population (RI classification used)	GFR equation used	Outcome Statistically significant/ clinical impact	References
Pazopanib	Control: TB < ULN, ALT <ULN Mild HI B1: TB < ULN, ALT > ULN; B2: ULN < TB < 1.5× ULN, ALT any Moderate HI: TB < 3× ULN, ALT any Severe HI: TB > 3× ULN, ALT any (ODWGI)	No	Mild HI: FDA approved dose of 800 mg per day. Moderate and severe HI tolerated dose 200 mg per day	Shibata et al. [139]
Eribulin	Normal Child A Child B	No	Mild, moderate HI: dose adjustment may not be considered	Witteveen et al. [140], Devriese et al. [141]
Abiraterone	Normal Child A Child B Child C	No	Moderate and severe HI: higher AUC. Child B:no dose adjustment Child C:contraindicated	Marbury et al. [137]
TDM1	Normal Child A Child B	No	Transient trend of faster CL in HI. No dose adjustment.	Chunze et al. [142]

be enrolled in a phase 2/3 program, especially in tumor types where dysfunction is frequent (hepatocarcinoma and cirrhosis, renal cell carcinoma and nephrectomized patients).

In some instances and for pragmatic reasons, a stand-alone protocol would investigate the effect of renal and hepatic impairment on PKs of a drug in the same study. These studies take advantage of a more seamless and effective implementation in experienced phase I departments, an accelerated implementation of the program, and being able to combine PK and safety results of both organ dysfunction populations to better understand the pharmacology of the studied agent (e.g. abiraterone, erlotinib and veliparib) [125, 137, 143].

Key Expert Opinion Points

- Based on the new recommendations from the FDA's "Cancer Clinical Trial Eligibility Criteria: Patients with Organ Dysfunction or Prior or Concurrent", future organ dysfunction studies may be introduced in early stages of drug development as a sub-study of phase I clinical trial
- Accelerating anticancer drug development in patients with organ disfuction will provide them the same opportunities of accessibility of a novel therapeutic. For that, these patients may be included in the phase I trial stratified into multiple subgroups according to the underlying degrees of renal and hepatic dysfunction.
- Using PK/PD modeling allows to integrate data from dose-escalation phase, expansion phase and organ dysfunction cohorts for the determination of the most appropriate dose level for each functional status.
- Pharmacokinetic studies assisted by image-guided biodistribution techniques will improve the pharmacokinetic and pharmacodynamic characterization of drugs in special populations.

References

1. Webster AC, Nagler EV, Morton RL, Masson P. Chronic kidney disease. Lancet. 2017;389:1238–52.
2. Mehta RL, Kellum JA, Shah SV, Molitoris BA, Ronco C, Warnock DG, Levin A; Acute Kidney Injury Network. Acute Kidney Injury Network: report of an initiative to improve outcomes in acute kidney injury. Crit Care 2007;11(2): R31. PubMed PMID: 17331245; PubMed Central PMCID: PMC2206446.
3. Kidney Disease: Improving Global Outcomes (KDIGO) CKD-MBD Update Work Group. KDIGO 2017 clinical practice guideline update for the diagnosis, evaluation, prevention, and treatment of chronic kidney disease–mineral and bone disorder (CKD-MBD). Kidney Int Suppl. 2017;7:1–59.
4. Hill NR, Fatoba ST, Oke JL, Hirst JA, O'Callagan CA, Lasserson DS, et al. Global prevalence of Chronic Kidney Disease. A systematic review and meta-analysis. PLoS One. 2016, July 6; 11(7) e0158765. https://doi.org/10.1371/journal.pone.0158765. eCollection 2016.
5. Global Burden of Disease Study 2013 Collaborators. Global, regional, and national incidence, prevalence, and years lived with disability for 301 acute and chronic diseases and injuries in 188 countries, 1990–2013: a systematic analysis for the Global burden of disease study 2013.

Lancet. 2015 Aug 22;386(9995):743–800. https://doi.org/10.1016/S0140-6736(15)60692-4. Epub 2015 Jun 7. Review.
6. Neugarten J, Acharya A, Sibiger SR. Effect of gender on the progression of nondiabetic renal disease: a meta-analysis. J Am Soc Nephrol. 2000;11(2):319–29.
7. Samuels J, Ng CS, Nates J, Price K, Finkel K, Salahudeen A, et al. Small increases in serum creatinine are associated with prolonged ICU stay and increased hospital mortality in critically ill patients with cancer. Support Care Cancer. 2011;19(10):1527–32.
8. Janssen-Heijnen ML, Maas HA, Houteman S, Lemmens VE, Rutten HJ, Coeberg JW. Comorbidity in older surgical cancer patients: influence on patient care and outcome. Eur J Cancer. 2007;43(15):2179–93.
9. Saillard C, et al. Acute kidney injury in patients with cancer. N Engl J Med. 2017 Aug 3;377(5):499.
10. Jha V, Garcia-Garcia G, Iseki K, Li Z, Naicker S, Plattner B, et al. Chronic renal disease: global dimension and perspectives. Lancet. 2013 Jul 20;382:260–72.
11. Avarbock AB, et al. Lethal vascular leak syndrome after denileukin diftitox administration to a patient with cutaneous gamma/delta T-cell lymphoma and occult cirrhosis. Am J Hematol. 2008;83:593–5.
12. Sahni V, Choudhury D, Ahmed Z. Chemotherapy-associated renal dysfunction. Nat Rev Nephrol. 2009;5(8):450–62.
13. Eremina V, et al. VEGF inhibition and renal thrombotic microangiopathy. N Engl J Med. 2008;358(11):1129–36.
14. Usui J, et al. Clinicopathological spectrum of kidney diseases in cancer patients treated with vascular endothelial growth factor inhibitors: a report of 5 cases and review of literature. Hum Pathol. 2014;45:1918–27.
15. Rosner M, et al. Acute kidney injury in patients with cancer. NEJM. 2017;376(18):1770–81.
16. Glezerman IG, Edgar A. Jaimes. Chapter 11: chemotherapy and kidney injury. American Society of Nephrology 2016. https://www.asn-online.org/education/distancelearning/curricula/onco/Chapter11.pdf
17. Markowitz GS, et al. Collapsing focal segmental glomerulosclerosis following treatment with high-dose pamidronate. J Am Soc Nephrol. 2001;12(6):1164–72.
18. Stokes MB, et al. Glomerular disease related to anti-VEGF therapy. Kidney Int. 2008 Dec;74(11):1487–91.
19. Kumasaka R, et al. Side effects of the therapy: case 1. Nephrotic syndrome associated with gefitinib therapy. J Clin Oncol. 2004 Jun 15;22(12):2504–5.
20. Glezerman IG, Pietanza MC, Miller V, Seshan SV. Kidney tubular toxicity of maintenance pemetrexed therapy. Am J Kidney Dis. 2011 Nov;58(5):817–20.
21. Markowitz GS, Fine PL, Stack J, Kunis CL, Radharisshnan J, Palecki W, et al. Toxic acute tubular necrosis following treatment with zoledronate (Zometa). Kidney Int. 2003;64(1):281–9.
22. Izzedine H, et al. Acute tubular necrosis associated with mTOR inhibitor therapy: a real entity biopsy proven. Ann Oncol. 2013;24:2421–5.
23. Wanchoo R, et al. Renal effects of BRAF inhibitors: a systematic review by the Cancer and the Kidney International Network. Clin Kidney J. 2016;9(2):245–51.
24. Izzedine H, El-Fekih RK, Perazella MA. The renal effects of ALK inhibitors. Investig New Drugs. 2016;34:643–9.
25. Ciarimboli G, et al. Cisplatin nephrotoxicity is critically mediated via the human organic cation transporter 2. Am J Pathol. 2005;167:1477–84.
26. Zamlauski-Tucker MJ, et al. Ifosfamide metabolite chloroacetaldehyde causes Fanconi syndrome in the perfused rat kidney. Toxicol Appl Pharmacol. 1994;129:170–5.
27. Ciarimboli G, et al. New clues for nephrotoxicity induced by ifosfamide: preferential renal uptake via the human organic cation transporter 2. Mol Pharm. 2011;8:270–9.
28. Dietrich A, et al. Renal TRPathies. J Am Soc Nephrol. 2010;21:736–44.
29. Schrag D, et al. Cetuximab therapy and symptomatic hypomagnesemia. J Natl Cancer Inst. 2005;97:1221–4.

30. Muallem S, Moe OW. When eGF is offside, magnesium is wasted. J Clin Invest. 2007;117:2086–69.
31. van Cutsem E, et al. Open-label phase III trial of panitumumab plus best supportive care compared with best supportive care alone in patients with chemotherapy-refractory metastatic colorectal cancer. J Clin Oncol. 2007;25:1658–64.
32. Fung E, Anand S, Bhalla V. Pemetrexed-induced nephrogenic diabetes insipidus. Am J Kidney Dis. 2016 October;68(4):628–32.
33. Bressler RB, Huston DP. Water intoxication following moderate dose intravenous cyclophosphamide. Arch Intern Med. 1985;145:548–9.
34. Cutting HO. Inappropriate secretion of antidiuretic hormone secondary to vincristine therapy. Am J Med. 1971;51(2):269–71.
35. Azar I. Sunitinib-induced acute interstitial nephritis in a thrombocytopenic renal cell cancer patient. Case Rep Oncol Med. 2017;2017:6328204.
36. Perazella MA. Onco-nephrology: renal toxicities of chemotherapeutic agents. Clin J Am Soc Nephrol. 2012;7(10):1713–21.
37. Izzedine H, et al. Kidney injuries related to ipilimumab. Investig New Drugs. 2014 Aug;32:769–73.
38. Cortazar FB, et al. Clinicopathological features of acute kidney injury associated with immune checkpoint inhibitors. Kidney Int. 2016;90:638–47.
39. Shirali AC, et al. Association of acute interstitial nephritis with programmed cell death 1 inhibitor therapy in lung cancer patients. Am J Kidney Dis. 2016;68:287–91.
40. Widemann BC, Adamson PC. Understanding and managing methotrexate nephrotoxicity. Oncologist. 2006;11:694–703.
41. Perazella MA. Renal vulnerability to drug toxicity. Clin J Am Soc Nephrol. 2009;4(7):1275–83.
42. Choudhury D, Ahmed Z. Drug-associated renal dysfunction and injury. Nat Clin Pract Nephrol. 2006;2(2):80–91.
43. Humphreys BD, Siffer RJ, Magee CC. Renal failure associated with cancer and its treatment: an update. J Am Soc Nephrol. 2005;16(1):151–61.
44. Perazella MA, Moeckel GW. Nephrotoxicity from chemotherapeutic agents: clinical manifestations, pathobiology, and prevention/therapy. Semin Nephrol. 2010 Nov;30(6):570–81.
45. Pabla N, et al. Cisplatin nephrotoxicity: mechanisms and renoprotective strategies. Kidney Int. 2008 May;73(9):994–1007.
46. Kawai Y, et al. Relationship of intracellular calcium and oxygen radicals to Cisplatin-related renal cell injury. J Pharmacol Sci. 2006;100:65–72.
47. Ramesh G, Reeves WB. TNFR2-mediated apoptosis and necrosis in cisplatin-induced acute renal failure. Am J Physiol Renal Physiol. 2003;285:F610–8.
48. Faubel S, et al. Caspase-1-deficient mice are protected against cisplatin-induced apoptosis and acute tubular necrosis. Kidney Int. 2004 Dec;66(6):2202–13.
49. Hutchens MP, et al. Estrogen protects renal endothelial barrier function from ischemia-reperfusion in vitro and in vivo. Am J Physiol Renal. 2012;303:F377–85.
50. Nolin TD, et al. Emerging evidence of the impact of kidney disease on drug metabolism and transport. Clin Pharmacol Ther. 2008;83:898–903.
51. Sun H, et al. Effects of renal failure on drug transport and metabolism. Pharmacol Ther 2006 Jan;109(1–2):1–11. Epub 2005 Aug 8.
52. Zhang Y, Zhang L, Abraham S, Apparaju S, Wu TC, Strong JM, et al. Assessment of the impact of renal impairment on systemic exposure of new molecular entities: evaluation of recent new drug applications. Clin Pharmacol Ther. 2009;85(3):305–11.
53. Matzke GR, Comstock TJ. Influence of renal function and dialysis on drug disposition. In: Burton ME, Shaw LM, Schentag JJ, Evans WE, editors. Applied pharmacokinetics and pharmacodynamics: principles of therapeutic drug monitoring. 4th ed. Philadelphia: Lippincott Williams & Wilkins; 2006. p. 187–212.
54. Schwartz GJ, Furth SL. Glomerular filtration rate measurement and estimation in chronic kidney disease. Pediatr Nephrol. 2007;22(11):1839–48.

55. Sandilands EA, Dhaun N, Dear JW, Webb DJ. Measurement of renal function in patients with chronic kidney disease. Br J Clin Pharmacol. 2013;76(4):504–15.
56. Perrone RD, Steinman TI, Beck GJ, Skibinski CI, Royal HD, Lawlor M, et al. Utility of radioisotopic filtration markers in chronic renal insufficiency: simultaneous comparison of 125I-iothalamate, 169Yb-DTPA, 99mTc-DTPA, and inulin. Am J Kidney Dis. 1990;16(3):224–35.
57. Gaspari F, Perico N, Matalone M, Signorini O, Azzollini N, Mister M, et al. Precision of plasma clearance of iohexol for estimation of GFR in patients with renal disease. J Am Soc Nephrol. 1998;9(2):310–3.
58. Levey AS, Greene T, Schluchter MD, Cleary PA, Teschan PE, Lorenz RA, et al. Glomerular filtration rate measurements in clinical trials: modification of diet in renal disease study group and the diabetes control and complications trial research group. J Am Soc Nephrol. 1993;4(5):1159–71.
59. Stevens LA, Coresh J, Greene T, Levey AS. Assessing kidney function-measured and estimated glomerular filtration rate. NEJM. 2006;354(23):2473–83.
60. Gross A, et al. Simultaneous administration of a cocktail of markers to measure renal drug elimination pathways: absence of a pharmacokinetic interaction between Fluconazole and sinistrin, p-aminohippuric acidand pindolol. J Clin Pharmacol. 2001;51:547–55.
61. Deutz NE, Safar A, Schutzler S, Memelink R, Ferrando A, Spencer H, et al. Muscle protein synthesis in cancer patients can be stimulated with a specially formulated medical food. Clin Nutr. 2011 December;30(6):759–68.
62. De Campos-Ferraz, et al. An overview of amines as nutritional supplements to counteract cancer cachexia. J Cachexia Sarcopenia Muscle. 2014;5(2):105–10.
63. O'Callagan CA, Shine B, Lasserson DS. Chronic kidney disease: a large-scale population-based study of the effects of introducing the CKD-EPI formula for eGFR reporting. BMJ Open. 2011;1(2):e000308. https://doi.org/10.1136/bmjopen-2011-000308.
64. Murata K, Baumann NA, Saenger AK, Larson TS, Rule AD, Lieske JC. Relative performance of the MDRD and CKD-EPI equations for estimating glomerular filtration rate among patients with varied clinical presentations. Clin J Am Soc Nephrol. 2011;6(8):1963–72.
65. 17 December 2015 EMA/CHMP/83874/2014 Committee for Medicinal Products for Human use (CHMP). Guideline on the evaluation of the pharmacokinetics of medicinal products in patients with decreased renal function. https://www.ema.europa.eu/en/documents/scientific-guideline/guideline-evaluation-pharmacokinetics-medicinal-products-patients-decreased-renal-function_en.pdf
66. Tett SE, Kirkpatrick CM, Gross AS, McLachlan AJ. Principles and clinical application of assessing alterations in renal elimination pathways. Clin Pharmacokinet. 2003;42(14):1193–211.
67. Beumer JH, Ding F, Tawbi H, Lin Y, Viluh D, Chatterjee I, et al. Effect of renal dysfunction on toxicity in three decades of cancer therapy evaluation program–sponsored single-agent phase I studies. J Clin Oncol. 2016;34(2):110–6.
68. Field KM, Dow C, Michael M. Part I: Liver function in oncology: biochemistry and beyond. Lancet Oncol. 2008;9(11):1092–101.
69. Mansfield AS, Rudeck MA, Vulih D, Smith GL, Jo HP, Percy IS. The effect of hepatic impairment on outcomes in phase 1 clinical trials in cancer subjects. Clin Cancer Res. 2016;22(22):5472–9.
70. Hope VD, Eramova I, Capurro D, Donoghoe MC. Prevalence and estimation of hepatitis B and C infections in the WHO European Region: a review of data focusing on the countries outside the European Union and the European Free Trade Association. Epidemiol Infect. 2014;142(2):270–86.
71. European Association for the Study of Liver. EASL clinical practical guidelines: management of alcoholic liver disease. J Hepatol 2012 Aug; 57(399–420).
72. Vernon G, Baranova A, Younossi ZM. Systematic review: the epidemiology and natural history of non-alcoholic fatty liver disease and non-alcoholic steatohepatitis in adults. Aliment Pharmacol Ther. 2011;34(3):274–85.

73. Villano JL, et al. Abraxane induced life-threatening toxicities with metastatic breast cancer and hepatic insufficiency. Investig New Drugs. 2006;24:455–6.
74. Hill JM, Loeb E, MacLellan A, Hill NO, Khan A, King JJ. Clinical studies of platinum coordination compounds in the treatment of various malignant diseases. Cancer Chemother Rep. 1975;59:647–59.
75. Mando OG. Imatinib-induced fatal acute liver failure. World J Gastroenterol. 2007;13: 6608–11.
76. Mindikoglu AL, Regev A, Bejarano PA, Martinez EJ, Jeffers LJ, Schiff ER. Imatinib mesylate (gleevec) hepatotoxicity. Dig Dis Sci. 2007;52:598–601.
77. Slavin RE, Dias MA, Saral R. Cytosine arabinoside induced gastrointestinal toxic alterations in sequential chemotherapeutic protocols: a clinical-pathologic study of 33 patients. Cancer. 1978;42:1747–59.
78. Robinson K, Lambiase L, Li J, Monteiro C, Schiff M. Fatal cholestatic liver failure associated with gemcitabine therapy. Dig Dis Sci. 2003;48:1804–8.
79. Tran A, Housset C, Boboc B, Tourani JM, Carnot F, Berthelot P. Etoposide (VP 16-213) induced hepatitis. Report of three cases following standard-dose treatment. J Hepatol. 1991;12(1):36–9.
80. Asbury RF, Rosenthal SN, Descalzi ME, Ratcliffe RL, Arseneau JC. Hepatic veno-occlusive disease due to DTIC. Cancer. 1980;45:2670–4.
81. Friedman HS, et al Chapter 13 Nonclassic alkylating agents. Cancer chemotherapy and biotherapy Second edition 1996 edited by Bruce A. Chabner and Dan L. Longo. Pages 333–356 (DTIC).
82. Scheithauer W, McKendrick J, Begbie S, et al. Oral capecitabine as an alternative to iv 5-fluorouracil-based adjuvant therapy for colon cancer: safety results of a randomized, phase III trial. Ann Oncol. 2003;14:1735–43.
83. Van Cutsem E, Twelves C, Cassidy J, et al. Oral capecitabine compared with intravenous fluorouracil plus leucovorin in patients with metastatic colorectal cancer: results of a large phase III study. J Clin Oncol. 2001;19:4097–106.
84. Chu E, Allegra CJ. Chapter 6 Antifolates. Cancer chemotherapy and biotherapy. Second edition 1996 edited by Bruce A. Chabner and Dan L. Longo pages 109–148 (methotrexate).
85. Morris-Stiff G, Tan YM, Vauthey JN. Hepatic complications following preoperative chemotherapy with oxaliplatin or irinotecan for hepatic colorectal metastases. Eur J Surg Oncol. 2008;34:609–14.
86. Doroshow JH, et al. Pharmacology of oxaliplatin in solid tumor patients with hepatic dysfunction: a preliminary report of the national cancer institute working group. Sem Oncol. 2003a Aug;30(4 suppl 15):14–9.
87. Doroshow JH, Synold TW, Gandara D, et al. Pharmacology of oxaliplatin in solid tumor patients with hepatic dysfunction: a preliminary report of the National Cancer Institute Organ Dysfunction Working Group. Semin Oncol. 2003b;30(suppl 15):14–9.
88. Rubbia-Brandt L, Audard V, Sartoretti P, et al. Severe hepatic sinusoidal obstruction associated with oxaliplatin-based chemotherapy in patients with metastatic colorectal cancer. Ann Oncol. 2004;15:460–6.
89. Vauthey JN, Pawlik TM, Ribero D, et al. Chemotherapy regimen predicts steatohepatitis and an increase in 90-day mortality after surgery for hepatic colorectal metastases. J Clin Oncol. 2006;24:2065–72.
90. Iorga A, Dara L, Kaplowitz N. A drug-induced liver injury: cascade of events leading to cell death, apoptosis or necrosis. Int J Mol Sci. 2017;18(5). pii: E1018.
91. Suzuki A, Takahashi T, Okuno Y, Seko S, Fukuda Y, Nakamura K, et al. Liver damage in patients with colony-stimulating factor-producing tumors. Am J Med. 1993;94(2):125–32.
92. Rivory LP, Slaviero KA, Clarke SJ. Hepatic cytochrome P450 3A drug metabolism is reduced in cancer patients who have an acute-phase response. Br J Cancer. 2002;87(3):277–80.
93. Petrovic V, Teng S, Piquette-Miller M. Regulation of drug transporters during infection and inflammation. Mol Interv. 2007;7(2):99–111.

94. Le Couteur DG, Fraser R, Hilmer S, Rivory LP, McLean AJ. The hepatic sinusoid in aging and cirrhosis: effects on hepatic substrate disposition and drug clearance. Clin Pharmacokinet. 2005;44(2):187–200.
95. Hung DY, Chang P, Cheung K, McWhinney B, Masci PP, Weiss M, et al. Cationic drug pharmacokinetics in diseased livers determined by fibrosis index, hepatic protein content, microsomal activity, and nature of drug. Pharmacol Exp Ther. 2002;301(3):1079–87.
96. George J, Murray M, Byth K, Farrell GC. Differential alterations of cytochrome P450 proteins in livers from patients with severe chronic liver disease. Hepatology. 1995a;21(1):120–8.
97. George J, Liddle C, Murray M, Byth K, Farrell GC. Pre-translational regulation of cytochrome P450 genes is responsible for disease specific changes of individual P450 enzymes among patients with cirrhosis. Biochem Pharmacol. 1995b;49(7):873–81.
98. Furlan V, Demirdjian S, Bourdon O, Magdalou J, Taburet AM. Glucuronidation of drugs by hepatic microsomes derived from healthy and cirrhotic human livers. J Pharmacol Exp Ther. 1999 May;289(2):1169–75.
99. Elbekai RH, Korashy HM, El-Kadi OS. The effect of liver cirrhosis on the regulation and expression of drug metabolising enzymes. Curr Drug Metab. 2004 Apr;5(2):157–67.
100. Kullak-Ublick GA, Beuers U, Paumgartner G. Molecular and functional characterization of bile acid transport in human hepatoblastoma Hep G2 cells. Hepatology. 1996 May;23(5):1053–60.
101. Briz O, Serrano MA, Rebollo N, Hangenbuch B, Meier PJ, Koepsell H, et al. Carriers involved in targeting the cytostatic bile acid-cisplatin derivatives cis-diammine-chloro-cholylglycinateplatinum (II) and cis-diammine-bisursodeoxycholate-platinum(II) toward liver cells. Mol Pharmacol. 2002 Apr;61(4):853–60.
102. Figg WD, Dukes GE, Lesesne HR, Carson SW, Songer SS, Pritchard JF, et al. Comparison of quantitative methods to assess hepatic function: Pugh's classification, indocyanine green, antipyrine, and dextromethorphan. Pharmacotherapy. 1995 Nov–Dec;15(6): 693–700.
103. Tang HS, Hu OY. Assessment of liver function using a novel galactose single point method. Digestion. 1992;52(3-4):222–31.
104. Testa R, Caglieri S, Risso D, Arzani L, Campo N, Alvarez S, et al. Monoethylglycinexylidide formation measurement as a hepatic function test to assess severity of chronic liver disease. Am J Gastroenterol. 1997 Dec;92(12):2268–73.
105. Faybik P, Hetz H. Plasma disappearance rate of indocyanine green in liver dysfunction. Transplant Proc. 2006 Apr;38(3):801–2.
106. Molino G, Avagnina P, Belforte G, Bircher J. Assessment of the hepatic circulation in humans: new concepts based on evidence derived from a D-sorbitol clearance method. J Lab Clin Med. 1998;131(5):393–405.
107. Engel G, Hofmann U, Heidemann H, Cosme J, Eichelbaum M. Antipyrine as a probe for human oxidative metabolism: identification of the cytochrome P50 enzymes catalyzing 4-hydroxyantipyrine, 3-hydroxymethylantipyrine, and norantipyrine formation. Clin Pharmacol Ther. 1996 Jun;59:613–23.
108. Villeneuve JP, Pichette P. Cytochrome P450 and liver diseases. Curr Drug Metab. 2004;5:273–5.
109. Rogers JF, Rocci ML, Haughey DB, Bertino JS. An evaluation of the suitability of intravenous midazolam as an in vivo marker for hepatic cytochrome P4503A activity. Clin Pharmacol Ther. 2003 Mar;73(3):153–8.
110. Oellerich M, Armstrong VW. The MEGX test: a tool for the real-time assessment of hepatic function. Ther Drug Monit. 2001 Apr;23(2):81–92.
111. Orlando R, Piccoli P, De Martin S, Padrini R, Floreani M, Palatini P. Cytochrome P450 1A2 is a major determinant of lidocaine metabolism in vivo. Clin Pharmacol Ther. 2004 Jan;75(1):80–8.
112. Durand F, Valla D. Assessment of the prognosis of cirrhosis: child–pugh versus MELD. J Hepatol. 2005;42(Suppl(1)):S100–7.

113. Pugh RN, Murray-Lyon IM, Dawson JL, Pietroni MC, Williams R. Transection of the oesophagus for bleeding oesophageal varices. Br J Surg. 1973;60:646–9.
114. Fernandez-Esparrach G, Sanchez-Fuevo A, Ginès P, Uriz J, Quintó L, Ventura PJ, et al. A prognostic model for predicting survival in cirrhosis with ascites. J Hepatol. 2001;34(1): 46–52.
115. Longheval G, Vereerstraeten P, Thiry P, Delhaye M, Moine O, Deviere J, et al. Predictive models of short- and long-term survival in patients with nonbiliary cirrhosis. Liver Transpl. 2003;9(3):260–7.
116. Malinchoc M, Kamath PS, Gordon FD, Peine CJ, Rank J, ter Borg PC. A model to predict poor survival in patients undergoing transjugular intrahepatic portosystemic shunts. Hepatology. 2000;31(4):864–71.
117. Wiesner RH, McDiarmid SV, Kamath PS, Edwards EB, Malinchoc M, Kremers WK, et al. MELD and PELD: application of survival models to liver allocation. Liver Transpl. 2001;7(7):567–80.
118. Amitrano L, Guardascione MA, Bennato R, Manguso F, Balzano A. MELD score and hepatocellular carcinoma identify patients at different risk of short-term mortality among cirrhotics bleeding from esophageal varices. J Hepatol. 2005 Jun;42(6):820–5.
119. Evans LT, Kim WR, Poterucha JJ, Kamath PS. Spontaneous bacterial peritonitis in asymptomatic outpatients with cirrhotic ascites. Hepatology. 2003 Apr;37(4):897–901.
120. Schmidt LE, Larsen FS. MELD score as a predictor of liver failure and death in patients with acetaminophen-induced liver failure. Hepatology. 2007 Mar;45(3):789–96.
121. Taylor RM, et al. Acute Liver Failure study Group. Fulminant hepatitis A virus infection in the United States: incidence, prognosis an outcomes. Hepatology. 2006;44:1589–97.
122. Dunn W, et al. MELD accurately predicts mortality in patients with alcoholic hepatitis. Hepatology. 2005;41:353–8.
123. Cholongitas E, Senzolo M, Patch D, Kwong K, Niolopoulou V, Leandro G, et al. Risk factors, sequential organ failure assessment and model for end-stage liver disease scores for predicting short-term mortality in cirrhotic patients admitted to intensive care unit. Aliment Pharmacol Ther. 2006 Apr 1;23(7):883–93.
124. Csonka D, Hazell K, Waldron E, Lorenzo S, Duval V, Trandafir L, et al. Phase-1, open-label, single dose study of the pharmacokinetics of buparlisib in subjects with mild to severe hepatic impairment. J Clin Pharmacol. 2016;56(3):316–23.
125. Miller AA, Murry DJ, Owzar K, Hollis DR, Lewis LD, Kindler HL, et al. Phase I and pharmacokinetic study of erlotinib for solid tumors in patients with hepatic or renal dysfunction: CALGB 60101. J Clin Oncol. 2007 Jul 20;25(21):3055–60.
126. Siegel-Lakhai WS, Crul M, De Porre P, Zhang S, Chang I, Boot H, et al. Clinical and pharmacologic study of the farnesyltransferase inhibitor tipifarnib in cancer patients with normal or mildly or moderately impaired hepatic function. J Clin Oncol. 2006;24(28):4558–64.
127. Yang HC, et al. Models of chronic kidney disease. Drug Discov Today Dis Models. 2010;7(1–2):13–9. https://doi.org/10.1016/j.ddmod.2010.08.002.
128. CHMP/EWP/89249/2004 Guidelines on the clinical investigation of the pharmacokinetics of therapeutic proteins. https://www.ema.europa.eu/en/documents/scientific-guideline/guideline-clinical-investigation-pharmacokinetics-therapeutic-proteins_en.pdf
129. Pharmacokinetics in Patients with Impaired Renal Function — Study Design, Data Analysis, and Impact on Dosing and Labeling U.S. Department of Health and Human Services Food and Drug Administration Center for Drug Evaluation and Research (CDER) March 2010. Clin Pharmacol. https://www.fda.gov/media/78573/download
130. Dobbs NA, Twelves CJ. Anthracycline doses in patients with liver dysfunction: do UK oncologists follow current recommendations? Br J Cancer. 1998;77(7):1145–8.
131. Arbuck SG, et al. Etoposide pharmacokinetics in patients with normal and abnormal organ function. JCO. 1986;4(11):1690–5.
132. D'Incalci M, et al. Pharmacokinetics of etoposide in patients with abnormal renal and hepatic function. CCR. 1986;46:2566–71.

133. Calvert AH, et al. Phase I studies with carboplatin at the Royal Marsden Hospital. Cancer Treat Rev. 1985 Sep;12(Suppl A):51–7.
134. Tan AR, et al. Pharmacokinetics of eribulin mesylate in cancer patients with normal and impaired renal function. Cancer Chemother Pharmacol. 2015;76:1051–61.
135. Takimoto CH. Dose-escalating and pharmacological study of oxaliplatin in adult cancer patients with impaired renal function: a National Cancer Institute Organ Dysfunction Woeking Group study. J Clin Oncol. 2003 Jul 15;21(14):2664–72.
136. Gibbons J, et al. Phase I and pharmacokinetic study of imatinib mesylate in patients with advanced malignancies and varying degrees of renal dysfunction: a study by the national cancer institute organ dysfunction working group. J Clin Oncol. 2008 Feb 1;26(4):570–6. https://doi.org/10.1200/JCO.2007.13.3819.
137. Marbury T, et al. Single-dose pharmacokinetic studies of abiraterone acetate in men with hepatic or renal impairment. J Clin Pharmacol. 2014;54(7):732–41.
138. Synold TW, et al. Dose-escalating and pharmacologic study of oxaliplatin in adult cancer patients with impaired hepatic function: a national cancer institute organ dysfunction working group study. Clin Cancer Res. 2007;13:3660–6.
139. Shibata SI, et al. Phase 1 study of pazopanib in patients with advanced solid tumors and hepatic dysfunction: a national cancer institute organ dysfunction working group study. Clin Cancer Res. 2013;19(13):3631–9.
140. Witteveen P, et al. Eribulin mesylate pharmacokinetics in patients with hepatic impairment. J Clin Oncol 2010 28:15_suppl, 2582. https://ascopubs.org/doi/abs/10.1200/jco.2010.28.15_suppl.2582
141. Devriese LA, et al. Pharmacokinetics of eribulin mesylate in patients with solid tumors and hepatic impairment. Cancer Chemother Pharmacol 2012 Dec;70(6):823–32. https://doi.org/10.1007/s00280-012-1976-x. Epub 2012 Sep 26.
142. Chunze Li C, et al. A phase I pharmacokinetic study of trastuzumab emtansine (T-DM1) in patients with human epidermal growth factor receptor 2-positive metastatic breast cancer and normal or reduced hepatic function. Clin Pharmacokinet. 2017 Sep;56(9):1069–80. https://doi.org/10.1007/s40262-016-0496-y.
143. Tawbi HAH, et al. Early phase I study of the PARP inhibitor veliparib (ABT-888) alone or in combination with carboplatin/paclitaxel (CP) in patients with varying degrees of hepatic or renal dysfunction: a study of the NCI-Organ Dysfunction Working Group (ODG). JCO 2014;32(15) suppl 2572. https://ascopubs.org/doi/abs/10.1200/jco.2014.32.15_suppl.2572

Index

T. A. Yap et al. (eds.), *Phase I Oncology Drug Development*,
https://doi.org/10.1007/978-3-030-47682-3

D

The manufacturer's authorised representative in the EU is Springer Nature Customer Service Centre GmbH, Europaplatz 3, 69115 Heidelberg, Germany. If you have any concerns regarding our products, please contact ProductSafety@springernature.com

Printed and bound by CPI Group (UK) Ltd, Croydon, CR0 4YY
30/09/2026
02225498-0014